METHODS IN MOLECULAR BIOLOGY

Series Editor
John M. Walker
School of Life Sciences
University of Hertfordshire
Hatfield, Hertfordshire, AL10 9AB, UK

For further volumes:
http://www.springer.com/series/7651

Basophils and Mast Cells

Methods and Protocols

Edited by

Bernhard F. Gibbs

Medway School of Pharmacy, The University of Kent, Chatham Maritime, Kent, UK

Franco H. Falcone

Division of Molecular and Cellular Science, The School of Pharmacy,
The University of Nottingham, Nottingham, UK

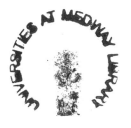

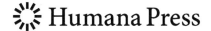

Editors
Bernhard F. Gibbs
Medway School of Pharmacy
The University of Kent
Chatham Maritime
Kent, UK

Franco H. Falcone
Division of Molecular and Cellular Science
The School of Pharmacy
The University of Nottingham
Nottingham, UK

ISSN 1064-3745   ISSN 1940-6029 (electronic)
ISBN 978-1-4939-1172-1 ISBN 978-1-4939-1173-8 (eBook)
DOI 10.1007/978-1-4939-1173-8
Springer New York Heidelberg Dordrecht London

Library of Congress Control Number: 2014944733

Preface

According to the latest epidemiological findings, it appears that allergic diseases will soon be affecting over 40% of the population in both Europe and elsewhere. There is, therefore, an overwhelming unmet need to unravel the immunological causes of allergic inflammation and to improve anti-allergic therapies. In recent years, it has come to light that mast cells and their blood-borne basophil counterparts not only contribute significantly to the symptoms of allergy but also play a role in supporting the underlying tendency of the immune system to respond in a pro-allergic manner. This immunomodulatory function has particularly led to a resurgence into basophil research and may one day finally uncover the biological role for this enigmatic and rare cell type which so readily releases a number of major inflammatory and immunomodulatory chemical mediators within very short periods of time. Moreover, the discovery that both mast cells and basophils potentially contribute to a variety of diseases, such as urticaria, cancer, and autoimmune diseases, as well as physiological functions, has increased the need for improved tools for researching these cells (*see* Chapter 1).

One of the most problematic features of mast cells and basophils is their striking differences in behavior and response to various stimulating agents and drugs depending on their location and the species from which they are studied. This limits, to some extent, our ability to extrapolate findings from, for example, mouse to human, but also tissue to tissue and the use of tumor mast cell and basophil lines. It is therefore imperative that better tools for the isolation of these cells from primary tissues are forthcoming. This indeed has been the case in recent years, and we now present a book which, we feel, will significantly help anyone conducting research into these cells from the most practical point of view: definitive lab-based protocols targeted to those who actually do the work!

Whether you are planning to purify basophils or mast cells from peripheral blood (Chapter 2) or tissues (Chapter 3), or if you want to culture them from precursors from buffy coat blood (Chapter 4) or bone marrow (Chapter 5), you'll find well-tested protocols in this book. Other chapters discuss the use of mast cells in organotypic skin models (Chapter 6), the difficulty of counting basophils (Chapter 7), how to stain mast cells and basophils in tissues (Chapter 9), as well as how to assess mediator release (Chapter 10) and signal transduction (Chapter 15). Also discussed is the suitability of using mast cell or basophil-like cell lines as surrogates for primary mast cells and basophils (Chapter 8) and the use of reporter cell lines (Chapter 13) for the detection of allergen-specific IgE in serum samples. Chapter 12 presents protocols which can be used to measure mast cell migration by microscopy. Chapter 14 describes protocols that can be used for gene silencing of mast cells and basophils, two cell types that are notoriously difficult to transfect.

Researchers more interested in ex vivo or in vivo analysis will find protocols for human basophil activation tests (BATs) in Chapter 11, for mast cell phenotyping (Chapter 16), or the study of murine basophils by flow cytometry in Chapter 17. Chapter 18 closes with in vivo models that can be used for the analysis of mast cell functions.

Our book is written by leading research scientists in the field of basophil and mast cell biology. The impetus for this consortium of authors was given by the recently established

EU/ESF-BMBS COST Action BM1007 "Mast Cells and Basophils—Targets for Innovative Therapies" which we would like to acknowledge for providing the ideal platform for scholarly collaboration in this field.

We sincerely hope that this methodology book will provide you with all the necessary tools for your research into mast cells and basophils, and we wish you every success in the quest to shed more light on these fascinating cell types.

Chatham Maritime, UK
Nottingham, UK

Bernhard F. Gibbs
Franco H. Falcone

Contents

Contributors

MARCOS J.C. ALCOCER • *School of Biosciences, The University of Nottingham, Nottingham, UK*

CORNELIA AMALINEI • *Grigore T. Popa University of Medicine and Pharmacy and Institute of Legal Medicine, Iasi, Romania*

METIN ARTUC • *Klinik für Dermatologie, Venerologie, und Allergologie, Allergie-Centrum-Charité, Charité, Berlin, Germany*

MAGDA BABINA • *Klinik für Dermatologie, Venerologie, und Allergologie, Allergie-Centrum-Charité, Charité, Berlin, Germany*

MONIKA BAMBOUSKOVÁ • *Laboratory of Signal Transduction, Institute of Molecular Genetics, v.v.i., Academy of Sciences of the Czech Republic, Prague, Czech Republic*

ELENA BORZOVA - *BMRC, University of East Anglia, Norwich, UK; Department of Clinical Allergology, Russian Medical Academy of Postgraduate Education, Moscow, Russia*

CHRIS H. BRIDTS • *Department of Immunology and Allergology, University of Antwerp, Wilrijk, Belgium*

LUC S. DE CLERCK • *Department of Immunology and Rheumatology, University of Antwerp, Wilrijk, Belgium*

CLEMENS A. DAHINDEN • *Institute of Immunology, University Hospital Bern, Inselspital, Bern, Switzerland*

PAVEL DRÁBER • *Laboratory of Biology of Cytoskeleton, Institute of Molecular Genetics, v.v.i., Academy of Sciences of the Czech Republic, Prague, Czech Republic*

PETR DRÁBER • *Laboratory of Signal Transduction, Institute of Molecular Genetics, v.v.i., Academy of Sciences of the Czech Republic, Prague, Czech Republic*

DIDIER G. EBO • *Department of Immunology and Allergology, University of Antwerp, Wilrijk, Belgium*

LUÍS ESCRIBANO • *Spanish Mastocytosis Network (REMA), Salamanca, Spain; Centro de Investigación del Cáncer, Salamanca, Spain*

FRANCO H. FALCONE • *Division of Molecular and Cellular Science, The School of Pharmacy, The University of Nottingham, Nottingham, UK*

SIDSEL FALKENCRONE • *Department of Dermatology, Odense University Hospital, Odense, Denmark*

JASMINE FARRINGTON • *Department of Biomedical Science, University of Sheffield, Sheffield, UK*

BERNHARD F. GIBBS • *Medway School of Pharmacy, The University of Kent, Chatham Maritime, Kent, UK*

VLADIMIR ANDREY GIMÉNEZ-RIVERA • *Department of Dermatology and Allergy, Charité - Universitätsmedizin Berlin, Berlin, Germany*

SVEN GUHL • *Klinik für Dermatologie, Venerologie, und Allergologie, Allergie-Centrum-Charité, Charité, Berlin, Germany*

MARGO M. HAGENDORENS • *Department of Immunology and Allergology, University of Antwerp, Wilrijk, Belgium*

ZUZANA HÁJKOVÁ • *Laboratory of Biology of Cytoskeleton, Institute of Molecular Genetics, v.v.i., Academy of Sciences of the Czech Republic, Prague, Czech Republic*

HANS JÜRGEN HOFFMANN • *Department of Clinical Medicine, University of Aarhus, Aarhus N, Denmark; The Department of Pulmonary Medicine, Aarhus University Hospital, Aarhus C, Denmark*

BETTINA M. JENSEN • *Allergy Clinic, Dept. 22, 1. floor, Gentofte Hospital, Hellerup, Denmark*

JONGHUI KIM • *Klinik für Dermatologie, Venerologie, und Allergologie, Allergie-Centrum-Charité, Charité, Berlin, Germany*

EDWARD F. KNOL • *Departments of Immunology, University Medical Center Utrecht, Utrecht, The Netherlands; Departments of Dermatology/Allergology, University Medical Center Utrecht, Utrecht, The Netherlands*

CHRISTEL MERTENS • *Department of Immunology and Allergology, University of Antwerp, Wilrijk, Belgium*

MARTIN METZ • *Department of Dermatology and Allergy, Charité - Universitätsmedizin Berlin, Berlin, Germany*

JOSÉ MÁRIO MORGADO • *Instituto de Estudios de Mastocitosis de Castilla La Mancha, Toledo, Spain; Spanish Mastocytosis Network (REMA), Toledo, Spain*

RYOSUKE NAKAMURA • *National Institute of Health Sciences, Tokyo, Japan*

ANA OLIVERA • *Mast Cell Biology Section, Laboratory of Allergic Diseases, National Institute of Allergy and Infectious Diseases, National Institutes of Health, Bethesda, MD, USA*

EGLE PASSANTE • *School of Pharmacy and Biomedical Sciences, University of Central Lancashire, Preston, UK*

PETER T. PEACHELL • *Academic Unit of Respiratory Medicine, The Medical School, University of Sheffield, Sheffield, UK*

JUAN RIVERA • *Molecular Immunology Section, Laboratory of Molecular Immunogenetics, National Institute of Arthritis and Musculoskeletal and Skin Diseases, National Institutes of Health, Bethesda, MD, USA*

VITO SABATO • *Department of Immunology and Allergology, University of Antwerp, Wilrijk, Belgium*

LAURA SÁNCHEZ-MUÑOZ • *Instituto de Estudios de Mastocitosis de Castilla La Mancha, Toledo, Spain; Spanish Mastocytosis Network (REMA), Toledo, Spain*

CHRISTIAN SCHWARTZ • *Department of Infection Biology, University Clinic Erlangen and Friedrich-Alexander-University Erlangen-Nuremberg (FAU), Erlangen, Germany*

ELIZABETH P. SEWARD • *Department of Biomedical Science, University of Sheffield, Sheffield, UK*

FRANK SIEBENHAAR • *Department of Dermatology and Allergy, Charité - Universitätsmedizin Berlin, Berlin, Germany*

PER S. SKOV • *Allergy Clinic, Dept. 22, 1. floor, Gentofte Hospital, Hellerup, Denmark*

VADIM V. SUMBAYEV • *Medway School of Pharmacy, University of Kent, Kent, UK*

EMILY J. SWINDLE • *Faculty of Medicine, Academic Unit of Clinical and Experimental Sciences, Southampton General Hospital, University of Southampton, Southampton, UK*

CRISTINA TEODÓSIO • *Spanish Mastocytosis Network (REMA), Salamanca, Spain; Centro de Investigación del Cáncer, Salamanca, Spain*

DAVID VOEHRINGER • *Department of Infection Biology, University Clinic Erlangen and Friedrich-Alexander-University Erlangen-Nuremberg (FAU), Erlangen, Germany*

ANDREW F. WALLS • *Clinical and Experimental Sciences, Faculty of Medicine, University of Southampton, Southampton, UK*

DANIEL WAN • *School of Pharmacy, The University of Nottingham, Nottingham, UK*

XIAOWEI WANG • *School of Biosciences, The University of Nottingham, Nottingham, UK*

TORSTEN ZUBERBIER • *Klinik für Dermatologie, Venerologie, und Allergologie, Allergie-Centrum-Charité, Charité, Berlin, Germany*

Part I

Introduction & Historical Background

Chapter 1

Paradigm Shifts in Mast Cell and Basophil Biology and Function: An Emerging View of Immune Regulation in Health and Disease

Ana Olivera and Juan Rivera

Abstract

The physiological role of the mast cell and basophil has for many years remained enigmatic. In this chapter we briefly summarize some of the more recent studies that shed new light on the role of mast cells and basophils in health and disease. What we gain from these studies is a new appreciation for mast cells and basophils as sentinels in host defense and a further understanding that dysregulation of mast cell and basophil function can be a component of various diseases other than allergies. Perhaps, the most important insight reaped from this work is the increasing awareness that mast cells and basophils can function as immunoregulatory cells that modulate the immune response in health and disease. Collectively, the recent knowledge provides new challenges and opportunities towards the development of novel therapeutic strategies to augment host protection and modify disease through manipulation of mast cell and basophil function.

Key words Allergy, Atherosclerosis, Autoimmunity, Basophils, Cancer, Dermatitis, Immunoglobulin E, Infection, Mast cells, Proteases

1 Introduction

It is more than a century since mast cells and subsequently basophils were described by Paul Ehrlich based on the staining of their "metachromatic" granules with basic aniline dyes [1–4]. For many years, thereafter, the biological role of mast cells and basophils has remained enigmatic. Mast cells are known to be localized around blood vessels in connective tissues but they are not part of the perivascular system [5]. These cells are long-term tissue residents with slow turnover; they fully differentiate in tissues but still retain the ability to proliferate and replenish themselves [6]. On the other hand, the basophil was for many years viewed as a blood "mast cell" and because of its rarity (~1 % of blood leukocytes) had long been considered as a redundant cell type or possibly a circulating precursor of tissue mast cells [7]. Features in common to both cell types include the presence of preformed metachromatic granules,

Bernhard F. Gibbs and Franco H. Falcone (eds.), *Basophils and Mast Cells: Methods and Protocols*, Methods in Molecular Biology, vol. 1192, DOI 10.1007/978-1-4939-1173-8_1, © Springer Science+Business Media New York 2014

as described by Paul Ehrlich [1–5, 8], that contain a vast array of releasable allergic mediators [9], the surface expression of the high affinity receptor for IgE [5, 10], and the ability to similarly synthesize T helper 2-polarizing cytokines and chemokines de novo [5, 10, 11]; characteristics that have served to cement the view of a common biological function. Nonetheless, beyond the difference in where the cells are localized in vivo, there are distinct features of both cell types: Basophil maturation occurs in the bone marrow and not in peripheral tissues as seen for mast cells; unlike mast cells, basophils do not proliferate after maturation; and the life-span of a mast cell can be weeks (perhaps months) whereas that of a basophil is normally measured in days. Moreover, both murine and human basophils express intracellular and cell surface molecules that are distinct from those expressed on a mast cells [7, 12]. These differences suggest discrete in vivo functions for these cells but only recently have we begun to appreciate their specific roles. This new awareness arises in large part as a result of novel discoveries on previously unrecognized roles for both mast cells and basophils in health and disease [7, 13].

In this introductory chapter, we can only capture a few of these recent discoveries. For the sake of brevity, we cannot summarize the vast recent literature that has contributed to all the new insights in this field, but we hope the examples presented herein set the tenor for the following chapters, which will provide additional details. The rapidly expanding awareness of a role for mast cells and basophils in innate immunity and as immunomodulatory cells [14] has driven much of this new investigation. While there is still some controversy on some of the specific roles assigned to these cells [15, 16], there is an increasing appreciation that mast cells and basophils play a role in immune protection and, as important players in the immune system, can also become dysregulated and contribute to diseases, other than allergic disease. Such discoveries underlie a shifting paradigm in mast cell and basophil biology and function.

2   Novel Roles for Mast Cells and Basophils: Protecting the Host

2.1   An Unexpected Protective Role of Mast Cells in Atopic Dermatitis

Contact dermatitis is a common form of skin inflammation that may appear after exposure to an irritant or, usually, an allergen. In mice, studies on allergic contact dermatitis are normally conducted using contact hypersensitivity models (CHS) (*see* Chapter 18), also known as delayed-type hypersensitivity reactions (DTH) [17]. In these models, mice are sensitized and consequently challenged epicutaneously with a hapten such as dinitrofluorobenzene (DNFB), oxazolone, fluorescein isothiocyanate (FITC), or trinitrochlorobenzene (TNCB). This elicits a local immune reaction with characteristics of allergic contact dermatitis. In contrast to these models that normally employ a single challenge, other models use periodic challenges with these haptens, producing a chronic inflammatory response that is more akin to human atopic dermatitis [18]. The role of mast cells in CHS or delayed-type IV hypersensitivity reaction is still controversial because depending on the type of mast cell-deficient mice or the model of CHS, the elicitation of the inflammatory response was reduced, enhanced, or unchanged [15, 16, 19–21]. This may not be surprising considering the immunomodulatory functions of mast cells (discussed in more detail in a following section) and the variety of protocols and models used to elicit CHS (with different types of haptens, concentrations of hapten, solvent, sites of sensitization, and times during the course of CHS measuring inflammation), which may affect some aspects of the immune response. In fact, Norman et al. showed that the mast cell-deficient $Kit^{w/w-v}$ mice had a more severe response than their wild-type counterparts (mast cell sufficient) after elicitation with high doses of oxazolone, but when low doses of this irritant were used the $Kit^{w/w-v}$ mice had reduced responses [22]. These experiments are important as they reflect how the strength of the stimulus elicits an immune response that may require that mast cells serve a dual role (protective versus exacerbating). Similar to the strength of stimulus, all other factors mentioned above may differentially promote the type of immune response, what particular immune cells are involved, and which pro- or anti-inflammatory components are induced in the local environment and, thus, which mast cell responses are elicited and their specific role in the inflammatory process.

In models of chronic skin inflammation that show hallmarks of human atopic dermatitis (including barrier abnormalities, infiltration of mast cells and eosinophils, elevated IL-4 and IgE, and a predominant Th2-type of inflammation [23] with a late phase Th-1 component (Hershko and Rivera, unpublished observation)), mast cells have a predominant role dampening inflammation [21]. Instead of a single challenge, oxazolone applied repeatedly over the course of 20–25 days caused chronic skin inflammation that was markedly exacerbated in mast cell-deficient $Kit^{W-sh/W-sh}$ mice [21]. Interestingly, the suppression of inflammation by mast cells was dependent on their production of IL-2 (a cytokine not normally associated with the biological function of mast cells in vivo), since the enhanced disease in $Kit^{W-sh/W-sh}$ mice was reduced when the mice were engrafted with wild-type mast cells, but not with IL-2-deficient mast cells. The view of IL-2-mediated suppression in atopic dermatitis was further supported by a similarly exacerbated skin inflammation in IL-2-deficient mice or in wild-type mice treated with anti-CD25 antibody (which binds and transiently inactivates the IL-2 receptor). Of particular interest, however, was that the rescue of the suppressive role of mast cells in $Kit^{W-sh/W-sh}$ mice after engraftment of wild-type mast cells was observed even when these cells were not engrafted at the site of inflammation (by intradermal reconstitution). Engraftment distal to the local site (by i.v. reconstitution, which results in engraftment in the spleen, lymph nodes, and other tissues other than the skin) was sufficient to promote the protective effect and dampen the inflammation. Several lines of evidence suggested that suppression of skin inflammation by mast cells occurred in the spleen: In $Kit^{W-sh/W-sh}$ mice engrafted with wild-type mast cells, production of IL-2 by these cells was observed in the spleen. In addition, the numbers of mast cells increased in this organ (together with the skin and lymph nodes) after induction of chronic inflammation and the increase of mast cells in the spleen showed a marked association with increased disease intensity. Thus, as the inflammation in the skin worsened more mast cells were recruited to the spleen and this recruitment plateaued at a point where disease intensity entered a steady state. At the local site of inflammation expansion of regulatory T cells (Tregs) was observed in wild-type mice. In contrast, in $Kit^{W-sh/W-sh}$ mice reconstituted with IL-2-deficient mast cells, Treg expansion was reduced but could be rescued by reconstitution of $Kit^{W-sh/W-sh}$ with wild-type mast cells. These findings suggested that the recruitment of mast cells to the spleen during oxazolone-induced chronic allergic dermatitis played an important role in regulating Treg expansion and increased the numbers of these cells at the local site of inflammation. It is interesting that systemic rather than local mast cell production of IL-2 (in the skin) led to Treg expansion, but one might speculate that such circumstances might allow mast cells to play a dual role in both promoting (at the local site) and preventing (by distal regulation) inflammation.

The protective role for mast cells in DTH reactions was also manifested when DTH was elicited secondarily to the inflammatory response induced by either UVB irradiation [24] or mosquito bites [25]. In the latter study, downregulation of the skin inflammatory response by mast cells was attributed to their production of IL-10 at a distal site, likely in the lymph nodes since $Kit^{W-sh/W-sh}$ mice showed reduced IL-10 production in the lymph node compared to wild-type mice or mast cell-reconstituted $Kit^{W-sh/W-sh}$ mice [25]. IL-10-mediated mast cell-dependent suppression was also found in long-term DTH responses (up to 15 days after a single epicutaneous challenge with a hapten) or after UVB chronic irradiation. Reconstitution experiments using IL-10-deficient mast cells in $Kit^{w/wv}$ mice demonstrated a requirement for mast cell-produced IL-10 in these models [26]. Thus, although the cytokine involved in suppressing inflammation differs depending on the type of model studied, overall, the findings demonstrate an anti-inflammatory role of mast cells in long-term DTH [26], late stages of chronic allergic dermatitis [21] or short-term DTH responses secondary to another inflammatory stimulus like UVB-irradiation [24] or mosquito bites [25]. These findings reveal an unsuspected role for mast cells in controlling the inflammatory response and thus one must consider if manipulation of the ability of mast cells to produce such cytokines may be of potential interest in controlling skin diseases in humans.

2.2 Protection by Basophils to Reinfection (Hookworms, Ticks)

The innate immune contribution of mast cells to protection to infection by various species of parasites (reviewed in [13, 16, 27]) has long been recognized. Interestingly, however, even though peripheral basophilia during parasite infections has been described [28], the actual involvement of basophils in parasite-elicited T-helper type 2 responses and their role in parasite expulsion had not been fully appreciated. This was, in large part, due to the erroneous belief that mice did not have basophils and thus studies in mouse models were hampered by this notion. Subsequent recognition that indeed basophils were present in mice [29–31], and the discovery of antibodies that depleted basophils in vivo [7] as well as the development of basophil-null [32] and basophil ablation mouse models [33] ushered in a new era of investigation on the role of these cells in health and disease. While basophils comprise only about 1 % of circulating leukocytes, they are the major innate immune cell producing IL-4 after helminth infection [34–36]. At the moment, it is unclear under what circumstances the IL-4 producing role of basophils is essential for host protection versus situations where IL-4 production by basophils may play a contributory role in Th2-mediated immunity. Evidence of the latter role is provided by models of basophil deficiency [32, 33], or transient depletion of basophils by injection of anti-FcεRI or anti-CD200R3 mAbs [37], which demonstrated no effect on the immune response and the expulsion of the *Nippostrongylus brasiliensis* (*N. brasiliensis*) following initial infection, but showed a contributory role in worm expulsion when Th2 cells were absent [38]. These findings suggested that during the initial infection the role of basophils is redundant. During a secondary infection to *N. brasiliensis*, however, the presence of basophils seemed critical for the expulsion of this helminth, regardless of the presence or absence of mast cells or CD4 T cells, which were both required for protection during the initial infection [32]. The mechanisms governing basophil-mediated protection against reinfection are not well understood. Nonetheless, because IL-4 and IL-13 are important for Th2 cell polarization, effector cell recruitment, and tissue responses to worm infection [39], and basophils can abundantly secrete both cytokines during these infections [34, 35, 38, 40], part of the protection may be mediated through the production of IL-4/IL-13 [32]. This concept is partly supported by the lack of recruitment of eosinophils to mediastinal lymph nodes in the absence of basophils [32] and by the requirement of STAT6 (which is activated by IL-4Rα) for worm expulsion during repeated infections [37]. A less well-appreciated function of basophils (most clearly demonstrated in the mouse) is their capacity to express MHC class II and other surface molecules, like the B cell survival and activation factor (BAFF) [41–43], which may confer the ability to prime naïve T cells into Th2 cells and also increase humoral responses through support of B cell differentiation and survival. The expression of such molecules in human basophils is less well defined, yet some evidence for basophil MHC class II expression (HLA-DR) has emerged from studies of the role of basophils in systemic lupus erythematosus (discussed below) [44–46]. While the role of such molecules on basophils is not completely understood, they may play a role during parasite infections and help contribute to basophil-induced protection [37, 47].

A role for basophils in the protection against tick re-infestation was also recently demonstrated. These studies used antibody-mediated depletion of basophils and an elegantly engineered mouse that allows for diphtheria toxin-induced, basophil-specific ablation [33]. After repeated infestations many animals develop resistance to ticks but the nature of this anti-tick immunity was unclear. Wada and colleagues showed that upon repeated infestation, engorgement of these ecto-parasites is diminished and is associated with recruitment of basophils to the tick-feeding site. This resistance to reinfection was transferred by sera of previously tick-infected animals, indicating the importance of a component of the humoral immune response. Furthermore, they showed that the presence of immunoglobulin Fc receptors on the basophils was required [33]. While the specific mechanism for the basophil-mediated protective effect and which basophil-effector molecules involved have not been investigated, these findings also demonstrate that basophils function in protection to reinfection by parasites. Further studies will be needed to investigate how basophils mediate this protection and to determine if these findings can be extended to other species of parasites and to parasite infections of humans.

2.3 The Protective Effect of Mast Cell and Basophil Proteases

An area of considerable interest that has emerged from studies of the protective role of mast cells and basophils is that of the role of mast cell proteases in host defense. While the release of mast cell proteases (MCP) from activated mast cells or basophils is known to promote inflammation in certain pathological conditions, such as asthma or arthritis, their role is not restricted to only these pro-inflammatory functions [48]. In many circumstances their actions have been shown to be protective instead of harmful, contributing to the Yin-Yang of protective and harmful consequences of mast cell and basophil-derived products.

Proteases cleave a variety of functionally diverse protein substrates through recognition of specific peptide sequences. Cleavage can result in protein activation or inhibition and thus it is not surprising that the overall physiopathological impact of mast cell proteases depends on the environmental circumstances in which they are released. When mice are exposed to venoms from certain honeybees, snakes, lizards, and scorpions, mast cell carboxypeptidase 3 (CPA3) and other mast cell proteases are essential for limiting the toxicity, morbidity, and mortality. These venoms contain toxins (i.e., sarafotoxins and helodermin in snake and lizard venoms, respectively) that share structural similarities with endogenous mammalian peptides (endothelin-1 and VIP, respectively) and bind their corresponding receptors in mast cells thus causing them to degranulate [49, 50]. While mast cell degranulation causes changes in vascular permeability, local inflammation, and anaphylaxis, the symptoms to intradermal injection of these venoms were more severe and even lethal in mice lacking mast cells, CPA3, or the corresponding peptide receptors, indicating that mast cell CPA3-mediated proteolytic degradation of these toxins benefits the host [49, 51].

Importantly, the control of toxicity by mast cells is not limited to animal venoms. These cells can protect against hypothermia, diarrhea, and death induced by an injection of endothelin-1 [50] or VIP [49]; findings that may have implications in multiple pathologies, such as sepsis, where any of these or other vasoactive peptides are elevated. Certain models of moderate to moderately severe sepsis have revealed a protective function of mast cells using kit-dependent mast cell-deficient mouse models [52, 53], and the findings suggest that these protective effects may be mediated by mast cell-derived cytokines and/or mast cell proteases. For example, an interesting study in a model of severe septic peritonitis by cecal ligation and puncture [54] showed that the peptide neurotensin, which is increased and contributes to hypotension and mortality in this model, can be degraded by activated mast cells [54, 55] and can cause a reduction in the levels of neurotensin diminishing its negative effects during sepsis [54]. These authors identified neurolysin as the main mast cell protease involved in the degradation of neurotensin [54]. Similarly, other studies described a protective role for mast cell-derived mMCP4 in eliminating TNF, which can promote inflammation [53, 56], during moderately severe septic peritonitis [56]. Others have shown an essential role for mMCP6 in the clearance of *K. pneumoniae* injected intraperitoneally [57]. In addition to the models of peritonitis, mast cell-derived mMCP4 was shown to play a key role in restricting inflammation in the brain after trauma [58], and mMCP4 [59] and CPA [60], presumably derived from mast cells or basophils, were found to reduce lung inflammation during allergic asthma by degrading, respectively, IL-33 and IL-13 [59]. Thus, an emerging view from such studies is that mast cell and basophil proteases can serve not only to promote inflammation but may be essential in limiting toxicity and infection.

3   Unexpected Physiopathological Roles of Mast Cells and Basophils

3.1   Adverse Effects of Mast Cell Protection in Atopic Dermatitis: The Atopic March

Recent studies in our lab indicated that mice subjected to chronic allergic dermatitis induced by repeated exposure to a hapten were more susceptible to airway inflammation induced by a different allergen [61], a phenomenon that resembles the increased incidence and severity of asthma after AD in humans commonly known as the atopic march [62]. Thus, as postulated, occurrence of atopic dermatitis in early life increases susceptibility and/or severity of asthma or other allergies in later life. As described in the previous section, our findings indicated that mast cells suppressed skin inflammation in a chronic allergic dermatitis model [21] and thus it was of interest to determine if in such a model one might observe a relationship between atopic dermatitis and allergic asthma. Interestingly, the findings indicated an enhanced sensitivity to the inhaled allergen following the resolution of dermatitis, which was dependent on mast cells since an enhanced asthmatic response was not seen in mice lacking mast cells ($Kit^{W-sh/W-sh}$) but was recovered when such mice were reconstituted with bone marrow-derived mast cells prior to the induction of dermatitis [61]. In fact, the findings showed that the increased airway reactivity was associated with a persistent increase in the overall number of mast cells after the induction and resolution of atopic dermatitis. However, how an increase in mast cell numbers results in enhanced sensitivity to an oral challenge is unclear. Similar to their role in suppressing allergic chronic dermatitis, their potentiating effect in airway sensitivity did not appear to be consequence of a direct effector function in the local environment because mast cell numbers were not increased in the lung but only in distal sites such as the skin, lymph nodes, and spleen. This was particularly obvious in $Kit^{W-sh/W-sh}$ mice that were intradermally reconstituted with mast cells, since they showed increased airway hypersensitivity following atopic dermatitis even though no mast cells could be detected in the lungs [61].

The mechanism(s) underlying this distal effect of mast cells on airway reactivity is unclear. Nonetheless, it was previously shown that activation of mast cells in the skin at the time of immunization was effective in enhancing an antibody response to vaccine antigens [63] presumably by recruiting or activating dendritic cells and/or lymphocytes to the lymph nodes [64, 65]. Similarly, mast cells that are elevated in numbers after AD may potentially promote interactions with dendritic cells or T cells (discussed further below) in the lymph nodes to facilitate an immune response to an inhaled challenge. Regardless, the idea that mast cells can suppress allergic dermatitis while promoting airway hypersensitivity highlights the plasticity of the mast cell [66], which is likely influenced by the overall pathological environment of the disease. Consistent with this view, while mast cells produced IL-2 in the spleen during

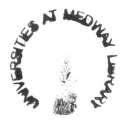

chronic dermatitis [21], after resolution of the dermatitis they no longer produced IL-2 and induction of this cytokine was not detected after provocation of asthma [61]. This change in phenotype suggests that such transformations ultimately shape the type of response by the mast cell and thus its role in health and disease.

3.2 An Unexpected Role for Mast Cells in Obesity

Obesity is a condition characterized by excess adiposity, metabolic dysregulation in white adipose tissue, and a chronic low-grade inflammation in various organs, thereby increasing the incidence of insulin resistance, diabetes, cardiovascular disease, and other diseases [67]. Although the exact mechanisms involved in the progression of this condition and the specific contribution of immune cell types are not clear, it is generally accepted that nutrient excess causes vascular changes in the tissue, infiltration of immune cells, and chronic overload of macrophages, which then causes metabolic dysfunction in the adipocytes, as well as induction of inflammatory cytokine production by immune cells. Mast cells, which are present in adipose tissue, as well as other innate and adaptive immune cells, have been implicated in the initiation and progression of obesity [67–69]. Interestingly, increase in the epididymal fat tissue and other fat depots in mice with diet-induced obesity correlates with increased mast cell numbers in these tissues [70–72]. In humans, the white adipose tissue of obese subjects contains higher numbers of mast cells than that from lean donors and these cells are localized in the proximity of blood vessels [71], particularly in diabetic individuals [73]. Furthermore, these cells were also found preferentially localized in fibrosis bundles and their presence correlated, as in mice [71], with macrophage accumulation and endothelial cell inflammation [73]. In obesity-related glomerulopathy, mast cells infiltrate renal tubulointerstitial regions and their presence is associated with tubular atrophy and interstitial fibrosis [74]. These mast cells had a higher tryptase or chymase content [71, 73] than those in normal individuals and might be activated in this disease, since subjects with body mass index ≥32 kg/mm^2 had significantly higher serum tryptase concentrations than lean individuals in two independent studies [71, 75]. In contrast, this correlation was not found in a smaller cohort study of children [76], and thus, whether the absence of correlation may be due to a smaller cohort or to age-dependent factors or other unknown variables is not clear. Regardless, adipose tissue has been described as a reservoir of committed mast cell progenitors with the endowed potential to home to peripheral tissues [77]. Thus, the possibility exists that nutrient overload may directly or indirectly affect the differentiation of these progenitors into mature mast cells and promote their activation or homing to other tissues.

A mouse study that demonstrates a role for mast cells in obesity employed two models of Kit-dependent mast cell-deficient mice, $Kit^{W-sh/W-sh}$ and $Kit^{W/Wv}$, fed with a Western-type diet consisting of high fats and sugar [71]. These mice gained significantly less body weight than wild-type congenic controls on the same diet [71, 72]. The lower weight gain was accompanied by significantly lower concentrations of serum leptin, insulin, and various cytokines and these mice had a higher resting metabolic rate and higher glucose tolerance and insulin sensitivity than WT mice [71]. The adoptive transfer of wild-type bone marrow-derived mast cells in such mast cell-deficient mice caused a gain in body weight as well as recovery of most of the aforementioned parameters. While reconstitution of the mast cell-deficient mice with mast cells from TNF-deficient mice resulted in a similar weight gain as mice reconstituted with wild-type mast cells, mice reconstituted with mast cells from IL-6 or INF γ-deficient mice had poor weight gain, indicating that mast cell-derived IL-6 and INF γ play a role in obesity progression, but not TNF. Mast cell stabilizing drugs, such as cromolyn and ketotifen, also prevented diet-induced obesity and improved preestablished obesity and diabetes in mice that had consumed a Western diet for 12 weeks, suggesting a role for mast cells not only in the onset but also in the progression of obesity [71]. A caveat of this work is that the discovery of a role for mast cells in diet-induced obesity was almost entirely based on Kit-dependent mast cell-deficient mouse models, which clearly have mast cell-unrelated defects [15, 16]. Moreover, it should be noted that the efficacy and selectivity of cromolyn at inhibiting mast cell functions has been questioned [78]. Yet, taken together with the correlative studies in other mouse models and in humans, this study makes a strong argument for the role of mast cells in the promotion of obesity.

As mentioned above, there is evidence of a requirement for mast cell cytokines (IL-6 and IFN γ) in promoting obesity but the exact mechanism by which these products might regulate obesity is not understood. Given the involvement of mast-derived products in immune cell recruitment, activation, and in the production of cytokines that can affect the surrounding endothelial cells, fibroblasts, and smooth muscle cells, the consequences of accumulating mast cells in adipocyte tissues may be many fold [79]. While the production of cytokines by mast cells may contribute to the proinflammatory nature of obesity, it should be noted that the production of prostanoids by mast cells may also promote adipocyte dysfunction not only by inhibiting lipolysis, but also by promoting fat deposition. Thus, palmitic acid, a common and abundant fatty acid in Western-style diets, was shown to induce PGE2 production by mast cells [80], a lipid product that has anti-lipolytic responses in adipocytes [81]. In addition, another mast cell-derived prostanoid product, PGJ2, a metabolite of PGD2, was found to activate PPAR γ, which mediates differentiation of adipocytes [72]. Thus, collectively these mast cell products may all contribute to enhance fat deposition.

3.3 Mast Cells in Atherosclerosis

Atherosclerosis is a progressive disease defined by the appearance of lesions or plaques in the walls of large and mid-size arteries, and often is the underlying cause of cardiovascular disease. The pathogenesis of atherosclerosis involves the accumulation of lipids from blood in the subendothelial region of the arterial wall and a complex interplay between endothelial, vascular, and inflammatory cells that leads to the progression of the artherosclerotic plaque into a rupture-prone unstable plaque that is the main cause for the complications of artherosclerosis. A number of inflammatory cells including macrophages, T cells, dendritic cells and, relatively recently, mast cells have been suggested to be involved in the initiation and/or progression of the disease [82]. Mast cells are usually found in the perivascular area of vessel walls and are more abundant in the intima and adventitia of atherosclerotic plaques in mice and humans and in intraplaque neovessels in humans. These MCs contain higher tryptase and chymase [83–86], and their presence and content correlate with disease progression and plaque hemorrhage, destabilization, and lipidosis [69, 85]. While cause and effect has not been clearly demonstrated there is considerable correlation between mast cell activation or the presence of mast cell-derived products and atherosclerotic plaque progression [82, 87]. Moreover, the functional importance of mast cells in the progression of plaque formation was demonstrated by use of the mast cell-deficient mouse, $Kit^{w/wv}$. Crossing of these mice with two atherosclerotic mouse models, the LDLr$^{-/-}$ mouse [88, 89] and the ApoE$^{-/-}$ mice [90], which develop atherosclerosis upon feeding with a high fat diet or spontaneously, respectively, attenuated the progression of atherosclerosis. This manifested as a decrease in lipid deposition, lesion size, and immune cell infiltration in arterial walls [88, 89], a phenotype that could be reversed by adoptive transfer of wild-type bone marrow-derived mast cells, strongly suggesting a cause and effect relationship between mast cells and atherosclerosis progression in this model [89]. However, when mast cells from IL-6 or IFN γ-deficient mice were used in the adoptive transfer experiments, the atherosclerotic phenotype was not restored thus implicating these mast cell-produced cytokines in the development of the disease [89]. Similar conclusions were drawn from studies in ApoE$^{-/-}$/$Kit^{w/wv}$ mice fed with a high fat diet for 6 months to accelerate the disease [90]. These mice showed a diminished development of atherosclerotic lesions and reduced hepatic steatosis, but also reduced serum levels of LDL and HDL and considerable elevation of the cytokines IL-6 and IL-10 in the earlier phase of the disease [90].

Potentially mast cells could contribute to the development of atherosclerosis at many points in this process [82, 91]. Some studies have suggested that mast cell-derived products can promote the recruitment of inflammatory cells to the developing atherosclerotic plaque by inducing vascular permeability [92] and the expression of adhesion molecules by the endothelium [89, 93]. Mast cell-derived proteases may also degrade the various components of the extracellular matrices in the plaque, destabilizing the plaque [87]. Others have shown that mast cell-derived IL-6 or IFN γ promotes apoptosis of smooth muscle cells, which together with microvessel formation triggered by mast cell products promote the development of arterial aneurysms [94].

The triggers for mast cell activity in this disease are not well understood. It is possible that the lipid components, such as oxidized LDL molecules, induce mast cell degranulation and leukocyte adhesion [64]. Oxidized LDL-IgG complexes have been detected in atherogenic lesions, and they were found to induce pro-inflammatory cytokine production by mast cells [95]. Recently, IgE was reported to be required for atherosclerosis development since ApoE$^{-/-}$/FcεRIα-deficient mice had reduced atherosclerosis, and IgE was found to be elevated in patients with myocardial infarction or unstable angina pectoris. However, the contribution of IgE was primarily due to effects on macrophage apoptosis, and the possible role of mast cells in these mice was not investigated [96]. Nonetheless, the collective studies provide evidence of a contributory role for mast cells in this disease.

3.4 Mast Cells in Tumor Growth and Development

The connection between inflammation and the development of cancer is widely appreciated [97]. Although lymphocytes have taken the center stage, and the presence of high numbers of Tregs in tumors has been associated with a dampening of the immune response in this environment [98], a contributory role for mast cells in tumor development is also beginning to emerge. A number of studies in human cancers and mouse tumor models established an association between the location and numbers of mast cells (as well as mast cell protease content in the tumors) and the stage of malignancy, microvessel density or prognosis and recurrence of tumors. This, together with the findings of mast cell-derived cytokines in the developing tumors, has suggested a role for mast cells in promoting the development of tumors [99–111]. Tumor-derived SCF [112] and tumor-induced cytokines [113], for example TNF [102], are thought to be involved in the recruitment and responsiveness of mast cells to particular types of tumors, although it is not known whether such factors have a general role in mast cell biology and function in most tumors. An evolving view, based on numerous studies, is that at early stages of malignancy mast cells are recruited to the tumor where they proliferate and are activated to produce mediators that promote tumor vessel formation, recruitment of immune cells, and immunosuppression, all of which would favor tumor progression. As the tumor evolves and becomes more aggressive, the tumor environment does not support mast cell proliferation/recruitment within the tumor and tumor growth becomes more independent of mast cells. However, not all tumors show a positive correlation with mast cells but instead some show no correlation or a negative correlation, which would be more consistent with an immunomodulatory or immunoregulatory role of mast cells on the progression of the tumor [105, 106, 108, 114]. Given the plasticity of mast cells to differentiate and respond differently depending on environmental cues, it is not surprising that the role of mast cells may vary depending on the type of tumor and the stage of tumor development.

The role of mast cells as promoters of tumor growth has primarily been demonstrated in Kit-dependent mast cell-deficient mouse models, including $Kit^{w/wv}$ [115] and $Kit^{W-sh/W-sh}$ mice [106, 113, 116–119]. Implantation of a variety of tumor types in these mice showed reduced numbers of tumors and reduced size of tumors for orthotopically implanted B16 melanoma cells [115, 118], pancreatic ductal adenocarcinoma [116], Lewis lung carcinoma [119], prostate adenocarcinomas [106], and urothelial carcinoma cells expressing HY antigens [117]. That mast cells were important for tumor development was demonstrated by injection of mast cells derived from wild-type syngenic mice into the mast cell-deficient mice, which reversed this phenotype enhancing tumor growth and numbers. A similar reduction in tumor growth and vascularization was observed when an inducible mouse model of Myc-promoted pancreatic β-cell and skin tumorigenesis was crossed with the mast cell-deficient $Kit^{W-sh/W-sh}$ mouse [113] as well as in a mouse model of polyposis lethally irradiated and reconstituted with marrows of $Kit^{W-sh/W-sh}$, CD34-, or CD43-deficient mice that are unable to differentiate mast cells or recruit their precursors to peripheral sites [102]. Studies in these models have also revealed some clues about how mast cells may regulate tumor development, although the exact mechanisms are unclear. Nonetheless, reconstitution of mast cell-deficient mice with mMCP9-deficient mast cells, unlike reconstitution with wild-type mast cells, failed to rescue the development of well-differentiated, slow-growing prostate cell adenocarcinomas in these mice, suggesting that mMCP9 plays a role in advancing the development of this type of tumor probably by promoting cell migration and invasion [106]. Other studies have suggested a role for mast cell-derived TNF in the proliferation of adenomatous polyps [102], and a possible immunoregulatory effect of mast cells in enhancing immunosuppression thus reducing protective anti-tumor immunity [117]. It is likely that mast cells may employ multiple mechanisms depending on the environment and tumor type.

It is important to stress, however, that the role of mast cells, even in mouse models, is not unidirectional, since they may influence tumorigenesis in many other ways. For example, it was shown that even though the presence of mast cells promoted early stage prostate cancer in a mouse model, paradoxically, targeting mast cells in a tumor-prone transgenic adenocarcinoma of the mouse prostate resulted in a more aggressive tumor, indicating a suppressive function for mast cells in this latter circumstance [106]. Another recent study suggests that reduction of mast cell (and possibly other cells) TNF production by mast cell-derived PGD2 restricts vascular permeability and inflammation in the tumor environment [119]. In this study the authors reconstituted $Kit^{W-sh/W-sh}$ mice with PGD2-deficient mast cells and found increased size and number of lung carcinoma cell tumors. This effect was counteracted by reconstitution of $Kit^{W-sh/W-sh}$ mice with mast cells deficient in both PGD2 and TNF production [119]. Other studies unraveling a suppressive role for mast cells in the evolution into aggressive tumors include a genetic model of early stage of intestinal neoplasia (*APC-Min* mouse) that when crossed with a mast cell-deficient mouse showed more numerous and larger tumors [120]. These findings exemplify the complexity of the potential role of mast cells in tumor growth and development. While one might consider the potential targeting of mast cells to treat cancer, this may be restricted to certain types and stages of tumors. Of considerable concern is that targeting of mast cells may worsen the disease given the dual and opposing roles for these cells in some tumors [106]. Thus, it is essential to understand the underlying mechanisms by which mast cells can promote versus inhibit tumor development. An important cautionary note on the aforementioned studies is the consideration that Kit itself is a factor that may be dysregulated within the tumor cells in some types of cancer [121], and thus the results using Kit-dependent mast cell-deficient models should be further validated for a better understanding of the role of mast cells in cancer.

3.5   Mast Cells and Basophils in Autoimmune Diseases

The ability of mast cells to respond to IgE and IgG immune complexes and inflammatory stimuli, and to secrete mediators that affect immune and nonimmune cells [9] positions them as likely contributors in the development of autoimmune disease. Although the potential contribution of mast cells in autoimmune diseases has been long recognized, their specific role in disease progression is still not well defined [122]. In animal models, this is in part due to nonuniformity in the experimental approaches to induce autoimmune diseases or differences intrinsic to the mouse models used. While many of such models share a somewhat similar clinical manifestation of disease, they may still differ in the cell types involved, the exact sequence of events required for disease development, and the underlying mechanisms allowing for disease development. In addition, the interpretation of the contribution of mast cells using mast cell-deficient models has, in instances, been hampered by the known defects in these models.

For more than two decades there have been reports on the contributory role of mast cells in rheumatoid arthritis (RA) and multiple sclerosis (MS). For RA, the overall picture, using different approaches, generally supports the concept that mast cell activity exacerbates the inflammatory process and severity of this disease, although this effect may not always manifest or be predominant due to the redundancy of the immune system, depending on the specific characteristics of the human disease or the animal model under study. The findings are somewhat more ambiguous in MS as there is considerable divergence in the experimental approaches, the mouse models used, and the influence of dietary, other environmental, and genetic factors may be key in this disease. Thus, studies on the role of mast cells in mouse models of MS (experimental autoimmune encephalomyelitis, EAE) have resulted in a differing of opinion on the role of these cells in this disease (reviewed in [15, 16, 122, 123]). Importantly, it should be noted that the baseline environment and the type or strength of the stimulus used to induce MS in mouse models may reveal or mask a role for mast cells in this disease [122]. This view is highly consistent with the aforementioned plasticity of mast cells as influenced by the environment in which they reside.

Rheumatoid arthritis (RA) is an autoimmune disorder characterized by chronic inflammation of the joints, with synovial hyperplasia, cartilage destruction, bone erosion, and changes in joint function. An association between the inflamed joint and the presence of mast cells has long been recognized. MCs and MC-derived products are elevated in the synovial fluid and synovial tissue of RA patients [124–127] and in the arthritic lesions of mice [128–130], suggesting their participation in joint inflammation. In addition, mast cell stabilizers such as nedocromil, tranilast, cromolyn, or salbutamol have been shown effective in reducing neutrophil infiltration and clinical scores of arthritis in collagen-induced and K/BxN serum-induced arthritis in mice [128, 130, 131] and treatment of some arthritis patients with anti-histaminic or anti-serotoninergic drugs was reported as effective in reducing arthritic attacks [124]. Such studies support the concept of a contributory role of mast cells in this inflammatory condition. In addition, the inhibitor of the tyrosine kinase KIT, imatinib mesylate (Gleevec), which induces apoptosis in rheumatoid synovial mast cells [132], was reported to be efficacious in reducing arthritic swelling and pain and other markers of disease in two out of three patients with severe RA [133]. While further studies are required to determine if the effect is indeed mast cell specific (given the off target effects of such inhibitors), collectively the studies to date provide some level of confidence in a role for mast cells in RA. Unfortunately, the results from mast cell-deficient mouse models used to address the specific role of mast cells in arthritis have not been clear-cut. While the $Kit^{W/W-v}$ mast cell-deficient mouse is resistant to arthritis induction by K/BxN serum transfer [131, 134–137] and to anticollagen monoclonal antibody and LPS-induced arthritis [138], the $Kit^{W-sh/W-sh}$ mast cell-deficient mice or mice in which mast cells are eradicated by insertion of Cre recombinase in the carboxypeptidase A3 locus

(Cre-Master) were fully susceptible to collagen- [139], anticollagen- and LPS- [138], and K/BxN-induced arthritis [134, 140]. The defect in the development of arthritis in $Kit^{W/W-v}$ mice can be restored by reconstitution of the mice with wild-type bone marrow-derived mast cells. It has been reasoned that the results obtained in the $Kit^{W/W-v}$ may be attributed to a more prominent role for mast cells in the context of differences in the numbers of neutrophils in these mice relative to $Kit^{W-sh/W-sh}$ mice [15, 134]. Nevertheless, these studies have been helpful as they not only clarify some aspects of the mechanisms of action of mast cells in this model, but also serve to unravel the harmful role of mast cells that may be obscured in other models by either the redundancy with other immune cells or by the potential opposing effects of mast cells to promote or protect against disease progression. This may be of relevance when considering the targeting of mast cells in disease.

Several mast cell products have been implicated in the pathogenesis of arthritis, although some are not necessarily produced only by mast cells. Thus, mice lacking histidine decarboxylase, the enzyme producing histamine [141], mice deficient in the tryptases mMCP7 [142], mMCP6 [142, 143], which appears to be expressed in all synovial mast cells as demonstrated in the K/BxN serum-transfer-induced arthritic synovium [143], or mMCP4 [144], showed markedly reduced scores of arthritis in various models. In addition, mice deficient in the cytokine IL-1, which is produced by mast cells via the activation of FcγRIIIA in autoantibody-induced arthritis, also had reduced arthritis [135]. Many stimuli have been proposed to activate mast cell degranulation or cytokine production in the environment of the arthritic synovium [135]. Autoantibody-induced arthritis was shown to require FcγRIIIA [134, 135, 145] and the complement receptor C5aR, which may be needed for the release of neutrophil chemoattractants into the synovium [136], while in collagen-induced arthritis models the IL33 receptor in mast cells [146] has been implicated. Interestingly, in RA patients the presence of high IgE that is complexed with anti-IgE has been reported [147]. Thus, in some cases of RA mast cell or basophil contribution may be a consequence of FcεRI activation.

The role of basophil in autoimmunity has not been as extensively investigated. Nonetheless, one classic example where these cells can promote autoimmunity is in the well-described case of autoimmune chronic urticaria where patients generate IgG autoantibodies directed to the FcεRIα chain [148]. More recently, we uncovered a previously unrecognized role for basophils in the pathogenesis of systemic lupus erythematosus (SLE), a complex autoimmune disease affecting multiple target organs and characterized by the presence of autoreactive antibodies [148]. Using Lyn kinase-deficient mice, which develop a lupus-like disease in late life, we demonstrated the presence of elevated levels of autoreactive IgE. The high levels of autoreactive IgE were required for the development of the lupus phenotype in the Lyn-deficient mice as demonstrated by the reduced kidney disease when the IgE locus was also genetically deleted in these mice [44]. The link between autoreactive IgE and progression of autoimmune disease is not restricted to this animal model of lupus, since it is observed in another lupus models in which deletion of the IgE locus reduces mortality and onset of nephritis (Dema and Rivera, unpublished observations). More importantly, studies in human SLE cohorts of more than 200 individuals showed that a high percentage (>50 %) of patients have high levels of autoreactive IgEs and this correlates with increased disease activity and lupus nephritis ([44]; Dema, Charles, Rivera, unpublished observations). The presence of auto-reactive IgE and the deposition of immunocomplexes in the kidney of Lyn-deficient mice were dependent on IL-4, since these were absent in Lyn-deficient mice also carrying a deletion in the IL-4 gene. Notably, investigation of the underlying mechanism leading to increased IL-4 and to the presence of circulating auto-reactive IgE led us to uncover that basophils (and not mast cells) were activated in these mice and produced large amounts of IL-4. In fact, depletion of basophils prevented the increased IL-4 levels, markedly reduced the presence of autoreactive IgE, and reversed a Th2-bias found in the Lyn-deficient mice as well as the glomerulo-nephritis seen at late stages of the disease. This, together with the finding that autoreactive IgE-containing IgG immune complexes can activate basophils to produce IL-4, demonstrated that baso-phils can serve as amplifiers of autoimmunity, whereby their activation by IgE-containing immune complexes results in increased B cell-mediated autoantibody production (mechanistic details provided in the next section). These findings clearly link the basophil to the promotion of autoimmune disease, such as SLE, and raise the question of whether basophils may play a role in the immuno-modulation of other autoimmune diseases.

4 The Immunomodulatory Role of Mast Cells and Basophils

Given the contributory, rather than essential, nature of mast cells and basophils in many of the aforementioned protective and exacerbating roles, perhaps it is not surprising that these cells exert immunoregulatory function. A regulatory role for mast cells was inferred by Paul Ehrlich when he named them "Mastzellen" in the belief that they provided nutritional function because of their high content of granules. The role of mast cells in modulating the immune response has long been recognized due, in part, to the effects of mast cell granule mediators on other immune cells [149]. However, until recently the molecular basis by which mast cells or basophils exerted such influence on the immune system was inadequately investigated. In this section, we briefly summarize some of the recent work with a primary focus on how mast cells influence and are in turn influenced by T cells. In addition, we briefly summarize what we are learning about the role of basophils in modulating B cell function and the humoral response.

4.1 Recent Advances in Mast Cell Immune Modulation

The idea that mast cells and T cells can communicate is supported by the presence of a diverse array of molecules on their cell surface that can mediate their cross talk [150]. Mast cells can also be found close to T cells in inflamed tissues as well as in lymphoid organs [19, 151–153]. Recent studies have shown that mast cells and activated T cells can interact via ICAM-1 (CD54) and LFA-1 (CD11a) expressed, respectively, on their cell surface, an interaction that enhances FcεRI-mediated mast cell degranulation [154]. Mast cells can also influence T-effector cells as they are able to act as antigen-presenting cells [155]. Expression of MHC class II molecules (MHC-II) by mast cells can be induced by treatment with LPS and IFN-γ [156]. While such MHC-II bearing mast cells failed to stimulate naïve T cells, they effectively supported activated T-effectors and caused expansion of regulatory T cells (Tregs). This antigen-presenting role of mast cells is further supported by the demonstration that treatment of peritoneal cell-derived mast cells (PCMCs) with IFN-γ and IL-4 also induced expression of MHC-II molecules. In this case the authors found that these MHC-II competent PCMCs were able to present antigen to effector T cells causing their activation, proliferation, and the formation of an immunological synapse between the PCMC and the T cell [157]. Antigen presentation by mast cells is not limited to MHC class II, as it was recently reported that MHC-I-dependent cross presentation of mast cells to CD8$^+$ T cells caused increased CD8$^+$ T cell proliferation and effector functions [158]. While it is clear that such interactions can have reciprocal effects on both mast cells and T cell effector functions, a mechanistic understanding of the processes underlying these events is currently limited.

Perhaps, where a considerable advance has been made towards understanding mechanisms associated with Treg and mast cell interactions is in the discovery of OX40 and OX40L interactions, respectively, between these cells [159–165]. It was first reported that this interaction results in the suppression of MC degranulation [161]. A consequence of this interaction was impaired influx of extracellular Ca^{2+} after FcεRI stimulation of mast cells. It was demonstrated that this suppression of Ca^{2+} influx was a result of increased cAMP generation in the mast cells after OX40L engagement. Use of reagents that inhibited cAMP generation in mast cells restored normal Ca^{2+} influx and normal degranulation even in the presence of Tregs. In addition, OX40-deficient Tregs failed to induce cAMP production in mast cells or suppress Ca^{2+} influx and degranulation. Further mechanistic studies demonstrated that soluble OX40 could effectively block Treg-mediated suppression of mast cells and that in mast cells the suppressive effects of OX40L engagement were mediated through dampening of Fyn-dependent signals [163, 164].

However, the interaction of Tregs with mast cells via the OX40-OX40L axis also has consequences on Treg function. Piconese and colleagues demonstrated [162] that mast cells can abrogate Treg suppressive activity upon OX40/OX40L interaction. This was dependent, at least in part, on IL-6 production and resulted in an increase in IL-17 producing T cells. These results suggest that in some inflammatory conditions one might find the presence of mast cells in close proximity to Tregs and Th-17 cells. Consistent with this view, in the EAE mouse model of multiple sclerosis, mast cells were found to localize with Tregs and Th-17 cells. Similarly, these cell types could be identified in the BAL fluid of OTII transgenic mice challenged with ovalbumin intranasally. While there are numerous other examples where mast cells have been shown to play a role in regulating Treg and T-effector function, the findings briefly highlighted herein begin to unravel the mechanisms involved and promote the view that such interactions may play a key role in regulating the immune response in health and disease.

4.2 Basophils and B Cells: Boosting the Humoral Response

While mast cell interactions with B cells were recently described to enhance B cell proliferation and differentiation [166], in the past few years there has been considerable focus on the role of basophils in influencing B cell biology and function and we will spotlight these studies herein. What is emerging from this recent work is that basophils can deliver help to B cells via both direct and indirect mechanisms.

As mentioned earlier in this chapter, under certain circumstances, basophils appear to migrate to the draining lymph nodes where they release IL-4 and induce Th2 cell differentiation [41, 42, 47, 167]. Th2 cell differentiation is essential for host defense to various pathogens and allergens through induction of protective IgG1 and IgE production by B cells. It is important to note, however, that basophils may not necessarily mediate Th2 cell differentiation alone but are likely to cooperate with dendritic cells [168, 169] and thus should not be considered as a replacement of dendritic cell function but may be more appropriately thought to augment dendritic cells in promoting Th2 cell differentiation. Thus, in this manner, basophils are likely to indirectly promote B cell function through cooperating with dendritic cells to increase T helper functions that amplify B cell responses.

Perhaps, a good example of more direct interdependence of basophils and B cells, in regulating humoral responses, is provided by the observation that immune surveillance is enhanced by IgD-mediated activation of B cell-stimulating programs in basophils [43]. IgD is secreted by plasmablasts in the mucosa where it can afford protection by binding to pathogens and other virulence factors. It also binds to basophils, via an unknown receptor, and crosslinking of basophil bound IgD was shown to cause the release of BAFF, IL-4, and IL-13 [43], which stimulates B cells to undergo IgM production as well as class switch recombination to IgG and IgA. In addition to IgD, other molecules like CD40L, which is expressed on basophils, provide further help for class switch recombination by engaging CD40 on B cells. Other examples of the direct interdependence of basophils and B cells are provided by in vivo and in vitro studies where depletion of basophils caused loss of plasmablasts in the spleen [44, 170]. These studies showed that basophil activation via IgE/Ag interactions causes a marked enhancement of plasma cell numbers with this increase being dependent on IL-4 and IL-6 [44, 170]. This is consistent with our recent finding (T. Ricks and J. Rivera, unpublished observation) that basophils localize to the plasmablast-enriched regions of the spleen in the *lyn*$^{-/-}$ mouse model, which has a basophilia that plays a role in amplification of autoantibody production and development of lupus [44, 171].

Finally, while the data suggests that both mouse and human basophils can augment memory responses of B cells and T cells [172–174], it is less clear if there are circumstances in which basophils alone can promote differentiation of naïve T and B cells. Nonetheless, it appears certain that basophils can now be viewed as important immunomodulatory cells with an apparent amplifying role in humoral responses.

5   Concluding Remarks

A number of points should be considered as the new era in mast cell and basophil biology and function further develops. A guiding principle can be garnered from the accumulating literature that not all mast cells are the same [66]. The intrinsic property of mast cells to develop in tissues provides a remarkable level of genomic and proteomic plasticity that makes a skin mast cell quite different from one residing in the spleen or in the joints (even though they are all considered connective tissue type mast cells). While basophils mature in the bone marrow, it is also apparent that their phenotype may be distinct when circulating in the blood versus recruited to the tissues. In mouse studies, minimal expression of MHC-II or BAFF was detected on blood basophils whereas upon recruitment to the lymph nodes these cells express considerable amounts of these molecules [44]. Thus, there is considerable danger in generalizing the findings on mast cell and basophil functions when studies are conducted with a limited sampling of mast cell or basophil types (or tissues) or by use of one or another mouse model.

Importantly, one should keep in mind that the immune system is highly regulated and finely tuned and, as such, even minor perturbations (like differences in stimuli strength or change in commensal flora) can result in markedly different responses [175]. Moreover, given that we accept a regulatory role for mast cells and basophils in immunity, the contributory (rather than essential) role of these cells positions them in a niche where their mode of activation, or the particular effector responses elicited, may be a determinant of the type or extent of inflammatory response initiated. Thus, arguments for or against a particular (patho)physiological role of mast cells and basophils should always be viewed in the context of the model or experiment. Of note is that even minor differences in the genetics (or alterations made to genes) of a presumed homogeneous population (such as seen in congenic mice) can cause marked variations in responses [176]. In our opinion, there is little uniformity in individual mouse responses (similar to what is seen in the study of humans) and thus only by large cohort samplings can one obtain the statistical power to provide a more general view of the (patho)physiological role of a given cell type or gene. However, such studies are both resource and labor intensive and frankly, not practical given the current fiscal constraints encompassing the worldwide scientific community. With this in mind it becomes important to translate basic laboratory discoveries to human health and disease. Finding correlates of human (patho)physiology provides the degree of confidence that justifies further dissection of a particular role for a cell, gene, or molecule in health and disease.

Regardless of these caveats, the enthusiasm for the expanding importance of mast cells and basophils in immunity is at an all-time high. It is a most heartening time to be a scientist in this field, as the rapid evolving technologies provide promise of future discoveries that advance a better understanding of mast cell and basophil biology and function. We envision that this new knowledge will translate into novel treatments for allergies and other diseases in which mast cells and basophils serve as effectors and modulators of the immune system.

References

1. Ehrlich P (1877) Beitrage zur Kenntnis der Anilinfarbungen und ihrer Verwendung in der mikroskopischen Technik. Arch Mikrosk Anat 13:263–277

2. Ehrlich P (1878) Beitrage zur Theorie und Praxis der histologischen Farbung. *6-17-1878*. Thesis, Leipzig University

3. Ehrlich P (1891) Farbenanalytische Untersuchungen zur Histologie und Klinik des Blutes. Hirschwald, Berlin

4. Ehrlich P, Lazarus A (1898) Die Anaemie, 1. Normale und pathologische Histologie des Blutes. Holder, Wien (revised and republished 1909)

5. Galli SJ (1993) New concepts about the mast cell. N Engl J Med 328:257–265

6. Metcalfe DD, Baram D, Mekori YA (1997) Mast cells. Physiol Rev 77:1033–1079

7. Karasuyama H, Mukai K, Obata K, Tsujimura Y, Wada T (2011) Nonredundant roles of basophils in immunity. Annu Rev Immunol 29:45–69

8. Dvorak AM, Nabel G, Pyne K, Cantor H, Dvorak HF, Galli SJ (1982) Ultrastructural

identification of the mouse basophil. Blood 59:1279–1285

9. Galli SJ, Kalesnikoff J, Grimbaldeston MA, Piliponsky AM, Williams CM, Tsai M (2005) Mast cells as "tunable" effector and immuno-regulatory cells: recent advances. Annu Rev Immunol 23:749–786

10. Kinet JP (1989) The high-affinity receptor for IgE. Curr Opin Immunol 2:499–505

11. Min B, Paul WE (2008) Basophils and type 2 immunity. Curr Opin Hematol 15:59–63

12. Falcone FH, Haas H, Gibbs BF (2000) The human basophil: a new appreciation of its role in immune responses. Blood 96:4028–4038

13. Galli SJ, Tsai M (2010) Mast cells in allergy and infection: versatile effector and regula-tory cells in innate and adaptive immunity. Eur J Immunol 40:1843–1851

14. Tsai M, Grimbaldeston M, Galli SJ (2011) Mast cells and immunoregulation/immuno-modulation. Adv Exp Med Biol 716:186–211

15. Reber LL, Marichal T, Galli SJ (2012) New models for analyzing mast cell functions in vivo. Trends Immunol 33:613–625

16. Rodewald HR, Feyerabend TB (2012) Widespread immunological functions of mast cells: fact or fiction? Immunity 37:13–24

17. Honda T, Egawa G, Grabbe S, Kabashima K (2013) Update of immune events in the murine contact hypersensitivity model: toward the understanding of allergic contact dermatitis. J Invest Dermatol 133:303–315

18. Matsumoto K, Mizukoshi K, Oyobikawa M, Ohshima H, Tagami H (2004) Establishment of an atopic dermatitis-like skin model in a hairless mouse by repeated elicitation of con-tact hypersensitivity that enables to conduct functional analyses of the stratum corneum with various non-invasive biophysical instru-ments. Skin Res Technol 10:122–129

19. Dudeck A, Dudeck J, Scholten J, Petzold A, Surianarayanan S, Köhler A, Peschke K, Vöhringer D, Waskow C, Krieg T, Müller W, Waisman A, Hartmann K, Gunzer M, Roers A (2011) Mast cells are key promoters of con-tact allergy that mediate the adjuvant effects of haptens. Immunity 34:973–984

20. Galli SJ, Nakae S, Tsai M (2005) Mast cells in the development of adaptive immune responses. Nat Immunol 6:135–142

21. Hershko AY, Suzuki R, Charles N, Alvarez-Errico D, Sargent JL, Laurence A, Rivera J (2011) Mast cell interleukin-2 production contributes to suppression of chronic allergic dermatitis. Immunity 35:562–571

22. Norman MU, Hwang J, Hulliger S, Bonder CS, Yamanouchi J, Santamaria P, Kubes P (2008) Mast cells regulate the magnitude and the cytokine microenvironment of the contact hypersensitivity response. Am J Pathol 172:1638–1649

23. Man MQ, Hatano Y, Lee SH, Man M, Chang S, Feingold KR, Leung DY, Holleran W, Uchida Y, Elias PM (2008) Characterization of a hapten-induced, murine model with multiple features of atopic dermatitis: struc-tural, immunologic, and biochemical changes following single versus multiple oxazolone challenges. J Invest Dermatol 128:79–86

24. Hart PH, Grimbaldeston MA, Swift GJ, Jaksic A, Noonan FP, Finlay-Jones JJ (1998) Dermal mast cells determine susceptibility to ultraviolet B-induced systemic suppression of contact hypersensitivity responses in mice. J Exp Med 187:2045–2053

25. Depinay N, Hacini F, Beghdadi W, Peronet R, Mecheri S (2006) Mast cell-dependent down-regulation of antigen-specific immune responses by mosquito bites. J Immunol 176:4141–4146

26. Grimbaldeston MA, Nakae S, Kalesnikoff J, Tsai M, Galli SJ (2007) Mast cell-derived interleukin 10 limits skin pathology in contact dermatitis and chronic irradiation with ultra-violet B. Nat Immunol 8:1095–1104

27. Abraham SN, St John AL (2010) Mast cell-orchestrated immunity to pathogens. Nat Rev Immunol 10:440–452

28. Costa JJ, Weller PF, Galli SJ (1997) The cells of the allergic response: mast cells, basophils, and eosinophils. JAMA 278:1815–1822

29. Dvorak AM, Seder RA, Paul WE, Kissell-Rainville S, Plaut M, Galli SJ (1993) Ultrastructural characteristics of Fc epsilon R-positive basophils in the spleen and bone marrow of mice immunized with goat anti-mouse IgD antibody. Lab Invest 68:708–715

30. Seder RA, Paul WE, Dvorak AM, Sharkis SJ, Kagey-Sobotka A, Niv Y, Finkelman FD, Barbieri SA, Galli SJ, Plaut M (1991) Mouse splenic and bone marrow cell populations that express high-affinity Fc epsilon receptors and produce interleukin 4 are highly enriched in basophils. Proc Natl Acad Sci U S A 88:2835–2839

31. Seder RA, Plaut M, Barbieri S, Urban J Jr, Finkelman FD, Paul WE (1991) Purified Fc epsilon R+ bone marrow and splenic non-B, non-T cells are highly enriched in the capacity to produce IL-4 in response to immobilized IgE, IgG2a, or ionomycin. J Immunol 147:903–909

32. Ohnmacht C, Schwartz C, Panzer M, Schiedewitz I, Naumann R, Voehringer D (2010) Basophils orchestrate chronic allergic dermatitis and protective immunity against helminths. Immunity 33:364–374

33. Wada T, Ishiwata K, Koseki H, Ishikura T, Ugajin T, Ohnuma N, Obata K, Ishikawa R, Yoshikawa S, Mukai K, Kawano Y, Minegishi Y, Yokozeki H, Watanabe N, Karasuyama H (2010) Selective ablation of basophils in mice

reveals their nonredundant role in acquired immunity against ticks. J Clin Invest 120: 2867–2875

34. Min B, Prout M, Hu-Li J, Zhu J, Jankovic D, Morgan ES, Urban JF Jr, Dvorak AM, Finkelman FD, LeGros G, Paul WE (2004) Basophils produce IL-4 and accumulate in tissues after infection with a Th2-inducing parasite. J Exp Med 200:507–517

35. van Panhuys N, Prout M, Forbes E, Min B, Paul WE, Le Gros G (2011) Basophils are the major producers of IL-4 during primary helminth infection. J Immunol 186: 2719–2728

36. Voehringer D, Shinkai K, Locksley RM (2004) Type 2 immunity reflects orchestrated recruitment of cells committed to IL-4 production. Immunity 20:267–277

37. Ohnmacht C, Voehringer D (2010) Basophils protect against reinfection with hookworms independently of mast cells and memory Th2 cells. J Immunol 184:344–350

38. Ohnmacht C, Voehringer D (2009) Basophil effector function and homeostasis during helminth infection. Blood 113:2816–2825

39. Voehringer D, Reese TA, Huang X, Shinkai K, Locksley RM (2006) Type 2 immunity is controlled by IL-4/IL-13 expression in hematopoietic non-eosinophil cells of the innate immune system. J Exp Med 203: 1435–1446

40. Lantz CS, Min B, Tsai M, Chatterjea D, Dranoff G, Galli SJ (2008) IL-3 is required for increases in blood basophils in nematode infection in mice and can enhance IgE-dependent IL-4 production by basophils in vitro. Lab Invest 88:1134–1142

41. Perrigoue JG, Saenz SA, Siracusa MC, Allenspach EJ, Taylor BC, Giacomin PR, Nair MG, Du Y, Zaph C, van Rooijen N, Comeau MR, Pearce EJ, Laufer TM, Artis D (2009) MHC class II-dependent basophil-CD4+ T cell interactions promote T(H)2 cytokine-dependent immunity. Nat Immunol 10: 697–705

42. Yoshimoto T, Yasuda K, Tanaka H, Nakahira M, Imai Y, Fujimori Y, Nakanishi K (2009) Basophils contribute to T(H)2-IgE responses in vivo via IL-4 production and presentation of peptide-MHC class II complexes to CD4+ T cells. Nat Immunol 10:706–712

43. Chen K, Xu W, Wilson M, He B, Miller NW, Bengtén E, Edholm ES, Santini PA, Rath P, Chiu A, Cattalini M, Litzman J, B Bussel J, Huang B, Meini A, Riesbeck K, Cunningham-Rundles C, Plebani A, Cerutti A (2009) Immunoglobulin D enhances immune surveillance by activating antimicrobial, proinflammatory and B cell-stimulating programs in basophils. Nat Immunol 10:889–898

44. Charles N, Hardwick D, Daugas E, Illei GG, Rivera J (2010) Basophils and the T helper 2 environment can promote the development of lupus nephritis. Nat Med 16:701–707

45. Charles N, Dema B, Rivera J (2012) Reply to: Basophils from humans with systemic lupus erythematosus do not express MHC-II. Nat Med 18:489–490

46. Charles N, Rivera J (2011) Basophils and autoreactive IgE in the pathogenesis of systemic lupus erythematosus. Curr Allergy Asthma Rep 11:378–387

47. Sokol CL, Chu NQ, Yu S, Nish SA, Laufer TM, Medzhitov R (2009) Basophils function as antigen-presenting cells for an allergen-induced T helper type 2 response. Nat Immunol 10:713–720

48. Caughey GH (2011) Mast cell proteases as protective and inflammatory mediators. Adv Exp Med Biol 716:212–234

49. Akahoshi M, Song CH, Piliponsky AM, Metz M, Guzzetta A, Abrink M, Schlenner SM, Feyerabend TB, Rodewald HR, Pejler G, Tsai M, Galli SJ (2011) Mast cell chymase reduces the toxicity of Gila monster venom, scorpion venom, and vasoactive intestinal polypeptide in mice. J Clin Invest 121:4180–4191

50. Maurer M, Wedemeyer J, Metz M, Piliponsky AM, Weller K, Chatterjea D, Clouthier DE, Yanagisawa MM, Tsai M, Galli SJ (2004) Mast cells promote homeostasis by limiting endothelin-1-induced toxicity. Nature 432: 512–516

51. Metz M, Piliponsky AM, Chen CC, Lammel V, Abrink M, Pejler G, Tsai M, Galli SJ (2006) Mast cells can enhance resistance to snake and honeybee venoms. Science 313:526–530

52. Malaviya R, Ikeda T, Ross E, Abraham SN (1996) Mast cell modulation of neutrophil influx and bacterial clearance at sites of infection through TNF-alpha. Nature 381:77–80

53. Piliponsky AM, Chen CC, Grimbaldeston MA, Burns-Guydish SM, Hardy J, Kalesnikoff J, Contag CH, Tsai M, Galli SJ (2010) Mast cell-derived TNF can exacerbate mortality during severe bacterial infections in C57BL/6-KitW-sh/W-sh mice. Am J Pathol 176:926–938

54. Piliponsky AM, Chen CC, Nishimura T, Metz M, Rios EJ, Dobner PR, Wada E, Wada K, Zacharias S, Mohanasundaram UM, Faix JD, Abrink M, Pejler G, Pearl RG, Tsai M, Galli SJ (2008) Neurotensin increases mortality and mast cells reduce neurotensin levels in a mouse model of sepsis. Nat Med 14: 392–398

55. Cochrane DE, Carraway RE, Boucher W, Feldberg RS (1991) Rapid degradation of neurotensin by stimulated rat mast cells. Peptides 12:1187–1194

56. Piliponsky AM, Chen CC, Rios EJ, Treuting PM, Lahiri A, Abrink M, Pejler G, Tsai M, Galli SJ (2012) The chymase mouse mast cell protease 4 degrades TNF, limits inflammation, and promotes survival in a model of sepsis. Am J Pathol 181:875–886

57. Thakurdas SM, Melicoff E, Sansores-Garcia L, Moreira DC, Petrova Y, Stevens RL, Adachi R (2007) The mast cell-restricted tryptase mMCP-6 has a critical immunoprotective role in bacterial infections. J Biol Chem 282:20809–20815

58. Hendrix S, Kramer P, Pehl D, Warnke K, Boato F, Nelissen S, Lemmens E, Pejler G, Metz M, Siebenhaar F, Maurer M (2013) Mast cells protect from post-traumatic brain inflammation by the mast cell-specific chymase mouse mast cell protease-4. FASEB J 27:920–929

59. Waern I, Lundequist A, Pejler G, Wernersson S (2013) Mast cell chymase modulates IL-33 levels and controls allergic sensitization in dust-mite induced airway inflammation. Mucosal Immunol 6(5):911–920

60. Waern I, Karlsson I, Thorpe M, Schlenner SM, Feyerabend TB, Rodewald HR, Åbrink M, Hellman L, Pejler G, Wernersson S (2012) Mast cells limit extracellular levels of IL-13 via a serglycin proteoglycan-serine protease axis. Biol Chem 393:1555–1567

61. Hershko AY, Charles N, Olivera A, Alvarez-Errico D, Rivera J (2012) Cutting edge: persistence of increased mast cell numbers in tissues links dermatitis to enhanced airway disease in a mouse model of atopy. J Immunol 188:531–535

62. Hahn EL, Bacharier LB (2005) The atopic march: the pattern of allergic disease development in childhood. Immunol Allergy Clin North Am 25:231–246, v

63. McLachlan JB, Shelburne CP, Hart JP, Pizzo SV, Goyal A, Brooking-Dixon R, Staats HF, Abraham SN (2008) Mast cell activators: a new class of highly effective vaccine adjuvants. Nat Med 14:536–541

64. Paananen K, Kovanen PT (1994) Proteolysis and fusion of low density lipoprotein particles independently strengthen their binding to exocytosed mast cell granules. J Biol Chem 269:2023–2031

65. Pulendran B, Ono SJ (2008) A shot in the arm for mast cells. Nat Med 14:489–490

66. Galli SJ, Borregaard N, Wynn TA (2011) Phenotypic and functional plasticity of cells of innate immunity: macrophages, mast cells and neutrophils. Nat Immunol 12:1035–1044

67. Chmelar J, Chung KJ, Chavakis T (2013) The role of innate immune cells in obese adipose tissue inflammation and development of insulin resistance. Thromb Haemost 109:399–406

68. Xu JM, Shi GP (2012) Emerging role of mast cells and macrophages in cardiovascular and metabolic diseases. Endocr Rev 33:71–108

69. Anand P, Singh B, Jaggi AS, Singh N (2012) Mast cells: an expanding pathophysiological role from allergy to other disorders. Naunyn Schmiedebergs Arch Pharmacol 385:657–670

70. Altintas MM, Nayer B, Walford EC, Johnson KB, Gaidosh G, Reiser J, De La Cruz-Munoz N, Ortega LM, Nayer A (2012) Leptin deficiency-induced obesity affects the density of mast cells in abdominal fat depots and lymph nodes in mice. Lipids Health Dis 11:21

71. Liu J, Divoux A, Sun J, Zhang J, Clement K, Glickman JN, Sukhova GK, Wolters PJ, Du J, Gorgun CZ, Doria A, Libby P, Blumberg RS, Kahn BB, Hotamisligil GS, Shi GP (2009) Genetic deficiency and pharmacological stabilization of mast cells reduce diet-induced obesity and diabetes in mice. Nat Med 15:940–945

72. Tanaka A, Nomura Y, Matsuda A, Ohmori K, Matsuda H (2011) Mast cells function as an alternative modulator of adipogenesis through 15-deoxy-delta-12, 14-prostaglandin J2. Am J Physiol Cell Physiol 301:C1360–C1367

73. Divoux A, Moutel S, Poitou C, Lacasa D, Veyrie N, Aissat A, Arock M, Guerre-Millo M, Clément K (2012) Mast cells in human adipose tissue: link with morbid obesity, inflammatory status, and diabetes. J Clin Endocrinol Metab 97:E1677–E1685

74. Wang X, Chen H, Zhang M, Liu Z (2012) Roles of Mast Cells and Monocyte Chemoattractant Protein-1 in the Renal Injury of Obesity-Related Glomerulopathy. Am J Med Sci 346(4):295–301

75. Fenger RV, Linneberg A, Vidal C, Vizcaino L, Husemoen LL, Aadahl M, Gonzalez-Quintela A (2012) Determinants of serum tryptase in a general population: the relationship of serum tryptase to obesity and asthma. Int Arch Allergy Immunol 157:151–158

76. Ward BR, Arslanian SA, Andreatta E, Schwartz LB (2012) Obesity is not linked to increased whole-body mast cell burden in children. J Allergy Clin Immunol 129:1164–1166

77. Poglio S, De Toni-Costes F, Arnaud E, Laharrague P, Espinosa E, Casteilla L, Cousin B (2010) Adipose tissue as a dedicated reservoir of functional mast cell progenitors. Stem Cells 28:2065–2072

78. Oka T, Kalesnikoff J, Starkl P, Tsai M, Galli SJ (2012) Evidence questioning cromolyn's effectiveness and selectivity as a 'mast cell stabilizer' in mice. Lab Invest 92:1472–1482

79. Shi MA, Shi GP (2012) Different roles of mast cells in obesity and diabetes: lessons from experimental animals and humans. Front Immunol 3:7

80. Iyer A, Lim J, Poudyal H, Reid RC, Suen JY, Webster J, Prins JB, Whitehead JP, Fairlie DP, Brown L (2012) An inhibitor of phospholipase A2 group IIA modulates adipocyte signaling and protects against diet-induced metabolic syndrome in rats. Diabetes 61:2320–2329

81. Kim S, Moustaid-Moussa N (2000) Secretory, endocrine and autocrine/paracrine function of the adipocyte. J Nutr 130:3110S–3115S

82. Weber C, Zernecke A, Libby P (2008) The multifaceted contributions of leukocyte subsets to atherosclerosis: lessons from mouse models. Nat Rev Immunol 8:802–815

83. Jeziorska M, McCollum C, Woolley DE (1997) Mast cell distribution, activation, and phenotype in atherosclerotic lesions of human carotid arteries. J Pathol 182:115–122

84. Kaartinen M, Penttila A, Kovanen PT (1994) Mast cells of two types differing in neutral protease composition in the human aortic intima. Demonstration of tryptase- and tryptase/chymase-containing mast cells in normal intimas, fatty streaks, and the shoulder region of atheromas. Arterioscler Thromb 14:966–972

85. Kovanen PT, Kaartinen M, Paavonen T (1995) Infiltrates of activated mast cells at the site of coronary atheromatous erosion or rupture in myocardial infarction. Circulation 92: 1084–1088

86. Ramalho LS, Oliveira LF, Cavellani CL, Ferraz ML, de Oliveira FA, Miranda Correa RR, de Paula Antunes Teixeira V, De Lima Pereira SA (2013) Role of mast cell chymase and tryptase in the progression of atherosclerosis: study in 44 autopsied cases. Ann Diagn Pathol 17:28–31

87. Bot I, Bot M, van Heiningen SH, van Santbrink PJ, Lankhuizen IM, Hartman P, Gruener S, Hilpert H, van Berkel TJ, Fingerle J, Biessen EA (2011) Mast cell chymase inhibition reduces atherosclerotic plaque progression and improves plaque stability in ApoE-/- mice. Cardiovasc Res 89:244–252

88. Heikkila HM, Trosien J, Metso J, Jauhiainen M, Pentikainen MO, Kovanen PT, Lindstedt KA (2010) Mast cells promote atherosclerosis by inducing both an atherogenic lipid profile and vascular inflammation. J Cell Biochem 109:615–623

89. Sun J, Sukhova GK, Wolters PJ, Yang M, Kitamoto S, Libby P, MacFarlane LA, Mallen-St Clair J, Shi GP (2007) Mast cells promote atherosclerosis by releasing proinflammatory cytokines. Nat Med 13:719–724

90. Smith DD, Tan X, Raveendran VV, Tawfik O, Stechschulte DJ, Dileepan KN (2012) Mast cell deficiency attenuates progression of atherosclerosis and hepatic steatosis in apolipoprotein E-null mice. Am J Physiol Heart Circ Physiol 302:H2612–H2621

91. Bot I, Biessen EA (2011) Mast cells in atherosclerosis. Thromb Haemost 106:820–826

92. Bot I, de Jager SC, Zernecke A, Lindstedt KA, van Berkel TJ, Weber C, Biessen EA (2007) Perivascular mast cells promote atherogenesis and induce plaque destabilization in apolipoprotein E-deficient mice. Circulation 115: 2516–2525

93. Zhang J, Alcaide P, Liu L, Sun J, He A, Luscinskas FW, Shi GP (2011) Regulation of endothelial cell adhesion molecule expression by mast cells, macrophages, and neutrophils. PLoS One 6:e14525

94. Sun J, Sukhova GK, Yang M, Wolters PJ, MacFarlane LA, Libby P, Sun C, Zhang Y, Liu J, Ennis TL, Knispel R, Xiong W, Thompson RW, Baxter BT, Shi GP (2007) Mast cells modulate the pathogenesis of elastase-induced abdominal aortic aneurysms in mice. J Clin Invest 117:3359–3368

95. Lappalainen J, Lindstedt KA, Oksjoki R, Kovanen PT (2011) OxLDL-IgG immune complexes induce expression and secretion of proatherogenic cytokines by cultured human mast cells. Atherosclerosis 214:357–363

96. Wang J, Cheng X, Xiang MX, Alanne-Kinnunen M, Wang JA, Chen H, He A, Sun X, Lin Y, Tang TT, Tu X, Sjöberg S, Sukhova GK, Liao YH, Conrad DH, Yu L, Kawakami T, Kovanen PT, Libby P, Shi GP (2011) IgE stimulates human and mouse arterial cell apoptosis and cytokine expression and promotes atherogenesis in Apoe-/- mice. J Clin Invest 121:3564–3577

97. Coussens LM, Zitvogel L, Palucka AK (2013) Neutralizing tumor-promoting chronic inflammation: a magic bullet? Science 339:286–291

98. Oleinika K, Nibbs RJ, Graham GJ, Fraser AR (2013) Suppression, subversion and escape: the role of regulatory T cells in cancer progression. Clin Exp Immunol 171:36–45

99. Chang DZ (2012) Mast cells in pancreatic ductal adenocarcinoma. Oncoimmunology 1: 754–755

100. Cheema VS, Ramesh V, Balamurali PD (2012) The relevance of mast cells in oral squamous cell carcinoma. J Clin Diagn Res 6:1803–1807

101. de Souza DA Jr, Toso VD, Campos MR, Lara VS, Oliver C, Jamur MC (2012) Expression of mast cell proteases correlates with mast cell maturation and angiogenesis during tumor progression. PLoS One 7:e40790

102. Gounaris E, Erdman SE, Restaino C, Gurish MF, Friend DS, Gounari F, Lee DM, Zhang G, Glickman JN, Shin K, Rao VP, Poutahidis T, Weissleder R, McNagny KM, Khazaie K (2007) Mast cells are an essential hematopoietic component for polyp development. Proc Natl Acad Sci U S A 104:19977–19982

103. Maltby S, Khazaie K, McNagny KM (2009) Mast cells in tumor growth: angiogenesis, tissue remodelling and immune-modulation. Biochim Biophys Acta 1796:19–26

104. Mangia A, Malfettone A, Rossi R, Paradiso A, Ranieri G, Simone G, Resta L (2011) Tissue remodelling in breast cancer: human mast cell tryptase as an initiator of myofibroblast differentiation. Histopathology 58:1096–1106

105. Nelissen S, Lemmens E, Geurts N, Kramer P, Maurer M, Hendriks J, Hendrix S (2013) The role of mast cells in neuroinflammation. Acta Neuropathol 125:637–650

106. Pittoni P, Tripodo C, Piconese S, Mauri G, Parenza M, Rigoni A, Sangaletti S, Colombo MP (2011) Mast cell targeting hampers prostate adenocarcinoma development but promotes the occurrence of highly malignant neuroendocrine cancers. Cancer Res 71: 5987–5997

107. Rabenhorst A, Schlaak M, Heukamp LC, Forster A, Theurich S, von Bergwelt-Baildon M, Büttner R, Kurschat P, Mauch C, Roers A, Hartmann K (2012) Mast cells play a protumorigenic role in primary cutaneous lymphoma. Blood 120:2042–2054

108. Ribatti D, Crivellato E (2011) Mast cells, angiogenesis and cancer. Adv Exp Med Biol 716:270–288

109. Souza LR, Fonseca-Silva T, Santos CC, Oliveira MV, Correa-Oliveira R, Guimaraes AL, De Paula AM (2010) Association of mast cell, eosinophil leucocyte and microvessel densities in actinic cheilitis and lip squamous cell carcinoma. Histopathology 57:796–805

110. Staser K, Yang FC, Clapp DW (2012) Pathogenesis of plexiform neurofibroma: tumor-stromal/hematopoietic interactions in tumor progression. Annu Rev Pathol 7: 469–495

111. Cai SW, Yang SZ, Gao J, Pan K, Chen JY, Wang YL, Wei LX, Dong JH (2011) Prognostic significance of mast cell count following curative resection for pancreatic ductal adenocarcinoma. Surgery 149:576–584

112. Huang B, Lei Z, Zhang GM, Li D, Song C, Li B, Liu Y, Yuan Y, Unkeless J, Xiong H, Feng ZH (2008) SCF-mediated mast cell infiltration and activation exacerbate the inflammation and immunosuppression in tumor microenvironment. Blood 112:1269–1279

113. Soucek L, Lawlor ER, Soto D, Shchors K, Swigart LB, Evan GI (2007) Mast cells are required for angiogenesis and macroscopic expansion of Myc-induced pancreatic islet tumors. Nat Med 13:1211–1218

114. Xia Q, Wu XJ, Zhou Q, Jing Z, Hou JH, Pan ZZ, Zhang XS (2011) No relationship between the distribution of mast cells and the survival of stage IIIB colon cancer patients. J Transl Med 9:88

115. Starkey JR, Crowle PK, Taubenberger S (1988) Mast-cell-deficient W/Wv mice exhibit a decreased rate of tumor angiogenesis. Int J Cancer 42:48–52

116. Chang DZ, Ma Y, Ji B, Wang H, Deng D, Liu Y, Logsdon CD, Hwu P (2011) Mast cells in tumor microenvironment promotes the in vivo growth of pancreatic ductal adenocarcinoma. Clin Cancer Res 17:7015–7023

117. Wasiuk A, Dalton DK, Schpero WL, Stan RV, Conejo-Garcia JR, Noelle RJ (2012) Mast cells impair the development of protective anti-tumor immunity. Cancer Immunol Immunother 61:2273–2282

118. Oldford SA, Haidl ID, Howatt MA, Leiva CA, Johnston B, Marshall JS (2010) A critical role for mast cells and mast cell-derived IL-6 in TLR2-mediated inhibition of tumor growth. J Immunol 185:7067–7076

119. Murata T, Aritake K, Matsumoto S, Kamauchi S, Nakagawa T, Hori M, Momotani E, Urade Y, Ozaki H (2011) Prostagladin D2 is a mast cell-derived antiangiogenic factor in lung carcinoma. Proc Natl Acad Sci U S A 108: 19802–19807

120. Sinnamon MJ, Carter KJ, Sims LP, Lafleur B, Fingleton B, Matrisian LM (2008) A protective role of mast cells in intestinal tumorigenesis. Carcinogenesis 29:880–886

121. Pittoni P, Piconese S, Tripodo C, Colombo MP (2011) Tumor-intrinsic and -extrinsic roles of c-Kit: mast cells as the primary off-target of tyrosine kinase inhibitors. Oncogene 30:757–769

122. Brown MA, Hatfield JK (2012) Mast Cells are Important Modifiers of Autoimmune Disease: With so Much Evidence, Why is There Still Controversy? Front Immunol 3:147

123. Costanza M, Colombo MP, Pedotti R (2012) Mast cells in the pathogenesis of multiple sclerosis and experimental autoimmune encephalomyelitis. Int J Mol Sci 13:15107–15125

124. Mican JM, Metcalfe DD (1990) Arthritis and mast cell activation. J Allergy Clin Immunol 86:677–683

125. Nakano S, Mishiro T, Takahara S, Yokoi H, Hamada D, Yukata K, Takata Y, Goto T, Egawa H, Yasuoka S, Furouchi H, Hirasaka K, Nikawa T, Yasui N (2007) Distinct expression of mast cell tryptase and protease activated receptor-2 in synovia of rheumatoid arthritis and osteoarthritis. Clin Rheumatol 26:1284–1292

126. Noordenbos T, Yeremenko N, Gofita I, van de Sande M, Tak PP, Cañete JD, Baeten D (2012) Interleukin-17-positive mast cells contribute to synovial inflammation in spondylarthritis. Arthritis Rheum 64:99–109

127. Tetlow LC, Woolley DE (1995) Distribution, activation and tryptase/chymase phenotype of mast cells in the rheumatoid lesion. Ann Rheum Dis 54:549–555

128. Pimentel TA, Sampaio AL, D'Acquisto F, Perretti M, Oliani SM (2011) An essential role for mast cells as modulators of neutrophils influx in collagen-induced arthritis in the mouse. Lab Invest 91:33–42

129. Shin K, Gurish MF, Friend DS, Pemberton AD, Thornton EM, Miller HR, Lee DM (2006) Lymphocyte-independent connective tissue mast cells populate murine synovium. Arthritis Rheum 54:2863–2871

130. Shiota N, Shimoura K, Okunishi H (2006) Pathophysiological role of mast cells in collagen-induced arthritis: study with a cysteinyl leukotriene receptor antagonist, montelukast. Eur J Pharmacol 548:158–166

131. Kneilling M, Hultner L, Pichler BJ, Mailhammer R, Morawietz L, Solomon S, Eichner M, Sabatino J, Biedermann T, Krenn V, Weber WA, Illges H, Haubner R, Röcken M (2007) Targeted mast cell silencing protects against joint destruction and angiogenesis in experimental arthritis in mice. Arthritis Rheum 56:1806–1816

132. Juurikivi A, Sandler C, Lindstedt KA, Kovanen PT, Juutilainen T, Leskinen MJ, Mäki T, Eklund KK (2005) Inhibition of c-kit tyrosine kinase by imatinib mesylate induces apoptosis in mast cells in rheumatoid synovia: a potential approach to the treatment of arthritis. Ann Rheum Dis 64:1126–1131

133. Eklund KK, Joensuu H (2003) Treatment of rheumatoid arthritis with imatinib mesylate: clinical improvement in three refractory cases. Ann Med 35:362–367

134. Mancardi DA, Jonsson F, Iannascoli B, Khun H, Van Rooijen N, Huerre M, Daëron M, Bruhns P (2011) Cutting Edge: The murine high-affinity IgG receptor FcgammaRIV is sufficient for autoantibody-induced arthritis. J Immunol 186:1899–1903

135. Nigrovic PA, Binstadt BA, Monach PA, Johnsen A, Gurish M, Iwakura Y, Benoist C, Mathis D, Lee DM (2007) Mast cells contribute to initiation of autoantibody-mediated arthritis via IL-1. Proc Natl Acad Sci U S A 104:2325–2330

136. Nigrovic PA, Malbec O, Lu B, Markiewski MM, Kepley C, Gerard N, Daëron M, Lee DM (2010) C5a receptor enables participation of mast cells in immune complex arthritis independently of Fcgamma receptor modulation. Arthritis Rheum 62:3322–3333

137. Tsuboi N, Ernandez T, Li X, Nishi H, Cullere X, Mekala D, Hazen M, Köhl J, Lee DM, Mayadas TN (2011) Regulation of human neutrophil Fcgamma receptor IIa by C5a receptor promotes inflammatory arthritis in mice. Arthritis Rheum 63:467–478

138. Zhou JS, Xing W, Friend DS, Austen KF, Katz HR (2007) Mast cell deficiency in Kit(W-sh) mice does not impair antibody-mediated arthritis. J Exp Med 204:2797–2802

139. Pitman N, Asquith DL, Murphy G, Liew FY, McInnes IB (2011) Collagen-induced arthritis is not impaired in mast cell-deficient mice. Ann Rheum Dis 70:1170–1171

140. Feyerabend TB, Weiser A, Tietz A, Stassen M, Harris N, Kopf M, Radermacher P, Möller P, Benoist C, Mathis D, Fehling HJ, Rodewald HR (2011) Cre-mediated cell ablation contests mast cell contribution in models of antibody- and T cell-mediated autoimmunity. Immunity 35:832–844

141. Rajasekaran N, Solomon S, Watanabe T, Ohtsu H, Gajda M, Bräuer R, Illges H (2009) Histidine decarboxylase but not histamine receptor 1 or 2 deficiency protects from K/BxN serum-induced arthritis. Int Immunol 21:1263–1268

142. McNeil HP, Shin K, Campbell IK, Wicks IP, Adachi R, Lee DM, Stevens RL (2008) The mouse mast cell-restricted tetramer-forming tryptases mouse mast cell protease 6 and mouse mast cell protease 7 are critical mediators in inflammatory arthritis. Arthritis Rheum 58:2338–2346

143. Shin K, Nigrovic PA, Crish J, Boilard E, McNeil HP, Larabee KS, Adachi R, Gurish MF, Gobezie R, Stevens RL, Lee DM (2009) Mast cells contribute to autoimmune inflammatory arthritis via their tryptase/heparin complexes. J Immunol 182:647–656

144. Magnusson SE, Pejler G, Kleinau S, Abrink M (2009) Mast cell chymase contributes to the antibody response and the severity of autoimmune arthritis. FASEB J 23:875–882

145. Ji H, Ohmura K, Mahmood U, Lee DM, Hofhuis FM, Boackle SA, Takahashi K, Holers VM, Walport M, Gerard C, Ezekowitz A, Carroll MC, Brenner M, Weissleder R, Verbeek JS, Duchatelle V, Degott C, Benoist C, Mathis D (2002) Arthritis critically dependent on innate immune system players. Immunity 16:157–168

146. Xu D, Jiang HR, Kewin P, Li Y, Mu R, Fraser AR, Pitman N, Kurowska-Stolarska M, McKenzie AN, McInnes IB, Liew FY (2008) IL-33 exacerbates antigen-induced arthritis by activating mast cells. Proc Natl Acad Sci U S A 105:10913–10918

147. Millauer N, Zuercher AW, Miescher SM, Gerber HA, Seitz M, Stadler BM (1999)

High IgE in rheumatoid arthritis (RA) patients is complexed with anti-IgE autoantibodies. Clin Exp Immunol 115:183–188

148. Kikuchi Y, Kaplan AP (2001) Mechanisms of autoimmune activation of basophils in chronic urticaria. J Allergy Clin Immunol 107:1056–1062

149. Miller JF (1975) Cellular basis of the immune response. Acta Endocrinol Suppl (Copenh) 194:55–76

150. Nakae S, Suto H, Iikura M, Kakurai M, Sedgwick JD, Tsai M, Galli SJ (2006) Mast cells enhance T cell activation: importance of mast cell costimulatory molecules and secreted TNF. J Immunol 176:2238–2248

151. Mekori YA (2004) The mastocyte: the "other" inflammatory cell in immunopathogenesis. J Allergy Clin Immunol 114:52–57

152. Bachelet I, Levi-Schaffer F, Mekori YA (2006) Mast cells: not only in allergy. Immunol Allergy Clin North Am 26:407–425

153. Kalesnikoff J, Galli SJ (2008) New developments in mast cell biology. Nat Immunol 9:1215–1223

154. Inamura N, Mekori YA, Bhattacharyya SP, Bianchine PJ, Metcalfe DD (1998) Induction and enhancement of Fc(epsilon)RI-dependent mast cell degranulation following coculture with activated T cells: dependency on ICAM-1- and leukocyte function-associated antigen (LFA)-1-mediated heterotypic aggregation. J Immunol 160:4026–4033

155. Frandji P, Tkaczyk C, Oskeritzian C, David B, Desaymard C, Mecheri S (1996) Exogenous and endogenous antigens are differentially presented by mast cells to CD4+ T lymphocytes. Eur J Immunol 26:2517–2528

156. Kambayashi T, Allenspach EJ, Chang JT, Zou T, Shoag JE, Reiner SL, Caton AJ, Koretzky GA (2009) Inducible MHC class II expression by mast cells supports effector and regulatory T cell activation. J Immunol 182:4686–4695

157. Gaudenzio N, Espagnolle N, Mars LT, Liblau R, Valitutti S, Espinosa E (2009) Cell-cell cooperation at the T helper cell/mast cell immunological synapse. Blood 114:4979–4988

158. Stelekati E, Bahri R, D'Orlando O, Orinska Z, Mittrucker HW, Langenhaun R, Glatzel M, Bollinger A, Paus R, Bulfone-Paus S (2009) Mast cell-mediated antigen presentation regulates CD8+ T cell effector functions. Immunity 31:665–676

159. Frossi B, D'Inca F, Crivellato E, Sibilano R, Gri G, Mongillo M, Danelli L, Maggi L, Pucillo CE (2011) Single-cell dynamics of mast cell-CD4+ CD25+ regulatory T cell interactions. Eur J Immunol 41:1872–1882

160. Frossi B, Gri G, Tripodo C, Pucillo C (2010) Exploring a regulatory role for mast cells: 'MCregs'? Trends Immunol 31:97–102

161. Gri G, Piconese S, Frossi B, Manfroi V, Merluzzi S, Tripodo C, Viola A, Odom S, Rivera J, Colombo MP, Pucillo CE (2008) CD4+CD25+ regulatory T cells suppress mast cell degranulation and allergic responses through OX40-OX40L interaction. Immunity 29:771–781

162. Piconese S, Gri G, Tripodo C, Musio S, Gorzanelli A, Frossi B, Pedotti R, Pucillo CE, Colombo MP (2009) Mast cells counteract regulatory T-cell suppression through interleukin-6 and OX40/OX40L axis toward Th17-cell differentiation. Blood 114:2639–2648

163. Sibilano R, Frossi B, Suzuki R, D'Inca F, Gri G, Piconese S, Colombo MP, Rivera J, Pucillo CE (2012) Modulation of FcepsilonRI-dependent mast cell response by OX40L via Fyn, PI3K, and RhoA. J Allergy Clin Immunol 130(751–760):e752

164. Sibilano R, Gri G, Frossi B, Tripodo C, Suzuki R, Rivera J, MacDonald AS, Pucillo CE (2011) Technical advance: soluble OX40 molecule mimics regulatory T cell modulatory activity on FcepsilonRI-dependent mast cell degranulation. J Leukoc Biol 90:831–838

165. Tripodo C, Gri G, Piccaluga PP, Frossi B, Guarnotta C, Piconese S, Franco G, Vetri V, Pucillo CE, Florena AM, Colombo MP, Pileri SA (2010) Mast cells and Th17 cells contribute to the lymphoma-associated pro-inflammatory microenvironment of angioimmunoblastic T-cell lymphoma. Am J Pathol 177:792–802

166. Merluzzi S, Frossi B, Gri G, Parusso S, Tripodo C, Pucillo C (2010) Mast cells enhance proliferation of B lymphocytes and drive their differentiation toward IgA-secreting plasma cells. Blood 115:2810–2817

167. Sokol CL, Barton GM, Farr AG, Medzhitov R (2008) A mechanism for the initiation of allergen-induced T helper type 2 responses. Nat Immunol 9:310–318

168. Tang H, Cao W, Kasturi SP, Ravindran R, Nakaya HI, Kundu K, Murthy N, Kepler TB, Malissen B, Pulendran B (2010) The T helper type 2 response to cysteine proteases requires dendritic cell-basophil cooperation via ROS-mediated signaling. Nat Immunol 11:608–617

169. Hammad H, Plantinga M, Deswarte K, Pouliot P, Willart MA, Kool M, Muskens F, Lambrecht BN (2010) Inflammatory dendritic cells–not basophils–are necessary and sufficient for induction of Th2 immunity to inhaled house dust mite allergen. J Exp Med 207:2097–2111

170. Rodriguez Gomez M, Talke Y, Goebel N, Hermann F, Reich B, Mack M (2010) Basophils support the survival of plasma cells in mice. J Immunol 185:7180–7185

171. Charles N, Watford WT, Ramos HL, Hellman L, Oettgen HC, Gomez G, Ryan JJ, O'Shea JJ, Rivera J (2009) Lyn kinase controls basophil GATA-3 transcription factor expression and induction of Th2 cell differentiation. Immunity 30:533–543

172. Denzel A, Maus UA, Rodriguez Gomez M, Moll C, Niedermeier M, Winter C, Maus R, Hollingshead S, Briles DE, Kunz-Schughart LA, Talke Y, Mack M (2008) Basophils enhance immunological memory responses. Nat Immunol 9:733–742

173. Wakahara K, Baba N, Van VQ, Begin P, Rubio M, Ferraro P, Panzini B, Wassef R, Lahaie R, Caussignac Y, Tamaz R, Richard C, Soucy G, Delespesse G, Sarfati M (2012) Human basophils interact with memory T cells to augment Th17 responses. Blood 120:4761–4771

174. Wakahara K, Van VQ, Baba N, Begin P, Rubio M, Delespesse G, Sarfati M (2013) Basophils are recruited to inflamed lungs and exacerbate memory Th2 responses in mice and humans. Allergy 68:180–189

175. Goldszmid RS, Trinchieri G (2012) The price of immunity. Nat Immunol 13:932–938

176. Rivera J, Tessarollo L (2008) Genetic background and the dilemma of translating mouse studies to humans. Immunity 28:1–4

Part II

Obtaining the Cells: Purification, Culture, Counting, and Cell Lines

Chapter 2

Purification of Basophils from Peripheral Human Blood

Franco H. Falcone and Bernhard F. Gibbs

Abstract

The purification of basophils from peripheral blood has represented a formidable challenge for researchers since they were discovered by Paul Ehrlich in 1879. From the first published attempts in the late 1960s, it took half a century to develop robust protocols able to provide sufficient numbers of pure, functionally unimpaired basophils. The existing protocols for basophil purification exploit those properties of basophils which distinguish them from other cell types such as their localization in blood, density, and the presence or absence of surface markers. Purification techniques have been used in various combinations and variations to achieve a common goal in mind: to obtain a pure population of human basophils in sufficient numbers for downstream studies. The arduous way leading up to the modern protocols is summarized in this historical retrospective. A fast protocol for purification of basophils to near homogeneity is also described.

Key words Basophils, Basophilic granulocytes, Cell separation, Elutriation, Immunomagnetic selection, Percoll, Ficoll

1 Introduction

1.1 A Brief History of Basophil Purification Protocols

Basophilic granulocytes are amongst the rarest leukocytes in human peripheral blood, making up less than 1 % of total white blood cell counts in healthy individuals. Their rarity, in combination with other factors, such as the lack of suitable selection markers and appropriate tools for purification, has hampered research with primary basophils for several decades [1]. While protocols for leukocyte cell separation were developed in the 1950s and 1960s, the first protocols attempting to obtain "pure" populations of basophils were published in 1967 and subsequent years. Many different protocols have been published since then, with varying degrees of success in terms of the recovery and purity obtained by these procedures.

An ideal purification protocol should fulfill most, if not all, of the following criteria: it should be fast (complete within a few hours of blood taking), have a high recovery and final purity (close to 100 %), not lead to activation or priming of the cells (i.e., not alter their phenotype), should not require expensive specialized equipment,

Bernhard F. Gibbs and Franco H. Falcone (eds.), *Basophils and Mast Cells: Methods and Protocols*, Methods in Molecular Biology, vol. 1192, DOI 10.1007/978-1-4939-1173-8_2, © Springer Science+Business Media New York 2014

and be financially affordable. Historically, most published protocols have failed one or more such criteria. Early protocols were characterized either by very low recoveries, low purities, or both.

Here, we shall briefly review how the protocols evolved from their modest origin as protocols for enrichment of basophils in the second half of the 1960s to sophisticated protocols resulting in near 100 % pure basophil preparations in the twenty-first century.

1.2 The 1960s and 1970s: First Attempts at Enriching Basophils

To the best of our knowledge, the first documented attempts to enrich human basophils were published in 1967 by Sampson and Archer [2] and one year later by Parwaresch [3]. The Parwaresch protocol describes the use of a specially shaped siliconized glass tube curved at the bottom and open at the top into which 2 mL of heparinized blood is filled and spun in a centrifuge. After centrifugation, the tip of the closed curved end at the bottom of the glass tube is cut open with a scalpel blade and the open tube slowly immersed vertically into a mercury bath. The mercury enters the glass tube from the small opening in the bottom and pushes the blood upwards towards the open end, from where fractions are collected onto microscope slides. The purity and recovery of the method are not reported, but are likely to have been very low. The Sampson protocol used dextran sedimentation of the buffy coat layer obtained from centrifuged blood followed by a centrifugation in an albumin solution with a specific gravity of 1.085, resulting in an enriched basophil population with a recovery of 25 % and purities ranging from 5 to 20 %. Higher purities of up to 50 % were obtained with blood from patients with chronic myeloid leukemia. Pruzansky and Patterson [4] described a two-step protocol in which leukocytes were first obtained by Ficoll–Sodium metrizoate density gradient centrifugation, and basophils selectively eluted from a glass bead column, resulting in 20 % pure basophils.

1.3 The 1980s: The 50 % Purity Barrier is Overcome but Recoveries Remain Low

In comparison with the relatively poor outcomes associated with the first published purification protocols, the next technique published by R.P. Day in 1972 [5] seemed well ahead of its time both in terms of its achieved recovery (74 %) and average purity (93 %). The protocol consisted of two sequential density gradient centrifugations in Hypaque/Ficoll (1.080 g/cm^3) and Hypaque (1.065 g/cm^3) respectively, from which a pellet was retrieved and separated in a third equilibrium density gradient centrifugation step (1.065 and 1.085 g/cm^3). Subsequent attempts by other laboratories however failed to reproduce these results [6–8], and did not achieve purities or recoveries beyond 40 %. For a while, no protocols seemed to be able to achieve purities higher than around 50 % [9–11].

A notable exception from this trend was the purification protocol published by Kauffmann et al., who were able to obtain 70 % average purity (recovery ranging from 8 to 20 %) in one single discontinuous Percoll gradient centrifugation step [12].

Purities only increased when protocols using adhesion to glass beads as a final step or multiple repeated density centrifugations were abandoned and replaced by other, more efficient selection methods. Weil and coauthors described a two-step positive selection protocol using flow cytometry and FITC-labeled anti-IgE antibodies, resulting in 97–99 % purity, but only 15 % recovery [13]. The disadvantage of this method was that, due to the nature of the selection, basophils could not be used for functional studies, as pointed out by Bjerke and coauthors [14].

Toll and coauthors published a three-step protocol consisting of Dextran sedimentation to remove erythrocytes, followed by Ficoll-Hypaque centrifugation [8]. The final step relied on an anti-IgE sepharose column which enabled affinity purification of basophils. Basophils bound to the anti-IgE sepharose were eluted by high buffer flow rates or mechanical agitation. The authors reported no functional impairment in histamine release tests and basophil purities ranging between 80 and 95 %, and a recovery of around 30 % [8]. However, IgE-based positive selection techniques and mechanical stress associated with elution by mechanical agitation are generally considered to increase the risk of degranulation [15].

A second flow cytometric procedure was published in 1986 by Pendy et al. [16]. Ficoll-purified leukocytes containing basophils were subjected to lactic acid stripping, a treatment which was shown by Pruzansky to dissociate IgE from its high affinity receptor [17]. Stripped basophils were then sensitized with FITC-labeled mouse anti-DNP IgE and sorted by flow cytometry. As expected, this positive selection protocol resulted in high purities (98–99 %) but low recoveries (29 %, range 18–35 %). Viability was partially affected (≥88 %). Functional data were not reported. Warner and colleagues reported a partial increase of the recovery by using a combination of Percoll gradient centrifugation and positive selection on Penicillin-sepharose after passive sensitization with Penicillin-specific IgE. The final purity obtained was 64 % (52–92 %) with a recovery of 48 % (28–64 %). There is no information regarding functionality; basophils were obtained from pre-screened donors with higher than average basophil numbers (>40,000/mL blood). Another flow cytometry protocol reported high purities (95–98 %) but these were obtained from chronic myeloid leukemia patients and umbilical cord blood, thus are not representative of what can be achieved from peripheral blood of healthy donors [18].

One of the main problems when purifying basophils is the accompanying high number of contaminating leukocytes. This issue was initially overcome by exploiting the expression of the high affinity IgE receptor on basophils, in combination with positive selection protocols. Positive selection however bears the risk of impairing basophil function. An alternative technology which can be used to remove the bulk of contaminants is the use of countercurrent centrifugal elutriation (*see* **Note 1**). Most protocols using elutriation reported basophil purities around 4–10 % after the elutriation step, although more recent protocols reported higher purities due to modified elutriation protocols, e.g., 17.7 % [19] or 12.6 % [20].

The first application of the principle of elutriation to the purification of basophils was published by De Boer in 1986 [21]. Percoll (density of 1,077 g/cm³) gradients were used as second step, followed by elutriation and a final Percoll centrifugation (1,067/1,075 %). Final purity is reported as 69 % (45–87 %) and the recovery 51 % (31–80 %) as judged by histamine content or 60 % by Alcian blue counts. The authors point to the fact that basophil purity appears to increase when Ficoll-Isopaque is used, possibly due to the phagocytic uptake of Isopaque [22]. The specific gravity of basophils was reported to range from 1.065 to 1.075 g/cm³, which is lower than the range for histamine containing cells in blood (1.065–1.085 g/cm³) reported by Graham [23].

Interestingly, in the same year Miroli and coauthors published a one-step Ficoll-Paque centrifugation protocol with a final purity of 9 % (range 6.4–12.5 %) and a recovery of 82 % (range 65–95 %) [24]. This protocol clearly shows the limitations of one-step protocols, but as pointed out by the authors, represents a good first step due to its low cost and robustness. The protocols published by Miroli and De Boer disagree, however, regarding the distribution of basophils in the various layers after centrifugation of blood on Ficoll-Paque.

The protocol published in 1989 by Lett-Brown et al. was the first attempt to use negative selection [25]. Leukocytes were obtained by Percoll density centrifugation and contaminating cells were partially removed using monoclonal antibodies to B-cell and T-cell antigens and subsequent removal of these cells with an anti-mouse immunoglobulin. This technique resulted in 75 % purity and 54 % recovery. Purified basophils appeared functionally unimpaired judging by low spontaneous release and normal histamine content of 1.1 pg/cell.

By the end of the 1980s, all the tools necessary for successful basophil purification were in place and had been tested in various combinations. The first real breakthroughs en route to obtaining pure basophils, however, only became possible after the development of new immunomagnetic selection techniques, as described in the next section.

1.4 The 1990s: Immunomagnetic Selection Makes First Breakthroughs Possible

As results obtainable by protocols published in the 1980s were still unsatisfactory in terms of achieved purity, recovery, or both, new purification techniques were tested in the 1990s. Schroeder and Hanrahan describe the use of neuraminidase-treated red blood cells coated with TNP hapten [26]. Basophils obtained by a Percoll gradient centrifugation were first incubated with anti-TNP purified mouse monoclonal IgE. The passively sensitized basophils were then incubated with the TNP-bearing red blood cells at 4 °C. The rosettes with attached basophils were isolated by another Percoll centrifugation, and red blood cells removed by hypotonic lysis. This protocol resulted in a mean purity of 83.5 % (range 66.8–92.6) and a recovery of 58 %, which compared very favorably with previous protocols. However, basophils obtained by this protocol were functionally impaired, as their maximum histamine release was only half of the basophils before rosetting. This may reflect both the positive selection procedure as well as the effects of hypotonic lysis on basophils.

Mul and coworkers improved the protocol by De Boer and Roos [21] by adding a final immunomagnetic purification step [27]. After Percoll centrifugation, cells underwent elutriation. The elutriation fraction containing basophils was again purified using a discontinuous Percoll gradient (1.068 and 1.075 g/cm^3), resulting in 70 % pure basophils. The cells obtained from the Percoll gradient were used for a final immunomagnetic negative selection step. Magnetic bead-cell rosettes were induced by coating beads with goat anti-mouse IgG and incubating the cells with mouse monoclonal antibodies to antigens expressed on contaminating cells (CD2, CD14, CD16, and CD19). Contaminating cells were then removed with a magnet. This protocol, albeit long and laborious from today's point of view, successfully increased the purities from 70 to 94.2 % (range: 87–98 %) with an excellent recovery of 80.2 % (range 72–85 %). The basophils were fully responsive to anti-IgE and fMLP stimulation.

Bjerke's protocol [14] also used immunomagnetic selection as the final step after Percoll gradient centrifugation (45.6 % pure), resulting in 97.8 % pure basophils with a recovery of 66.2 %, which were fully functional. This protocol, because of its brevity and the high purity and recovery achieved, can be considered the first major breakthrough in basophil purification. Around the same time, Mita et al. used a similar two-step protocol consisting of Percoll gradients followed by immunomagnetic selection which resulted in an average purity of at least 80 % [28].

Gibbs et al. obtained 67.3 % pure basophils using a three-step protocol consisting of Ficoll-Paque density centrifugation, elutriation, and negative immunomagnetic selection with Dynabeads [19]. Although basophil functionality was intact, the recovery was low (21.8 %). Very similar results were obtained with the same protocol by Falcone et al. [29]. A subsequent protocol published by the same group, using the first available commercial kit for basophil immunomagnetic selection, achieved a considerable improvement in terms of purity (97.6 %) and recovery (49.7 %), high viability (99.6 %), and unimpaired functionality [20]. Taken together, the main advantage of protocols including an elutriation step is that they allow the processing of larger volumes of blood, which would be cost-prohibitive for most laboratories if using Percoll and Immunomagnetic separation alone. The downside is that not many laboratories are equipped with a countercurrent centrifugal elutriator. Relatively high purities, albeit lower than in the aforementioned protocols, can also be achieved without elutriation, as shown by the protocol of McEuen, consisting of Percoll density centrifugation followed by immunomagnetic negative selection with a commercially available kit. This resulted in 82.4 % pure basophils (median: 95 %, range 35–100 %) and a mean recovery of 51.2 %. The highest purities were achieved in the samples in which the first step had achieved a 10 % or higher enrichment. Purities of 10 % or higher are routinely achieved by elutriation, again pointing to the benefits of this technique.

Flow cytometry was also employed by several protocols using this technology for the final purification step. Tanimoto and colleagues obtained a relatively high basophil purity of 84.7 % (range 77.3–90 %) by negative selection, but recoveries were low (16 %, range 11–19.9 %) [30]. A two-step protocol by Kepley et al. [31] consisting of Percoll density gradient centrifugation (32 % purity; range 20–45 %) followed by flow cytometry solely based on size and granularity, i.e., light scattering properties, resulted in 97 % purity (range 95–99 %). While this protocol had the advantage of not necessitating the use of expensive antibodies and resulted in unimpaired basophil functionality, it showed the characteristic problem of flow cytometry-based approaches: the low recovery (23 %; range 5–28 %). The four-step protocol published by Willheim [32] consisted of Ficoll-Paque centrifugation, elutriation, immunomagnetic cell sorting to remove contaminating monocytes, and fluorescent cell sorting after CDw17 and CD14 labeling (basophils were CD17$^+$/CD14$^-$). This protocol achieved the highest purities (99.4 %, range: 98.7–99.9 %) compared with any other protocol published before then. However, as could probably be expected from such a complex and laborious four-step protocol involving flow cytometry, recoveries were very low (mean 12.8 %, range 8–25 %).

1.5 The 2000s: New Emphasis on Rapid or Simplified Protocols

As the aims of obtaining almost homogeneous basophil populations with high recovery and pristine functionality had been achieved in the 1990s (although usually not together in the same protocol), protocols published in the 2000s focused on practical aspects such as duration of the protocol, simplicity of procedure, and preservation of basophil functionality (as reflected by the use of the terms "rapid" or "simplified" in the titles of the corresponding publications). The protocol by Tsang et al. [33] consists of Ficoll-Histopaque density centrifugation followed by immunomagnetic purification with a commercial kit, and results in 96.5 % (95–98 %) pure basophils with a mean yield of 40.8 % (21–56 %).

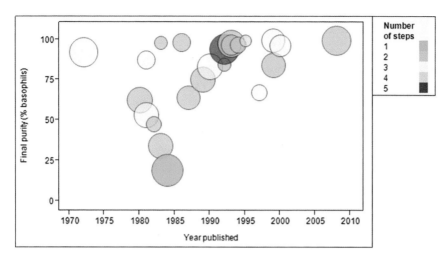

Fig. 1 Bubble plot showing the year of publication (*x*-axis), the final purity (*y*-axis), and the recovery (bubble diameter) of basophil purification protocols described in this chapter. The *color* indicates the number of steps in the protocol. Only protocols describing purification from peripheral blood of healthy donors were included

A more advanced version of this commercial kit, in combination with HetaSep precipitation, resulted in the rapid two-step purification protocol by Gibbs et al. [34] who obtained a mean purity of 99.3 % (range 97–100 %) with a mean recovery of 75.6 % (range 39–100 %). This is arguably the quickest protocol available to date, with viable, functional pure basophils obtained in less than 90 min.

Figure 1 summarizes the development of the purification protocols over the last 45 years. It is clear that with the exception of the early 1972 protocol [5], purities increased steadily over the years. Overall, there is no clear relationship between the number of steps in the protocol (indicated by the different colors) or the yield (diameter of bubbles) with the final purity (*y*-axis). However, it is also clear that protocols including flow cytometry, despite resulting in high final purities, have the lowest recoveries (means range 13–23 %) and are typically associated with reduced viability (~90 %). Whether the partial viability impairment is due to the obligatory red blood cell lysis step is not clear.

1.6   Concluding Remarks

Our short history of basophil purification has shown that a plethora of techniques has been developed for purification of human basophils. While some early techniques such as affinity chromatography for positive selection and adhesion to glass beads have now been abandoned, several techniques can be used in different combinations to obtain pure basophils. So how does one decide which protocol is the best?

The first question to answer is whether basophil purification is necessary at all. Some protocols allow assessment of basophil activation in whole blood or leukocyte preparations, e.g., when measuring the release of histamine, a preformed mediator which is to a large extent restricted to basophils in peripheral blood, or direct measurement of basophil activation via upregulation of surface activation markers such as CD63 or CD203c (*see* Chapter 11 regarding basophil activation tests). However certain applications, like signal transduction studies using Western Blotting, or gene transcription profiling using RT-PCR, will require highly purified cells, as well as high recovery.

Despite all these advances, the low number of basophils in peripheral blood of healthy donors still remains the limiting factor.

2   Materials

2.1   Reagents

All solutions should be sterile and used chilled unless stated otherwise.

1. EasySep™ Human Basophil Enrichment Kit (Stem Cell Technologies).
2. RoboSep Isolation buffer: DPBS without Ca^{2+}/Mg^{2+} with 2 % FBS (heat inactivated; v/v) and 1 mM EDTA (from 500 mM EDTA stock solution, pH 7.3) (Stem Cell Technologies).
3. HetaSep™ cell isolation medium (Stem Cell Technologies).
4. Accustain™ May-Grünwald stain 0.25 % w/v in Methanol (Sigma-Aldrich).
5. 3 % (v/v) Acetic Acid with Methylene Blue (Stem Cell Technologies).
6. 0.4 % (w/v) Trypan Blue (Stem Cell Technologies).

2.2   Supplies

1. 10 mL BD Vacutainer Sodium Heparin tubes (NH 170 I.U.).
2. 5 mL BD Falcon polystyrene round-bottom tubes.
3. Superfrost standard microscope slides.
4. Shandon Filter Cards (Fisher Thermo Scientific).
5. Shandon Cytoclip Stainless-Steel Slide Clip (Fisher Thermo Scientific).
6. Cytofunnels disposable, single (Fisher Thermo Scientific).

2.3   Equipment

1. EasySep™ Magnet for isolating up to 2.5×10^8 cells (Immunomagnetic column-free magnet) (Stem Cell Technologies).
2. CytoSpin 2, 3, or 4 Cytocentrifuge (Thermo Scientific Shandon).
3. Centrifuge.

3   Methods

3.1   Isolation
of Basophils
from Peripheral Blood

1. Collect peripheral blood by venepuncture in three or four blood collection tubes containing Na-heparin.

2. Pool the blood into a sterile 50 mL tube, add one part of HetaSep to five parts of blood then invert carefully, without shaking.

3. Split the HetaSep–blood mixture between three sterile 15 mL tubes and centrifuge at $110 \times g$ for 6 min with the brake off (*see* **Note 2**).

4. Let stand an additional 10 min at room temperature (*see* **Note 3**).

5. *Carefully* collect and pool the phases into a sterile 50 mL tube, containing the white blood cells without disturbing the red blood cell layer (*see* **Note 4**).

6. Top up the pooled upper phases to 50 mL with chilled RoboSep isolation buffer, and wash twice, using at least one wash at $120 \times g$, 10 min, followed by a second wash with chilled RoboSep buffer at $450 \times g$, 7 min (*see* **Note 5**).

7. After removing the supernatant, resuspend cell pellet in a total volume of 0.5 mL of chilled RoboSep buffer.

8. Mix 20 μL of cell suspension with 180 μL of 3 % acetic acid/methylene blue, and count cells in a Hemocytometer (*see* **Note 6**).

9. Carefully resuspend the cell pellet at 5×10^7 cells/mL or, if less than 25 million cells, a total volume of 0.5 mL of chilled RoboSep separation buffer and transfer to a sterile round-bottom 5 mL standard FACS tube (*see* **Note 7**).

10. Add 50 μL/mL of Human Basophil Enrichment Cocktail (i.e., for 500 μL, add 25 μL of cocktail), mix well, and let stand at RT or 4 °C for 10 min.

11. Resuspend EasySep® Nanoparticles by vigorously pipetting more than five times. Do not Vortex. Add 100 μL/mL (i.e., for 500 μL, add 50 μL of nanoparticles) of EasySep® Nanoparticles and mix well without vortexing.

12. Incubate at RT or 4 °C for 10 min.

13. Top-up suspension to 2.5 mL with separation buffer; gently resuspend the cells before transferring the tube containing the cell suspension to an Easy-Sep purple magnet and incubate for 5 min at RT.

14. Decant unbound cells into a fresh FACS tube. Do not feel tempted to shake or blot off any drops that may remain hanging from the mouth of the tube (*see* **Note 8**).

15. Remove the empty tube from the EasySep magnet and place the new tube (containing the supernatant from **step 14**) into the magnet. Set aside for 5 min at RT.

16. Repeat **steps 14** and **15** for a total of 3×5 min separations in the magnet. To improve recovery, at the expense of purity, only two isolations may be done.

17. Wash cells with isolation buffer or the desired assay medium.

18. Take aliquots for purity (cytospin staining using May–Grünwald's) and standard Trypan blue viability determination (*see* **Note 9**).

3.2 Preparation of Cytospins

1. Assemble cytofunnels with Filter Card and glass slide, which you have labeled with a pencil on the frosted area (*see* **Note 10**). Add 100 µL of cell suspension in cell culture medium containing FCS or RoboSep buffer (*see* **Note 11**).

2. Load cell suspension into cytofunnel and spin 1 min 500 rpm.

3. Disassemble cytospins units, allow slides to air-dry at RT for 10 min or until dry.

4. Cover whole slide with sufficient volume of May-Grünwald solution and stain for 3 min.

5. Pour off staining solution, rinse with deionized water, and allow to dry.

6. Examine cytospins under light microscope at 40× magnification or to see basophil morphology at 100× with oil immersion. Count a minimum of 500 cells for evaluation of purity. Basophils should appear fully granulated as shown in Fig. 2.

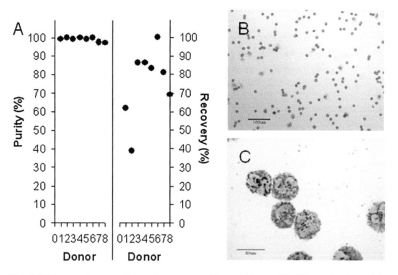

Fig. 2 (**a**) Percentage purity and recovery of basophils purified from fresh peripheral blood with the new two-step procedure (*n*=8). Recovery was determined by Alcian blue staining of cells both before and after magnetic cell sorting. Cytospin preparations stained with May–Grünwald stain showing 100 % pure basophils at 100× magnification (**b**) and at 1,000× magnification (**c**), showing that basophils are fully granulated. Reproduced from Gibbs et al. [34] with permission from John Wiley & Sons (RightsLink)

4   Notes

1. Elutriators are technical devices which allow the separation of particles with varying densities. Counter current centrifugal elutriators are special centrifuge-like devices manufactured by Beckman Instruments which allow a separation of a cell suspension into various fractions with different densities. The process of separation is considered to be gentle and does not require expensive reagents. The special design of the centrifuge results in the separation buffer flowing in the direction opposite to the centrifugal force. By stepwise increasing the flow rate (or decreasing the centrifugal force), cells are sequentially washed into collection tubes. It is not possible to obtain pure basophils by this protocol alone as their densities overlap in part with lymphocytes and neutrophils. However, it works well in generating a partially enriched population (>10 % purity in our hands) which can be used for, e.g., immunomagnetic selection.

2. Recovery from HetaSep is generally improved when using the minimal sized tube for total blood/HetaSep volumes; therefore, splitting a 30 mL sample between 3×15 mL tubes would be ideal.

3. The success of the separation can be influenced by several factors which are difficult to control, ranging from the ambient temperature to the status of the blood donor (e.g., fasting, or after a fatty meal), or the age of the blood sample. It is important to see a neat separation between the RBC layer and the WBC layer above.

4. We do this first using a sterile disposable cell culture 5 or 10 mL pipette followed by a pastette, making sure that the air is expelled before introducing into the liquid. You can also use pastettes only.

5. The slow centrifugation step is needed to remove the bulk of platelets.

6. This technique allows a so-called nucleated cell count. All cells dissolve but the cell nuclei remain intact, which are stained light blue by the methylene blue dye. This allows a quick count without interference from red blood cells which have no nuclei and are often difficult to distinguish from white blood cells in a hemocytometer in inexperienced hands.

7. 500 μL is the minimum volume for the purple EasySep magnet, but we recommend starting with at least 50 million cells (i.e., 1 mL at the recommended concentration of 50 million per mL) for optimal performance.

8. As this is a negative selection protocol, the unwanted cells will remain attached to the magnet via the magnetic beads. The decanted buffer should only contain basophils.

9. If necessary cell recovery can be determined using Alcian blue staining (which permits for rapid basophil-specific staining) in a hemocytometer, as described by Gilbert and Ornstein [35].

10. Do not use a marker pen. This will wash off during staining and ruin your cytospin.

11. Cytospins work best with at least 100,000 cells. However this would mean sacrificing a large number of purified basophils just for purity determination. We therefore routinely load fewer cells onto the cytospins. Alternatively, use the Alcian blue staining method described above.

Acknowledgements

This work was supported by the COST Action BM1007 Mast Cells and Basophils—Targets for Innovative Therapies.

References

1. Falcone FH, Haas H, Gibbs BF (2000) The human basophil: a new appreciation of its role in immune responses. Blood 96:4028–4038

2. Sampson D, Archer GT (1967) Release of histamine from human basophils. Blood 29:722–736

3. Parwaresch MR (1968) A new method for the enrichment of leukocytes, particularly of basophils. Blut 17:260–265

4. Pruzansky JJ, Patterson R (1970) Decrease in basophils after incubation with specific antigens of leukocytes from allergic donors. Int Arch Allergy Appl Immunol 38:522–526

5. Day RP (1972) Basophil leucocyte separation from human peripheral blood: a technique for their isolation in high purity and high yield. Clin Allergy 2:205–212

6. Ishizaka T, De Bernardo R, Tomioka H et al (1972) Identification of basophil granulocytes as a site of allergic histamine release. J Immunol 108:1000–1008

7. MacGlashan DW, Lichtenstein LM (1980) The purification of human basophils. J Immunol 124:2519–2521

8. Toll JB, Wikberg JE, Andersson RG (1981) Purification of human basophils by affinity chromatography on anti-IgE-sepharose 6 MB. Allergy 36:411–417

9. Pruzansky JJ, Patterson R (1981) Enrichment of human basophils. J Immunol Methods 44:183–190

10. Landry FJ, Findlay SR (1983) Purification of human basophils by negative selection. J Immunol Methods 63:329–336

11. Raghuprasad PK (1982) A rapid simple method of basophil purification by density centrifugation on Percoll. J Immunol 129:2128–2133

12. Kauffman HF, Levering PR, De Vries K (1983) A single centrifugation step method for the simultaneous separation of different leukocytes with special reference to basophilic leukocytes. J Immunol Methods 57:1–7

13. Weil GJ, Leiserson WM, Chused TM (1983) Isolation of human basophils by flow microfluorometry. J Immunol Methods 58:359–363

14. Bjerke T, Nielsen S, Helgestad J et al (1993) Purification of human blood basophils by negative selection using immunomagnetic beads. J Immunol Methods 157:49–56

15. Nielsen HV, Shah PM, Schiøtz PO (1998) Factors determining spontaneous histamine release from human basophils purified with Percoll gradients and Dynabeads. Allergy 53:302–306

16. Pendy LM, Arra SJ, Anselmino LM, Thomas LL (1986) A flow cytometric procedure for the isolation of antigenically responsive human basophils. J Immunol Methods 91:59–63

17. Pruzansky JJ, Grammer LC, Patterson R, Roberts M (1983) Dissociation of IgE from receptors on human basophils. I. Enhanced

passive sensitization for histamine release. J Immunol 131:1949–1953

18. Bodger MP, Newton LA (1987) The purification of human basophils: their immunophenotype and cytochemistry. Br J Haematol 67: 281–284

19. Gibbs BF, Noll T, Falcone FH et al (1997) A three-step procedure for the purification of human basophils from buffy coat blood. Inflamm Res 46:137–142

20. Haisch K, Gibbs BF, Körber H et al (1999) Purification of morphologically and functionally intact human basophils to near homogeneity. J Immunol Methods 226:129–137

21. De Boer M, Roos D (1986) Metabolic comparison between basophils and other leukocytes from human blood. J Immunol 136: 3447–3454

22. Splinter TA, Beudeker M, Van Beek A (1978) Changes in cell density induced by isopaque. Exp Cell Res 111:245–251

23. Graham HT, Lowry OH, Wheelwright F et al (1955) Distribution of histamine among leukocytes and platelets. Blood 10:467–481

24. Miroli AA, James BM, Spitz M (1986) Single step enrichment of human peripheral blood basophils by Ficoll-Paque centrifugation. J Immunol Methods 88:91–96

25. Lett-Brown MA, Robinson L, Juneja HS, Grant JA (1989) Purification of human basophils. Their response to anti-IgE. J Immunol Methods 117:163–167

26. Schroeder JT, Hanrahan LR (1990) Purification of human basophils using mouse monoclonal IgE. J Immunol Methods 133:269–277

27. Mul FP, Knol EF, Roos D (1992) An improved method for the purification of basophilic granulocytes from human blood. J Immunol Methods 149:207–214

28. Mita H, Akiyama K, Hayakawa T et al (1993) Purification of human blood basophils and leukotriene C4 generation following calcium ionophore stimulation. Prostaglandins Leukot Essent Fatty Acids 49:783–788

29. Falcone FH, Dahinden CA, Gibbs BF et al (1996) Human basophils release interleukin-4 after stimulation with *Schistosoma mansoni* egg antigen. Eur J Immunol 26:1147–1155

30. Tanimoto Y, Takahashi K, Takata M et al (1992) Purification of human blood basophils using negative selection by flow cytometry. Clin Exp Allergy 22:1015–1019

31. Kepley C, Craig S, Schwartz L (1994) Purification of human basophils by density and size alone. J Immunol Methods 175:1–9

32. Willheim M, Agis H, Sperr WR et al (1995) Purification of human basophils and mast cells by multistep separation technique and mAb to CDw17 and CD117/c-kit. J Immunol Methods 182:115–129

33. Tsang S, Hayashi M, Zheng X et al (2000) Simplified purification of human basophils. J Immunol Methods 233:13–20

34. Gibbs BF, Papenfuss K, Falcone FH (2008) A rapid two-step procedure for the purification of human peripheral blood basophils to near homogeneity. Clin Exp Allergy 38:480–485

35. Gilbert HS, Ornstein L (1975) Basophil counting with a new staining method using alcian blue. Blood 46:279–286

Chapter 3

Mast Cell Purification Protocols

Jasmine Farrington, Elizabeth P. Seward, and Peter T. Peachell

Abstract

Studying a tissue-specific mast cell can be of particular benefit given the heterogeneity that is known to exist among mast cells isolated or developed from different sources. Methods for isolating mast cells from a variety of tissues have been in existence for a number of years although, over time, these methodologies have been refined. We have had considerable experience studying mast cells isolated from human lung tissue. It is for this reason that, in this chapter, we provide detailed methods for the isolation and purification of human lung mast cells. However, it should be noted that the methods that are described in this chapter are generally applicable to the isolation of mast cells from different tissues and this will also be discussed.

Key words Mast cells, CD117, Dynabeads®

1 Introduction

Methods for the isolation of mast cells from animal and human tissues have been in existence for quite some time [1]. The methods that have been described show commonalities in that, in order to isolate mast cells, the tissue is physically and enzymatically disrupted. The details of the disruption can differ from method to method but nonetheless the principles are the same. This initial process leads to a mixed cell preparation of which mast cells comprise a proportion. Mast cells can be studied in a mixed cell preparation especially if straightforward functional studies are anticipated. For example, simple mediator release experiments are possible especially if stimuli (e.g., anti-IgE) are used and outputs (e.g., histamine) are measured that are likely to be mast cell specific. However, further purification may be necessary if more discrete biochemical studies are required.

In this chapter we describe in detail methods for the isolation and purification of human lung mast cells (HLMC). We also provide some general details to show how these methods are applicable to the isolation of mast cells from other tissues.

Bernhard F. Gibbs and Franco H. Falcone (eds.), *Basophils and Mast Cells: Methods and Protocols*, Methods in Molecular Biology, vol. 1192, DOI 10.1007/978-1-4939-1173-8_3, © Springer Science+Business Media New York 2014

2 Materials

2.1 Buffer and Culture Media

1. *Digestion buffer* is DMEM (with added HEPES and GlutaMAX) containing 2 % antibiotic–antimycotic solution, 1 % nonessential amino acids, and 10 % fetal calf serum (FCS).

2. *HBSS protein solution* contains 85 % HBSS, 2 % FCS, 10 % horse serum, and 1 % bovine serum albumin.

3. *HLMC culture medium* is used to culture purified mast cells and contains DMEM (with added HEPES and GlutaMAX) containing 1 % antibiotic-antimycotic solution, 1 % nonessential amino acids, and 10 % FCS and supplemented with 100 ng/mL human stem cell factor, 50 ng/mL IL-6, and 10 ng/mL IL-10.

2.2 Mast Cell Staining

1. Kimura stain (*see* **Note 1**) is used to stain mast cells and contains 11 mL of 0.05 % toluidine blue solution, 0.8 mL of 0.03 % light green SF yellowish dye, 0.5 mL of 4mg/ml Saponin in 50 % ethanol, and 5 mL of phosphate buffered saline at pH 6.4. The 0.05 % toluidine blue solution is prepared as follows: 0.05 g toluidine blue is dissolved in 50 mL 1.8 % NaCl solution, 22 mL ethanol, and 28 mL dH$_2$O.

2.3 Magnetic Cell Sorting

1. *Magnetic Dynabeads*® for mast cell purification are prepared as follows. The Dynabeads® which are conjugated to sheep anti-mouse IgG are coated with mouse anti-human CD117 antibody before use. 100 µL of bead mixture is rinsed three times in HBSS (+2 % FCS) using an MPC-1 magnet (Dynal). After the final wash, beads are resuspended in 0.4 mL of HBSS protein solution, 8 µL of mouse anti-human CD117 antibody is added, and the mixture is incubated at 4 °C for 2 h with continuous rotation. Beads are then washed three times using the MPC-1 magnet as described above and then resuspended in 100 µL of HBSS protein solution. To coated beads that are not used immediately, 0.1 % sodium azide is added as a preservative, and these can be stored for up 2 weeks at 4 °C. Before use, sodium azide is removed by washing the appropriate amount of beads three times in 8 mL of HBSS (+2 % FCS). The beads are then recovered by using the magnet. After the final wash the beads are resuspended in 1 mL of cold HBSS protein solution.

3 Methods

We obtain non-lesional tissue from surgical lung resections. This requires appropriate ethical approval. The tissue is then enzymatically digested using a modification of methods that have been described elsewhere ([2, 3]; *see* **Note 2**). Mast cells are isolated and further purified using the Dynal® magnetic bead system using methods similar to those described [4]. All procedures are carried out aseptically.

3.1 Tissue Dispersal and Digestion

1. Place lung tissue in a small amount of digestion buffer.

2. Chop tissue into small fragments using surgical scissors and rinse over 100 μm nylon gauze with DMEM (+2 % FCS).

3. Chop tissue fragments vigorously for a further 3–6 min to generate a consistent pulp. Throughout the chopping process, keep the tissue moist by adding DMEM (+2 % FCS).

4. Rinse the pulp twice over 100 μm gauze, and then transfer to a sterile pot containing 4 mL of digestion buffer per gram of chopped tissue.

5. Store chopped tissue overnight at 4 °C, with a loosely attached lid to allow oxygenation (*see* **Note 3**).

6. The following day, allow the tissue suspension to equilibrate to room temperature (19–22 °C) for 40 min before enzymatic digestion.

7. Once equilibrated, add the following enzymes to the tissue: cell culture-treated collagenase type I-A (3 mg/g of tissue) and hyaluronidase (3,76 mg/g of tissue; *see* **Note 4**). To aid disruption, place a sterile magnetic bead in the pot and stir the mixture gently for 75 min at 37 °C in a humidified CO_2 incubator.

8. After this incubation, obtain further physical disruption by plunging the mixture 30 times with a 50 mL syringe.

9. After physical and enzymatic disruption, filter the dispersed tissue three times by washing over 100 μm gauze.

10. Wash the dispersed cells three times with fresh DMEM (+2 % FCS) by centrifugation ($480 \times g$, 8 min) with volumes of 200–400, 100, and 50 mL of buffer for successive centrifugations.

11. After these washings, mast cell numbers are established. The mixed cell population is resuspended in typically 5–10 mL of buffer. Mast cells are identified using Kimura stain. Incubate an aliquot of the cells with the stain for 5 min (ratio of 1:10; for example, 10 μL cells: 90 μL stain) and count the cells using a hemocytometer (*see* **Note 5**).

3.2 Mast Cell Purification

1. Resuspend the mixed cell population in 4 mL of HBSS protein solution and incubate with continuous rotation for 30 min at 4 °C (*see* **Note 6**).

2. Make up the total volume of the cell suspension to 50–100 mL with cold (4 °C) HBSS (+2 % FCS).

3. Strain through 100 μm sterile cell filters (6–10 depending on the volume).

4. Centrifuge cells ($480 \times g$, 8 min).

5. In the meantime, wash an appropriate volume of coated Dynal beads in 8 mL of HBSS (+2 % FCS) using the MPC-1 magnet; after the wash, resuspend the beads in 1 mL of HBSS protein solution. The bead-to-mast cell ratio used is 5:1, which equates to 125 µL of bead suspension for 10×10^6 mast cells.

6. After centrifugation, resuspend the cells in 2 mL of HBSS protein solution mix with the beads and incubate with continuous rotation at 4 °C for 2 h.

7. After incubation, make up the bead-cell suspension to a total volume of 10 mL with cold HBSS (+2 % FCS) and transfer to a 15 mL tube.

8. Separate the mixture using an MPC-1 magnet by inserting the tube in the magnet for 3 min, discarding the supernatant, removing the tube from the magnet, and resuspending the magnetically adherent cells in 10 mL of HBSS (+2 % FCS).

9. Repeat this cycle for a total of three washes. The principle of the immunomagnetic bead separation is shown in Fig. 1 (*see* **Note** 7).

10. After the last wash, resuspend the isolated mast cells conjugated to the beads in 1 mL of HLMC culture medium with cytokines and count the cells using the Kimura stain. Additional culture medium can be added as appropriate.

11. Carry out full medium exchange within 3 days of the isolation and purification process, and, thereafter, exchange culture medium weekly.

12. Cells can be cultured for longer time periods in T12.5 culture flasks, at a density of 100,000–300,000 cells per mL at 37 °C, in a humidified CO_2 incubator. A full or half exchange of media and transfer to a new tissue culture flask is carried out every 7 days. Purity of the cultured mast cells is determined using the Kimura stain and further verified by using phycoerythrin (PE)-tagged anti-CD117 IgG_1 antibody (Miltenyi Biotec). Figure 2 shows an example of staining of mast cells with PE-tagged anti-CD117 following long-term culture.

4   Notes

1. In this chapter, a Kimura stain has been described for the detection of mast cells. However alternative stains can be used to detect mast cells including Alcian blue [5].

2. A number of alternative methods have been used for the digestion of human lung to obtain mast cells as well as those described in this chapter. These vary in the types of buffer used, enzyme

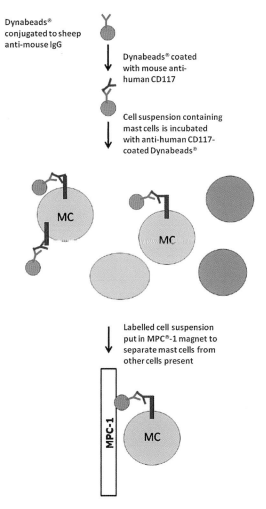

Dynabeads®
conjugated to sheep
anti-mouse IgG

Dynabeads® coated
with mouse anti-
human CD117

Cell suspension containing
mast cells is incubated
with anti-human CD117-
coated Dynabeads®

Labelled cell suspension
put in MPC®-1 magnet to
separate mast cells from
other cells present

Fig. 1 Schematic diagram showing mast cell (MC; *blue*) purification, utilizing Dynabeads® technology. Dynabeads® are conjugated to sheep anti-mouse IgG and then pre-coated with mouse anti-human CD117. The mixed cell population produced from the digestion step is then incubated with the coated beads. Mast cells (which express CD117 receptors) attach to the Dynabeads® and adhere to the magnetic particle concentrator (MPC-1) whereas other cells (shown in *green* and *purple*) do not. Contaminant cells are then washed away and mast cells recovered following removal from the magnetic field (adapted, with permission, from a diagram created by Claire Tree-Booker)

cocktails employed, and mechanisms of physical disruption. In principle similar protocols have been described for the isolation of mast cells from alternative tissues including human skin [6–8] and gut [9, 10] and from a variety of animal tissues [1].

3. This step aids the elimination of bacteria and other microorganisms, decreasing the likelihood of infection in cell preparations and cultures.

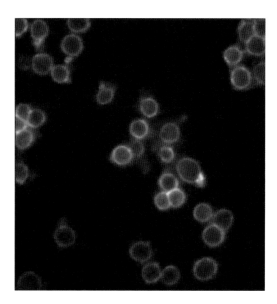

Fig. 2 Human lung mast cells stained with PE-tagged antibody to the mast cell surface antigen, CD117. The excitation wavelength was 488 nm and fluorescent images were taken at 578 nm. The picture shows live cells at 75 days post-isolation. The fluorescently tagged antibody labelled 98 % of the cells

4. Titrating the activity and suitability of various batches of collagenase and FCS can be quite a valuable investment in terms of ensuring good yields of functional mast cells.

5. These methods usually generate ~1×10^6 mast cells per g of lung tissue and the purity is between 5 and 15 %.

6. This stage acts as a blocking step to help prevent nonspecific protein binding.

7. Alternative methods have been described for the purification of mast cells including the use of discontinuous Percoll gradients, countercurrent elutriation (requires customization of a dedicated centrifuge and a specialized rotor head and chamber), and alternative immunomagnetic bead separation protocols. These methods are described elsewhere [11–15].

Acknowledgements

The authors are grateful to Mr. J. Rao, Mr. J. Edwards, Mr. D. Hopkinson, and Mr. A. Ahmed (Cardiothoracic Surgery) and Dr. S.K. Suvarna, Dr. P. Kitsanta, and Dr. J. Bury (Histopathology) at the Northern General Hospital, Sheffield, for their invaluable help in providing lung tissue specimens.

References

1. Ali H, Pearce FL (1985) Isolation and properties of cardiac and other mast cells from the rat and guinea-pig. Agents Actions 16:138–140

2. Cruse G, Kaur D, Yang W, Duffy SM, Brightling CE, Bradding P (2005) Activation of human lung mast cells by monomeric immunoglobulin E. Eur Respir J 25:858–863

3. Sanmugalingam D, Wardlaw AJ, Bradding P (2000) Adhesion of human lung mast cells to bronchial epithelium: evidence for a novel carbohydrate-mediated mechanism. J Leukoc Biol 68:38–46

4. Okayama Y, Hunt TC, Kassel O, Ashman LK, Church MK (1994) Assessment of the anti-c-kit monoclonal antibody YB5.B8 in affinity magnetic enrichment of human lung mast cells. J Immunol Methods 169:153–161

5. Gilbert HS, Ornstein L (1975) Basophil counting with a new staining method using alcian blue. Blood 46:279–286

6. Benyon RC, Lowman MA, Church MK (1987) Human skin mast cells: their dispersion, purification and secretory characterization. J Immunol 138:861–867

7. Lawrence ID, Warner JA, Cohan VL, Hubbard WC, Kagey-Sobotka A, Lichtenstein LM (1987) Purification and characterization of human skin mast cells. Evidence for human mast cell heterogeneity. J Immunol 139: 3062–3069

8. Bastan R, Peirce MJ, Peachell PT (2001) Regulation of immunoglobulin E-mediated secretion by protein phosphatases in human basophils and mast cells of skin and lung. Eur J Pharmacol 430:135–141

9. Lowman MA, Rees PH, Benyon RC, Church MK (1988) Human mast cell heterogeneity: histamine release from mast cells dispersed from skin, lung, adenoids, tonsils, and colon in response to IgE-dependent and nonimmunologic stimuli. J Allergy Clin Immunol 81:590–597

10. Fox CC, Dvorak AM, Peters SP, Kagey-Sobotka A, Lichtenstein LM (1985) Isolation and characterization of human intestinal mucosal mast cells. J Immunol 135:483–491

11. Weston MC, Anderson N, Peachell PT (1997) Effects of phosphodiesterase inhibitors on human lung mast cell and basophil function. Br J Pharmacol 121:287–295

12. Lewis A, Wan J, Baothman B, Monk PN, Suvarna SK, Peachell PT (2013) Heterogeneity in the responses of human lung mast cells to stem cell factor. Clin Exp Allergy 43:50–59

13. Church MK, Hiroi J (1987) Inhibition of IgE-dependent histamine release from human dispersed lung mast cells by anti-allergic drugs and salbutamol. Br J Pharmacol 90:421–429

14. Schulman ES, MacGlashan DW, Peters SP, Schleimer RP, Newball HH, Lichtenstein LM (1982) Human lung mast cells: purification and characterisation. J Immunol 129:2662–2667

15. Ishizaka T, Conrad DH, Schulman ES, Sterk AR, Ishizaka K (1983) Biochemical analysis of initial triggering events of IgE-mediated histamine release from human lung mast cells. J Immunol 130:2357–2362

Chapter 4

Generation of a Human Allergic Mast Cell Phenotype from CD133+ Stem Cells

Hans Jürgen Hoffmann

Abstract

Cultured human mast cells are a useful tool for research into innate immune responses as well as allergic mechanisms. Mast cells cultured from peripheral blood can provide information on immune mechanisms of known, selected individuals. With the method presented here eight million mast cells can be cultured from ca. one million stem cells purified from one unit (450 mL) of human peripheral blood. Culture with IgE and IL4 optimizes an allergic phenotype of the mast cells.

Key words Mast cell, Human stem cells, Buffy coat, Cultured mast cells, SCF, CD63, FcεRI

1 Introduction

Mast cells are tissue-resident cells first described by Ehrlich in 1878 that derive from bone marrow-derived hematopoietic stem cells. These CD34+ C117+ CD133+ cells released into circulation can be purified and cultured to resemble tissue mast cells. Mature mast cells contain large amounts of preformed heparin, histamine, and a number of cytokines, and continue to express the stem cell factor receptor CD117.

Mast cells are present in most tissues, characteristically proximal to blood vessels, nerves, and epithelia. Early work [1] identified two subtypes of mast cells based on the expression of chymase. Recent work has described distinguishable phenotypes of mast cells associated with anatomical compartments of the human lung [2] that were identified by protein markers (FcεRI, IL9-R, HDAC, and others). Mast cells can be purified from tissue or cultured from purified stem cells [3–6]. In both instances, they are dependent on SCF [7].

Bernhard F. Gibbs and Franco H. Falcone (eds.), *Basophils and Mast Cells: Methods and Protocols*, Methods in Molecular Biology, vol. 1192, DOI 10.1007/978-1-4939-1173-8_4, © Springer Science+Business Media New York 2014

2 Materials

2.1 Isolation and Culture of CD133⁺ Human Stem Cells

1. Human peripheral blood (100–450 mL), or fresh buffy coat, can be citrated or in EDTA (*see* **Note 1**).
2. Ficoll Paque (GE Health Care).
3. Sterile 50 mL tubes.
4. Sterile PBS.
5. Low-speed centrifuge.
6. AC133⁺ cell isolation kit (Miltenyi).
7. MACS buffer (Miltenyi).
8. LS Separation columns (Miltenyi).
9. StemSpan culture medium (Stem Cell Technologies, Vancouver, Canada).
10. Penicillin/streptomycin.
11. Foetal bovine serum (FBS).
12. Human recombinant stem cell factor (rhSCF) (R&D Systems, Abingdon, UK).
13. Human rhIL-3 (R&D Systems, Abingdon, UK).
14. Human rhIL-6 (R&D Systems, Abingdon, UK).
15. Recombinant IL-4 (Peprotech EC Ltd., London, UK).
16. Human monoclonal IgE, produced by various companies.
17. CM: Stem Span culture medium with IL-6 (50 ng/mL), SCF (100 ng/mL), and penicillin/streptomycin (100 µg/mL).

2.2 Reagents for Determining Mast Cell Purity and Reactivity

2.2.1 May–Grünwald–Giemsa Staining

1. May–Grünwald solution (Merck, Darmstadt, Germany).
2. Giemsa (Merck) diluted 1/10 in PBS, pH 6.4.
3. Microslides and cover slips.

2.2.2 Detection of Density of FcεRI, Mast Cell Reactivity, and Kit Surface Receptor Expression by Flow Cytometry

1. Polystyrene round-bottom tubes (5 mL).
2. PBS + 0.1 % BSA (4 °C).
3. Anti-CD63 FITC (Biolegend, San Diego, CA, clone H5C6).
4. CD203c PE (Biolegend, San Diego, CA, clone NP4D6).
5. Qifikit (Dako, Glostrup, Denmark).
6. Anti-human IgE (BD Pharmingen, San Jose, CA, clone G7-18).

3   Methods

All work is to be done in a sterile lab bench, except mast cell activation tests and staining (Subheadings 3.3 and 3.4).

3.1 Purification of CD133+ Stem Cells from Peripheral Blood

1. Bring Ficoll and PBS to room temperature (22 °C), and aliquot 13 mL Ficoll into a sterile 50 mL tube for each 24 mL blood to be processed (*see* **Note 2**).

2. Dilute blood with 0.25 volumes of PBS in a sterile flask, and carefully layer blood on the Ficoll layer (*see* **Note 3**). Centrifuge for 30 min at room temperature and $450 \times g$ without acceleration or brake to preserve the integrity of the gradient interface.

3. Using a sterile pipette or pastettete, remove the plasma layer above the interface. Collect PBMC at the interface and wash with 20 mL cold PBS for each gradient tube. Centrifuge for 5 min at 4 °C and $450 \times g$. Pool all cells into one 10 mL tube, wash them again in 10 mL MACS buffer, and count the number of leukocytes in the sample.

4. To count the cells, dilute 20 μL cells with 80 μL trypan blue, and count in a Bürker-Türk or Neubauer modified chamber. While counting, centrifuge as before (5 min, 4 °C, $450 \times g$).

5. Resuspend all cells in 300 μL MACS buffer (maximally 10^8 cells per 300 μL) in a 10 mL tube and chill on ice.

6. Add 100 μL Fc blocking reagent, and 100 μL CD133 microbeads per 300 μL cell suspension.

7. Incubate on ice for 2 min, and at 4 °C for 28 min. Dilute cells with 10 mL MACS buffer, and centrifuge for 5 min at 4 °C and $450 \times g$. Resuspend in 500 μL MACS buffer per 10^8 cells.

8. Wipe the MidiMACS with 70 % ethanol and place it in the sterile bench.

9. Fill each vial with 300 μL cells up to 10 mL with MACS buffer. Centrifuge for 5 min at $450 \times g$ and 4 °C. Pour off the supernatant and then resuspend the pellet in 5 mL MACS buffer.

10. Apply 3 mL MACS solution to an LS column in a MACS magnet. When the MACS solution has reached the top of the column, add the cell suspension. Collect the eluate in a clean tube. Wash the column with 3×5 mL MACS buffer, collecting the eluate each time. Remove the column from the magnet and pass 5 mL MACS buffer through to elute retained cells from the column. Count the number of cells in the eluate in a Bürker-Türk chamber or other hemocytometers. Centrifuge all tubes for 5 min at $450 \times g$ and 4 °C. There should be no visible pellet in the second last tube, and all CD133+ cells in the last tube.

3.2 Expansion of Stem Cells and Maturation of Mast Cells

1. Resuspend CD133⁺ stem cells in CM with IL-3 at $5 \cdot 10^5$ cells/mL and culture at 37 °C in a humidified CO_2 incubator.

2. Inspect the cultures twice a week for growth and sterility (*see* **Note 4**). If the medium appears spent, as indicated by an orange or even yellow color, add some more CM to continue supporting growth until the next medium change.

3. Change medium on a weekly basis. Transfer all cells and medium to a sterile centrifuge tube, and centrifuge for 5 min at $450 \times g$ and 4 °C. Remove the supernatant. Resuspend up the cell pellet in 1 mL CM and count in a Bürker-Türk chamber. Resuspend the cells at $5 \cdot 10^5$ cells/mL in the appropriate medium and transfer to a fresh well or flask of appropriate size.

4. IL-3 should be added for the first 3 weeks to expand cell lines. In weeks 4–6, the cells are cultured in CM only. In weeks 7–8, FBS (10 %), IL-4 (10 ng/mL), and IgE (80 kU/L) are added to mature mast cells (*see* **Note 5**).

5. At the end of the culture period, evaluate mast cell quality, purity, and reactivity as described in the next section.

3.3 Mast Cell Staining with May–Grünwald–Giemsa by Microscopy

1. Prepare a cytospin with 10^3–10^4 mast cells. Centrifuge at 1,000 rpm for 5 min. Air-dry until cells appear dry.

2. Stain with May–Grünwald solution for 4 min, and wash in PBS for 4 min.

3. Rinse in water, stain with Giemsa solution for 8 min, and rinse again in water.

4. Air-dry cytospins and examine mast cells in a light microscope to confirm the appearance of granules in the cytoplasm (Fig. 1).

3.4 Mast Cell Reactivity and Phenotyping by Flow Cytometry

1. Prepare five log dilutions of anti-IgE or (APC-labelled) anti-FcεRI antibody in PBS from 1 ng/10 µL as well as a blank tube (*see* **Note 6**).

2. Add 90 µL mast cell preparation containing at least 5,000 cells.

3. Incubate at 37 °C for 30 min.

4. Add antibodies to CD63 (FITC) and CD203c (PE) and incubate at 4 °C for 20 min (*see* **Note 4**).

5. Wash with 2 mL PBS, and centrifuge at $450 \times g$ and 4 °C.

6. Acquire data on a flow cytometer; plot a histogram of CD63 for all cells for all tubes, and set a threshold at 2 % of the blank. Plot the fraction of positive cells against anti-IgE or anti-FcεRI concentration (*see* **Note 7**).

7. Add titrated amounts of antibody to FcεRI, and CD117 to aliquots of mast cell culture. Use QiFikit according to the manufacturer's instructions to determine the density of receptors on cells.

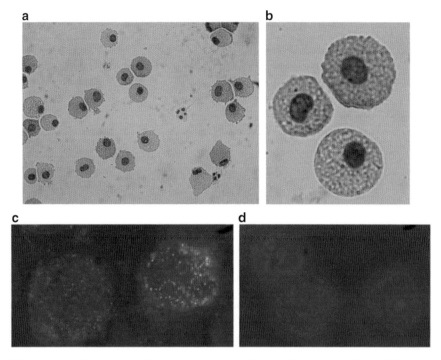

Fig. 1 CD133⁺ peripheral blood-derived mast cell, 7 weeks. (**a**) and (**b**) Human peripheral blood-derived mast cells (PBMC) cultured in serum-free StemSpan medium for 6 weeks and with 10 % FCS for 1 week. Stem cell factor, IL-6, and IL-3 were added to the media but IL-3 was omitted after the first week of culture. Cells stained with May–Grünwald–Giemsa show contents of cytoplasmic granules. (**c**) Cell surface expression of FcεRI α-chain by immunostaining with CRA-1 (*green*) or D. Isotype control. Cells counterstained with DAPI, 4′,6-diamidino-2-phenylindole, which is a fluorescent stain that binds strongly to nuclear DNA (*blue*) (reproduced from [4], with permission from Elsevier)

4   Notes

1. We have not purified CD133⁺ cells for mast cell culture from heparinized blood.

2. Typical yields of stem cells per mL blood are 3,800 for fresh blood, 2,500 for buffy coats, and blood 24 h old (unpublished observations).

3. This can take some practice. It is important to avoid disturbing the surface of the Ficoll layer. Find a comfortable and relaxed position, e.g., resting the elbow on the laminar flow bench edge. Use a pipetting aid which allows you to set the speed of dispensing to low, and use a constant flow rate, holding the tube at an angle of approx. 45–60°.

4. If there was a sign of contamination, the flask was removed or the well was emptied and cleansed with 70 % ethanol in water.

5. IgE can be obtained from myeloma, or as recombinant products. We have used recombinant human IgE [8].

6. Optimization of antibody concentrations should be performed by titration prior to the start of the experiment.

7. We use log SS (230V) and FS (40V) on a BD instrument to focus mast cells in the scatter plot. If APC-labelled anti-FcεRI is used to stimulate cells, the fraction of cells expressing FcεRI as well as the relationship between FcεRI expression and activation can be examined.

References

1. Irani AM, Schwartz LB (1994) Human mast cell heterogeneity. Allergy Proc 15:303–308

2. Andersson CK, Mori M, Bjermer L et al (2009) Novel site-specific mast cell subpopulations in the human lung. Thorax 64:297–305

3. Andersen HB, Holm M, Hetland TE et al (2008) Comparison of short term in vitro cultured human mast cells from different progenitors—peripheral blood-derived progenitors generate highly mature and functional mast cells. J Immunol Methods 336: 166–174

4. Holm M, Andersen HB, Hetland TE et al (2008) Seven week culture of functional human mast cells from buffy coat preparations. J Immunol Methods 336:213–221

5. Hoffmann HJ, Frandsen PM, Christensen LH et al (2012) Cultured human mast cells are heterogeneous for expression of the high-affinity IgE receptor FcεRI. Int Arch Allergy Immunol 157:246–250

6. Krohn IK, Lund G, Frandsen PM et al (2013) Mast cell FcεRI density and function dissociate from dependence on soluble IgE concentration at very low and very high IgE concentrations. J Asthma 50:117–121

7. Kirshenbaum AS, Goff JP, Kessler SW et al (1992) Effect of IL-3 and stem cell factor on the appearance of human basophils and mast cells from CD34+ pluripotent progenitor cells. J Immunol 148:772–777

8. Christensen LH, Holm J, Lund G et al (2008) Several distinct properties of the IgE repertoire determine effector cell degranulation in response to allergen challenge. J Allergy Clin Immunol 122:298–304

Chapter 5

Generation of Mast Cells from Murine Stem Cell Progenitors

Emily J. Swindle

Abstract

Mouse bone marrow-derived mast cells (mBMMCs) are an invaluable tool for the study of mast cell function from wild-type, knockout, and transgenic mice. This method describes the isolation of mast cell progenitors from the bone marrow of mouse femurs and their subsequent culture in an IL-3-rich culture medium. After 4 weeks, mBMMCs are obtained in high number and are of high purity. Assessment of their granularity by toluidine staining and IgE receptor expression by flow cytometry are also described. These cells are a useful tool in the determination of mast cell function in innate and adaptive immunity.

Key words Mast cell, BMMC, IgE, FcεRI, Degranulation

Abbreviations

BMMC   Bone marrow-derived mast cells
FcεRI   High-affinity IgE receptor

1 Introduction

Mouse mast cells develop from CD34+, CD117+ (Kit), CD13+, and FcεRI− cells which originate in the bone marrow. These mast cell progenitors (MCp) then migrate through the blood into peripheral tissue through the expression of $\alpha_V\beta_7$ integrin where their growth, development, and survival require the growth factor stem cell factor (SCF) [1]. There are two major phenotypes of mast cells depending on their location in specific tissue (connective or mucosal tissue) and the presence of granule-associated proteases (mouse mast cell protease (MCP)). Mouse connective tissue mast cells contain high levels of MCP4, 5, and 6, whereas mouse mucosal mast cells have MCP1 and 2 [2]. Bone marrow-derived mast

Bernhard F. Gibbs and Franco H. Falcone (eds.), *Basophils and Mast Cells: Methods and Protocols*, Methods in Molecular Biology, vol. 1192, DOI 10.1007/978-1-4939-1173-8_5, © Springer Science+Business Media New York 2014

cells (BMMCs) belong to the connective tissue type. They express the high-affinity IgE receptor (FcεRI), and can be passively sensitized with IgE and activated following antigen stimulation.

The following methods describe the isolation of stem cell progenitors from mouse bone marrow and the subsequent expansion and differentiation of these progenitors into mature mast cells in an IL-3 rich culture medium. After 4 weeks, mature BMMCs are obtained in high numbers (approx. 100 million cells per mouse (two femurs) and of high purity (>99 %). Assessment of the granularity and purity of these mast cell cultures are also described by toluidine blue staining and analysis of FcεRI and CD117 (Kit) receptor expression by flow cytometry, respectively. These methods can be used to obtain BMMCs from wild-type, knockout, and transgenic mice for further investigations into mast cell activation, chemotaxis, and adhesion.

2   Materials

2.1 Isolation of Mouse Bone Marrow Progenitors

1. Mouse (2–6 months old).
2. Scissors.
3. Forceps.
4. Ethanol solution (70 % in ddH$_2$O).
5. BMMC culture medium (1,000 mL): To 825 mL of RPMI 1640 add 100 mL of FCS (10 %) and the following L-glutamine (4 mM), penicillin/streptomycin (100 U/mL/100 µg/mL), HEPES (25 mM), sodium pyruvate (1 mM), nonessential amino acids (1×), β-mercaptoethanol (50 µM), and murine IL-3 (30 ng/mL, Peprotech). Mix thoroughly, filter through 0.2 µM filter, and store at 4 °C for up to 2 weeks. Prior to use pre-warm the culture medium at 37 °C.
6. Conical tube (20 mL).
7. Syringe needle (25 G).
8. Syringe (30 mL).
9. 6-Well plate.
10. Tissue culture flasks (125 cm^2).

2.2 Reagents for Determining BMMC Purity

2.2.1 Toluidine Staining

1. MOTA's fixative: To a 100 mL glass bottle add ddH$_2$O (50 mL) and lead acetate (basic, 4 g) and with continuous mixing add glacial acetic acid (1–2 mL) until the lead acetate is fully solubilized. Finally add the 100 % ethanol (50 mL) and store at room temperature for maximum of 2 months.
2. Toluidine blue solution: To a 50 mL conical tube add toluidine blue (0.25 g), ddH$_2$O (35 mL), and 100 % ethanol

(15 mL). Adjust the pH of the solution to less than 1 with HCl (1–2 mL) and store at room temperature.

3. Microslides and cover slips.

4. Permount mounting medium (Fisher Scientific).

5. Cytospin (Shandon).

2.2.2 Detection of FcεRI and Kit Surface Receptor Expression by Flow Cytometry

1. Polystyrene round-bottom tubes (5 mL).

2. PBS + 0.1 % BSA (4 °C).

3. Anti-mouse FcεRI-FITC (eBioscience, #11-5898).

4. Hamster IgG-FITC.

5. Anti-mouse CD117-PE (BD Pharmingen, # 555714).

6. Mouse IgG$_1$-PE.

3 Methods

3.1 Bone Marrow Cell Isolation and Mast Cell Culture

3.1.1 Isolation and Culture of Bone Marrow Progenitors

1. Using 70 % ethanol solution, sterilize scissors and forceps (*see* **Note 1**). Sacrifice a mouse and rinse in 70 % ethanol. Cut away the skin from around the back leg area and remove both femurs using the scissors and forceps. Place the femurs in BMMC culture medium (10 mL) (*see* **Note 2**).

2. Add BMMC culture medium (10 mL) to a well of a 6-well plate and place the femurs into the well. To another well, add 5 mL culture medium, fill a syringe with medium, and attach a 25 G needle to it. Using forceps, hold the femur and using the needle flush the bone marrow out of the femur into the culture medium (*see* **Note 3**).

3. Transfer the flushed bone marrow cells from the 6-well plate to a 125 cm^2 culture flask. Rinse the well with fresh medium (5 mL) and add this to the same culture flask. Add a further 40 mL of culture medium to the flask and culture the cells in an incubator for 3–4 days.

3.1.2 Expansion of Bone Marrow Cells and Maturation of BMMCs

After 3–4 days, change the medium of the bone marrow culture twice a week (e.g., Monday and Friday) by transferring the cell suspension to a sterile conical tube (50 mL) and centrifuge (300 × *g*, 5 min, room temperature). Remove the supernatant, resuspend the cell pellet in fresh culture medium (50 mL), and transfer to a new culture flask (T125 cm^2) (*see* **Note 4**). After 4 weeks, the culture consists of mature BMMCs. Before proceeding to use in experiments, the purity of the BMMCs is evaluated by toluidine blue staining of cytospin preparations (*see* section below) and FcεRI and CD117 expression by flow cytometry (*see* section below) (*see* **Note 5**).

3.2 Determination of BMMC Purity

3.2.1 Toluidine Blue Staining of Cytospin Preparations

1. Take 100,000 cells per sample and centrifuge ($300 \times g$, 5 min, room temperature).

2. Resuspend BMMC at 1×10^6/mL, transfer 100 µL of BMMC in duplicate to a cytospin chamber, and centrifuge at 500 rpm for 5 min (*see* **Note 6**).

3. Immerse cells (on microslide) in Mota's fixative (15 min, room temperature) and then gently wash with ddH$_2$O.

4. Allow to air-dry (15 min) and then immerse each slide in toluidine blue solution (20 min, room temperature).

5. Gently wash slide with ddH$_2$O, air-dry, and overlay with a cover slip using Permount.

6. Visualize cells under microscope for staining of granules by toluidine blue.

3.2.2 Surface Expression of FcεRI and CD117 (Kit) by Flow Cytometry

1. Take 50,000 cells per sample (two samples required, isotype and specific antibody) and centrifuge ($300 \times g$, 5 min, room temperature).

2. Resuspend cells at 0.5×10^6 cells/mL in pre-chilled PBS + 0.1 % BSA (4 °C) and transfer 100 µL aliquots into polystyrene round-bottom tubes (5 mL).

3. Add 1 µL of either anti-FcεRI-FITC and anti-CD117-PE or their respective isotype controls (hamster IgG-FITC and mouse IgG$_1$-PE) to each tube and incubate for 30 min at 4 °C in the dark (*see* **Note 7**).

4. Wash off excess antibodies by adding PBS + 0.1 % BSA (1 mL) to each tube and centrifuge ($300 \times g$, 5 min, 4 °C). Resuspend cell pellet in PBS + 0.1 % BSA (100 µL) and analyze 10,000 cells on a flow cytometer (*see* **Note 8**).

4 Notes

1. All procedures, including bone removal and femur lavage, are performed in a laminar flow hood. All reagents are sterilized by filtration and all surgical equipment sterilized by immersion in 70 % alcohol prior to use.

2. Remove as much attached muscle from the femurs as possible with scissors; this makes it easier to flush the bone.

3. The bone will become clear when the red marrow is removed.

4. It is important to replace the culture flasks every time the medium is changed to remove contaminating adherent cells. This is especially important in the first 2 weeks of culture when there are many adherent cells present. After 2 weeks of culture, adjust the cell density to 1×10^6/mL when the bone marrow cells start to proliferate.

5. The BMMCs should not be used after 7 weeks in culture as their reactivity begins to decrease.

6. A pale white spot should appear on slide indicating that cells have dried.

7. Prior optimization of antibody concentrations should be performed by titration prior to the start of the experiment.

8. Typically BMMC samples are greater than 99 % double positive for CD117 and FcεRI.

Acknowledgment

Financial support for work in the authors' laboratories was provided by the Faculty of Medicine, University of Southampton, and the Asthma, Allergy and Inflammation Research Charity.

References

1. Hallgren J, Gurish MF (2007) Pathways of murine mast cell development and trafficking: tracking the roots and routes of the mast cell. Immunol Rev 217:8–18

2. Stevens RL, Friend DS, McNeil HP, Schiller V, Ghildyal N, Austen KF (1997) Strain-specific and tissue-specific expression of mouse mast cell secretory granule proteases. Proc Natl Acad Sci U S A 91:128–132

Chapter 6

Integration of the Human Dermal Mast Cell into the Organotypic Co-culture Skin Model

Jonghui Kim, Sven Guhl, Magda Babina, Torsten Zuberbier, and Metin Artuc

Abstract

The organotypic co-culture skin model has been providing an advanced approach to the in vitro investigation of the skin. Mast cells, containing various mediators such as tryptase and chymase, are thought to contribute to many physiological and pathological events of the skin interactively with other cells. Here, we introduce an organotypic co-culture skin model which successfully integrates human dermal mast cells for further study of mast cell interactions with fibroblasts and keratinocytes.

Key words Organotypic co-culture skin model, Skin equivalent, Dermis equivalent, Human dermal mast cells, Fibroblasts, Keratinocytes

1 Introduction

The organotypic co-culture skin model, first introduced by Bell and co-workers in 1981 [1] and modified subsequently by others [2, 3], consisting of a fibroblast-populated dermis equivalent (DE) and superficial keratinocytic layer, has provided an advanced approach to in vitro investigations of the skin. Despite the strongly simplified composition of the organotypic co-culture system, it presents not only an in vivo-like morphologic pattern of epidermal differentiation, which is not seen in the standard 2D culture, but also a similar phenotypic expression of various epidermal differentiation markers which closely resemble the original tissue [4–7]. The organotypic skin model has become a powerful tool for investigations of cell interactions such as keratinocyte growth regulation [8], dynamics of basement membrane formation [9], and dermal-epidermal junction morphogenesis [10].

Mast cells (MCs) are bone marrow-derived cells, distributed widely throughout the body, particularly in the subepithelial tissue near blood vessel and nerves, and are thought to contribute to

Bernhard F. Gibbs and Franco H. Falcone (eds.), *Basophils and Mast Cells: Methods and Protocols*, Methods in Molecular Biology, vol. 1192, DOI 10.1007/978-1-4939-1173-8_6, © Springer Science+Business Media New York 2014

physiological and pathological events of the skin interactively with other cells. Some studies indicated that MCs enhance the proliferation of fibroblasts and may impede that of keratinocytes via their specific mediators tryptase and chymase [11–13]. Conversely, fibroblasts and keratinocytes also have effects on mast cell growth via growth factors such as stem cell factor (SCF), nerve growth factor, and granulocyte-macrophage colony-stimulating factor [14–17].

In order to further understand the interplay between MCs and other resident tissue cells, the development of a well-established organotypic co-culture skin model, integrating human dermal mast cells, would be desirable. Several studies used organotypic co-culture skin models, including other mast cells such as bone marrow-derived interleukin-3-independent murine mast cells (C1MC/C571 cell line) [18] and leukemic mast cells (HMC-1 cell line) [19, 20]. Later, the human dermal MCs, which are relatively more difficult to culture, were first integrated into the organotypic co-culture system by our group in 2002 [21] for further study of MC-keratinocyte interactions. However, this work required certain improvements, e.g., the fact that the keratinocytes themselves and also the organotypic co-cultures with mast cells were kept in medium containing serum (FBS) and cholera toxin, which was unfavorable.

Thus, we modified our previous work and could integrate the human dermal mast cells successfully into the serum-free and cholera toxin-free organotypic skin culture.

2 Materials

Prepare all materials for cell isolation and culture under sterile conditions, and store all solutions and media at 4 °C unless indicated otherwise.

2.1 Cell Isolation

1. Fetal calf serum (FCS): Heat inactivated for 30 min at 56 °C to inactivate heat-labile complement proteins.

2. Phosphate-buffered saline without Ca^{2+}/Mg^{2+} (PBS−).

3. Phosphate-buffered saline with Ca^{2+}/Mg^{2+} (PBS+).

4. Dispase solution: Dilute dispase type 1 (BD Bioscience) in PBS+ to a final concentration of 3 U/mL.

5. Dispersion medium: 5 mL of penicillin/streptomycin (penicillin 10,000 IU/streptomycin 10,000 μg/mL), 10 mL of FCS, 1.25 mg of amphotericin B (250 μg/mL), and 2.5 mL of $MgSO_4$ (1 M) in 500 mL of PBS+. Shortly before use, 10–15 mg of collagenase type IV (Worthington Biochem, Freehold, NJ, USA), 5–7.5 mg of Hyaluronidase type 1S (Sigma), and DNase 1 (End concentration in the dispersion medium 10 μg/mL) (Roche Applied Science, Basel, Switzerland) are diluted in 10 mL of the prepared solution.

6. 0.05 % Trypsin/0.01 % EDTA. Store aliquots at –20 °C.

7. Soybean trypsin inhibitor (SBTI): Dissolve 100 mg of SBTI in 100 mL PBS–. Store 10 mL aliquots at –20 °C.

8. Shaking water bath (37 °C).

9. Centrifuge (MinifugeRF, Heraeus, Germany).

10. Automated cell counter (CASY, Schärfe System GmbH, Germany).

11. Incubator (37 °C and 5 % CO_2).

2.2 Purification of Dermal Mast Cells

1. Sieves (mesh size 40, 100, and 300 μm).

2. Pre-separation filter (30 μm; Miltenyi Biotech).

3. MACS buffer: 500 mL of PBS–, 50 mL of FCS, 10 mL of EDTA (100 mM).

4. Sandoglobulin® (30,000 μg/mL; CSL Behring, Germany).

5. Human AB serum (Invitrogen).

6. Anti-human CD117 MicroBead kit (Miltenyi Biotech).

7. AutoMacs Miltenyi Biotech or another suitable MACS separator.

8. Trypan blue.

9. Acidic toluidine blue (0.1 % in 0.5 N HCl).

2.3 Cell Culture

1. Keratinocyte medium: KBM-Gold™ (Lonza) supplemented with KGM-Gold SingleQuots (Lonza).

2. Fibroblast medium: 500 mL of low-glucose Dulbecco's Modified Eagle Medium with L-glutamine (DMEM) (Gibco) supplemented with 5 mL of penicillin/streptomycin and 25 mL of FCS.

3. Stem cell factor (SCF) (50 μg/mL; Peprotech).

4. Interleukin-4 (IL-4) (20 μg/mL; Peprotech).

5. Mast cell medium: 500 mL of Iscove's basal medium supplemented with 5 mL of nonessential amino acids, 5 mL of penicillin/streptomycin, and 50 mL of FCS. Add SCF and IL-4 directly before use (end concentration 100 and 20 ng/mL, respectively).

6. Serum-free freezing medium (Promo Cell, cat. no. C-29910).

7. Dimethylsulfoxide (DMSO), cell culture grade.

8. Cryo 1 °C Freezing Chamber (Nalgene).

2.4 Organotypic Coculture

1. Collagen type I from rat tail (3.6 mg/mL; First Link Ltd, UK).

2. 10× concentrated low-glucose Dulbecco's modified Eagle medium without L-glutamine, NaHCO$_3$, and folic acid.

3. 1 M NaOH.

4. Matrigel™ Matrix (BD Biosciences).

5. Ascorbic acid, dissolved in distilled water at 50 mg/mL.

6. Metal grid (special made): $20 \times 20 \times 5$ mm (width $\times$ length $\times$ height).

7. Nylon mesh: Cut the nylon mesh into approximate squares of 20×20 mm. Wash and disinfect the small nylon mesh squares with 100 % ethanol and dry them in a laminar flow cabinet. Mix 1.1 mL of collagen type 1 and 50 mL of 0.03 N acetic acid and incubate the small nylon mesh squares with this mixture on a small Petri dish (diameter 5 cm) for 30 min at room temperature. Incubate them with approximately 25 mL of 0.1 % glutaraldehyde for a further 30 min at room temperature. Rinse them four times with PBS–. Store them in 70 % ethanol until used (*see* **Note 1**). Dry them in a laminar flow cabinet before use.

8. Organotypic culture medium: KBM-Gold™ supplemented with ascorbic acid (end concentration 50 µg/mL), SCF (end concentration 2.5 ng/mL), $CaCl_2$ (end concentration 1.3 mM), 0.1 % bovine serum albumin (BSA), and KGM-Gold SingleQuots except bovine pituitary extract.

2.5 Preparation of Frozen Sections

1. Liquid nitrogen container (Messer Griesheim).

2. Liquid nitrogen.

3. Cryomold 4557 (Tissue-Tek®, cat. no. 62534-25).

4. Cryotome FSE cryostat (Thermo Scientific).

5. Glass slides (Super Frost).

2.6 Immunohisto-chemistry

1. PAP-Pen (SCI, Germany).

2. Tris buffer (10×): Dissolve 9 g of Tris base, 68.5 g of Tris–HCl, and 87.5 g of NaCl in distilled water to a total volume of 1 L. Dilute 1 volume of the Tris buffer (10×) in 9 volumes of distilled water before use.

3. Peroxidase blocking reagent (Dako).

4. Avidin/Biotin kit (Vector Laboratories).

5. Fc receptor block solution: Mix 25 mL of RPMI 1640, 5 mL of FCS, and 50 µL of Sandoglobulin®. Store 1-mL aliquots at –20 °C until use.

6. Antibody-diluting solution: Dilute 2 mL of RPMI 1640 and 2 mL of FCS in 17.5 mL of distilled water. Store 1-mL aliquots at –20 °C until use.

7. Biotinylated secondary antibodies and streptavidin-HRP (Dako).

8. Dako AEC+ High Sensitivity Substrate Chromogen, Ready-to-Use (Dako).

9. Hematoxylin: Strain through paper filter before every use.

10. Mounting medium.

11. Anti-tryptase mouse monoclonal IgG1, $c = 0.2$ mg/mL (clone AA1).

12. Anti-cytokeratin 10 rabbit monoclonal IgG (clone EP1607IHCY).

13. Anti-transglutaminase 1 mouse monoclonal IgG2a (clone B.C1).

14. Anti-ß4 integrin mouse monoclonal IgG1 (clone ASC-8).

15. 5-bromo-2′-deoxyuridine (BrdU) (Sigma).

16. Anti-BrdU mouse monoclonal IgG1, $c = 1$ mg/mL (clone AB-3).

17. Anti-chymase antibody (Clone CC1).

3   Methods

Breast skin and foreskin, obtained from individuals undergoing breast-reduction surgery and circumcision, respectively, are the source of the tissue material. For the isolation of human dermal mast cells, keratinocytes and fibroblasts, we modified the method originally described by other investigators [22–25]. A skin equivalent (SE) has three parts: (1) acellular layer to avoid escaping cells from dermis equivalent to the culture medium, (2) the dermis equivalent containing fibroblasts and human dermal mast cells, and (3) the epidermal layer consisting of keratinocytes. Subsequently, the SE is airlifted and the level of the culture medium is adjusted leaving the epithelial cells exposed to the air. Half of the culture medium is renewed every 2 days for a further 10-day organotypic culture. Staining is obtained with a labeled streptavidin biotin method.

We utilize the serum-free keratinocyte growth medium (except bovine pituitary extract) which was first applied for the organotypic co-culture by Stark and co-workers [26]. According to our observation, all three cell species could be adapted well under this culture medium condition and we could obtain stable results.

All co-culture procedures should be carried out in a safety workbench and especially procedures with collagen and Matrigel™ Matrix on ice, unless otherwise specified.

3.1   Mast Cell Isolation, Purification, and Culture

1. Remove fat tissue from the skin tissue. Spread the skin tissue on a Petri dish (diameter 14 cm). Prepare the skin tissue by cutting it into an approximate quadrangle of 2×0.5 cm, and then cut these small pieces vertically at intervals of approximately 1–2 mm by leaving a slight connection on a 2-cm edge.

2. Incubate the prepared skin tissue overnight with the dispase solution in a 50-mL centrifuge tube at 4 °C.

3. Remove the epidermal layer thoroughly using tweezers (*see* **Note 2**).

4. Cut the dermis into small pieces with operating scissors as finely as possible, reducing to a soft doughy state (*see* **Notes 3** and **4**).

5. Incubate the dermis in a shaking water bath with the pre-warmed dispersion medium for approximately 60 min at 37 °C (*see* **Notes 5** and **6**).

6. Strain the solution with the leftover dermis and released cells through two sieves (mesh size 300 and 100 μm) (*see* **Note 7**). Centrifuge the filtrate at $250 \times g$ for 10 min at 4 °C to remove the dispersion medium (*see* **Note 8**).

7. Resuspend the cell pellet in PBS– and centrifuge at $250 \times g$ for 10 min at 4 °C.

8. Remove the supernatant, resuspend the cell pellet in MACS buffer, strain the suspension through a sieve (mesh size 40 μm), and centrifuge at $250 \times g$ for 10 min at 4 °C.

9. Remove the supernatant, resuspend the cell pellet in MACS buffer, and determine the cell number.

10. Strain the cell suspension through the pre-separation filter (30 μm) to remove cell clumps.

11. Centrifuge the cell suspension at $250 \times g$ for 10 min at 4 °C and remove the supernatant completely.

12. Resuspend the cell pellet in MACS buffer (350 μL per 10^8 cells), add human AB serum (150 μL per 10^8 cells) and Sandoglobulin® (10 μL per 10^8 cells), mix well, and incubate for 15 min at 4 °C.

13. Add CD117 MicroBeads (25 μL for every 500 μL cell suspension) and incubate for a further 11 min at 4 °C.

14. Wash the cells by adding MACS buffer, centrifuge at $250 \times g$ for 10 min at 4 °C, and remove the supernatant completely.

15. Resuspend the cell pellet at 10^8 cells per 500 μL of MACS buffer (*see* **Note 9**).

16. Place the column (large cell separation column) into the magnetic field of the suitable MACS separator. Choose the MACS column according to the number of the total cells (*see* **Note 10**).

17. Apply the cell suspension onto the column. Collect flow-through containing unlabeled cells (the negative fraction) (*see* **Note 11**).

18. Remove the column from the separator and place it in a collection tube.

19. Pipet the appropriate amount of MACS buffer onto the column and flush out the labeled cells by pushing the plunger into the column.

20. Add 10 mL of the Iscove basal medium to the suspension. Check the viability with trypan blue staining. Determine the number of the MCs with acidic toluidine blue.

21. Centrifuge at $250 \times g$ for 10 min at 4 °C, remove the supernatant, and resuspend the cell pellet in the mast cell medium at

1×10^6/mL. Add 2 μL of SCF and 2 μL of IL-4 for 1 mL of the cell suspension.

22. Place the culture into a humidified incubator with 5 % CO_2 at 37 °C.

23. Add 2 μL of SCF and 2 μL of IL-4 for 1 mL of the cell suspension twice a week.

24. During long-term culture, renew half of the medium once a week (semi-depletion) and add 1 μL of SCF and 1 μL of IL-4 for 1 mL of the cell suspension. Alternatively, add the same amount of SCF and IL-4 twice a week without medium renewal.

3.2 Fibroblast Isolation and Culture

1. Cut the de-epidermalized dermis with a scalpel into approximate squares of 3×3 mm and place in a culture dish (10 cm diameter) (*see* **Note 12**).

2. Leave the dish open under the safety workbench for up to 5 min so that the dermis pieces adhere to the surface of the dish.

3. Add the fibroblast medium by submerging the small dermis pieces in the medium, avoiding release from the dish.

4. Place the dishes in a humidified 37 °C incubator containing 5 % CO_2.

5. Change the medium every 3 days.

6. Trypsinize fibroblasts at confluence (*see* **Note 13**). For trypsinization of the fibroblasts, remove the culture medium and wash the cells with PBS– twice. Add 4 mL of 0.05 % trypsin/0.01 % EDTA and incubate for 3–5 min at 37 °C. Tap the culture flask gently to release the cells. Neutralize the trypsin with the same volume of the fibroblast medium. Determine the total number of fibroblasts and percent viability using trypan blue staining. Centrifuge the cell suspension at $250 \times g$ for 10 min at 4 °C. Remove the supernatant.

7. Seed 1×10^6 cells into a 175-cm² cell culture flask and add 20 mL of the fibroblast medium. Renew the medium every 3 days. Split or cryo-preserve the cells at confluence. For cryopreservation of the fibroblasts, resuspend the trypsinized fibroblasts in the precooled FCS-DMSO mixture (volume ratio of FCS:DMSO is 9:1) at 1×10^6/mL. Dispense 1 mL of the cell suspension into a cryogenic storage vial. Place the vial into a cryo 1 °C freezing chamber and store it at −80 °C overnight. Transfer the vial into liquid nitrogen or a cryogenic freezer.

3.3 Keratinocyte Isolation and Culture

1. Rinse the 10–15 small pieces of freed epidermis for a short time in PBS– (*see* **Note 14**).

2. Incubate them with 5 mL of 0.05 % trypsin/0.01 % EDTA for 15 min at room temperature.

3. Add the same volume of SBTI solution and mix gently for a short time.

4. Remove the epidermal layers by straining once through a sieve (mesh size 100 μm).

5. Determine the total number of keratinocytes and percent viability using trypan blue staining.

6. Centrifuge at $250 \times g$ for 10 min at 4 °C.

7. Remove the supernatant. Add PBS– and wash the cells slightly. Centrifuge once more at $250 \times g$ for 10 min at 4 °C.

8. Remove the supernatant and suspend 1×10^6 keratinocytes in 20 mL of the keratinocyte medium.

9. Place the cell suspension into a collagen-coated 175-cm^2 cell culture flask at 37 °C with 5 % CO_2 (*see* **Note 15**).

10. Renew the medium every 3 days. Split or cryo-preserve the cells at about 70–80 % confluence.

11. Trypsinization of the keratinocytes: Remove the culture medium and wash the cells with PBS– once. Add 4 mL of 0.05 % trypsin/0.01 % EDTA and incubate for 3–5 min at 37 °C. Tap the culture flask gently to release the cells. Neutralize the trypsin with the same volume of the SBTI solution. Determine the total number of fibroblasts and percent viability using trypan blue. Centrifuge the cell suspension at $250 \times g$ for 10 min at 4 °C. Remove supernatant.

12. Cryopreservation of the keratinocytes: Suspend the trypsinized keratinocytes in the serum-free freezing medium at 10×10^6/mL. Dispense 1 mL of the cell suspension into a cryogenic storage vial. Place the vial into a cryo 1 °C freezing chamber and store it at –80 °C overnight. Transfer the vial into liquid nitrogen or a cryogenic freezer.

3.4 Skin Equivalent (SE)

1. Prepare a suspension of fibroblasts and MCs together in pre-cooled FCS at 2.5×10^6/mL each.

2. Mix 10 volumes of collagen type I and 1 volume of 10× DMEM. Adjust the pH of the mixture to 7.0 by dropwise addition of 1 M NaOH prior to mixing with 1 volume of Matrigel™ Matrix. Leave the collagen-Matrigel mixture on ice for 20 min (*see* **Note 16**).

3. Coat the surface of a 24-well tissue culture plate with 200 μL of the previously prepared collagen-Matrigel mixture evenly and solidify at 37 °C for 10 min (*see* **Notes 17** and **18**).

4. Mix 100 μL of the fibroblast-MC suspension and 600 μL of the collagen-Matrigel mixture in a 2-mL Eppendorf tube. Pipet the mixture onto the 24-well tissue culture plate above the acellular collagen-Matrigel layer (*see* **Note 17**).

5. Solidify the mixture at 37 °C for 30 min. Then, add 1 mL of the keratinocyte medium with ascorbic acid (end concentration 50 μg/mL) and SCF (end concentration 12.5 ng/mL) and incubate at 37 °C for a further 30 min (*see* **Note 19**).

6. Prepare suspension of keratinocytes in a pre-warmed (37 °C) keratinocyte medium with ascorbic acid (end concentration 50 μg/mL) and SCF (end concentration 12.5 ng/mL) at 5.0×10^5 (*see* **Note 20**). Remove thoroughly the medium in the 24-well tissue culture plate and add carefully 1 mL of the prepared keratinocyte suspension. Incubate at 37 °C for 24 h.

3.5 Air-Lifting

1. Release the skin equivalent (SE) from the tissue culture plate and incubate at 37 °C until it contracts, shrinking by two-thirds of its diameter (*see* **Notes 21** and **22**).

2. Air-lift the contracted SE by placing it into the 6-well tissue culture plate on the metal grid covered by a previously prepared nylon mesh (*see* **Note 23**).

3. Add 5 mL of the organotypic culture medium, just to the level of the nylon mesh, leaving the epithelial cells exposed to the air (*see* **Note 24**).

4. Renew only half of the medium, by removing 2.5 mL and adding 2.5 mL of the organotypic culture medium every 2 days for a further 10-day organotypic culture (*see* **Notes 25** and **26**).

3.6 Preparation of Frozen Sections

1. Place the sample together with the nylon mesh on a glass object.

2. Wipe off excess medium around the sections using a paper towel, but do not touch the sample.

3. Cut away the uncovered part of the nylon mesh using a scalpel and tweezers.

4. Embed the sample in a tissue-freezing medium using Cryomold and freeze it with liquid nitrogen rapidly by touching only the bottom of the Cryomold for approximately 1 min (*see* **Notes 27–30**).

5. Cut frozen sections at 4–6 μm. Dry the sections at room temperature overnight; fix the section with ethanol or methanol if necessary. Store them at −80 °C until needed.

3.7 Immunohisto-chemistry

1. Draw a circle around the sections using a PAP pen to create a hydrophobic barrier (*see* **Note 31**).

2. Immerse sections in Tris buffer for 10 min. Do not allow the sections to become dry for the remaining procedure.

3. Block the endogenous peroxidase activity using peroxidase-blocking reagent for 10 min and wash in Tris buffer for 2×5 min (*see* **Note 32**).

4. Block endogenous biotin incubating the section with 0.001 % avidin D (w/v) in PBS for 10 min and wash in Tris buffer for 2×5 min.

5. Block the remaining biotin-binding sites on the avidin incubating the section with 0.001 % biotin (w/v) in PBS for 10 min and wash in Tris buffer for 2×5 min.

6. Block endogenous Fc receptor with the previously prepared Fc receptor block solution for 15 min.

7. Incubate the sections for 60 min at room temperature or overnight at 4 °C with diluted primary antibodies following the instruction of providers. Wash in Tris buffer for 2 × 5 min (*see* **Note 33**).

8. Incubate the sections for 10 min with biotinylated secondary antibodies and wash in Tris buffer for 2 × 5 min.

9. Incubate the sections for 10 min with streptavidin-HRP and wash in Tris buffer for 2 × 5 min.

10. Incubate the sections for 15 min with AEC substrate and wash in Tris buffer for 2 × 5 min.

11. Counterstain for 2 min with hematoxylin.

12. Wash under running tap water for 10 min and rinse with distilled water.

13. Add 1–2 drops of the mounting medium and place a cover glass over the section (*see* **Note 34**).

4   Notes

1. It is recommended to store the nylon mesh in ethanol at least for 1 day to prevent fungal contamination.

2. Because of the CD117-positive melanocytes, the epidermis should be completely removed. The dissected epidermis is used for the isolation of keratinocytes.

3. Even for experienced individuals, this procedure should take at least 30 min for 15 g skin tissue.

4. Put a small part of dermis aside for the subsequent isolation of fibroblasts.

5. The amount of the dispersion medium depends on the weight of the skin tissue, approximately 10 mL per gram of the skin tissue.

6. A 500-mL sterile PBS– bottle is suited for the incubation in a shaking water bath. Parafilm is also used to further seal the bottle to prevent contamination. The bottle is fixed on the bottom of the bath. The shaking frequency should be as high as possible, but without spilling the water.

7. In instances where substantial portions of the dermis remain, the dermis can be cut into small pieces again and the incubation with the used dispersion medium can be repeated.

8. We recommend using a 50 mL centrifuge tube until the blocking and magnetic labeling step and thereafter a 15 mL tube. Carry out the cell wash step by filling tubes to maximal volumes with PBS and MACS buffer, respectively.

9. Add 500 µL of MACS buffer, in case the number of cells is less than 10^8.

10. Our laboratory uses an autoMACS (Miltenyi, Germany) and we chose an autoMACS software program Possel-DS.

11. Fibroblasts can also be obtained from the negative fraction. Depending on the source of the skin, however, other dermal cell types can be included; wash the cells twice with PBS– and suspend the cells in the fibroblast medium. Place the suspension into a 175-cm^2 cell culture flask at 36 °C with 5 % CO_2. Renew the culture medium and continue to cultivate adherent fibroblasts.

12. The source of the tissue material is de-epithelialized dermis from the previous step (*see* Subheading 3.1).

13. Fibroblasts will migrate from the dermal tissue to the surface of the culture dishes.

14. The source of the tissue material is the dissociated epidermis from the previous step (*see* Subheading 3.1). A small piece means an approximate shape of 1×5 mm. If the skin tissue is cut as described above, small epidermal pieces can be harvested by removing the epidermal layer from the skin tissue.

15. Mix 140 µL of collagen type 1 and 10 mL of 0.03 N acetic acid. Coat the surface of a cell culture flask with the collagen solution evenly and leave it at room temperature for 30 min. Wash with PBS– for 3×5 min.

16. Because of the contraction of the mixture, it is necessary to keep the stated time. Considering the contraction and the loss, 1 volume should be between 70 and 80 µL for one sample.

17. Try to pipet directly onto the bottom of the wells, not onto the wall. The collagen-Matrigel mixture is very sticky and easily solidifies at room temperature.

18. It is important not to allow the formation of air bubbles. So pipet only in one stroke and do not touch it again.

19. Ascorbic acid in the phase seems to improve the viability of MCs.

20. Only keratinocytes of the second passage are used for the organotypic co-culture.

21. The SE is separated from the 24-well culture plate physically, starting with a 10 µL Eppendorf pipette tip at the side wall of the well and making a gentle stroke along the side wall. It can be repeated if the gel is not released completely.

22. Duration depends on the collagen density and the number of cells that DE contains. In the given condition, it takes approximately 3 h. The contraction is essential for the subsequent development of the epidermal structure.

23. For the air-lifting of the contracted SE, a special-made thin stainless iron plate of 0.5×7.0 cm with a right-angle bend at 0.8-cm point from one end is used. The SE is spooned up using the bent part and put on the metal grid covered by a prepared nylon mesh.

24. The epidermal layer should be kept free from the medium to the end of the organotypic culture. Otherwise, the epidermal layer will not be developed well.

25. Mix the medium using a 1-mL pipette before removing the medium (4–5 strokes).

26. Add BrdU at a final concentration of 50 µM by the last medium renewal.

27. The paraffin section includes some problems with the organotypic culture because of its fragility, e.g., a structure deformation by the fixation and the separation of the epidermal layer from the DE during the treatment.

28. The sample should be completely surrounded with the tissue-freezing medium, without air bubbles lying in the middle of the medium level.

29. Fill a small Dewar flask with liquid nitrogen. Freeze the sample with liquid nitrogen as rapidly as possible by touching only the bottom of the Cryomold for approximately 1 min—an edge of the Cryomold is fixed with a 30-cm wire for easy handling. Do not allow the freezing medium to touch the liquid nitrogen because of the formation of bubbles.

30. Other freezing techniques, e.g., placing in a cryostat microtome, lead to a structure deformation. Also, the rapid freezing with liquid nitrogen makes the tissue-freezing medium more solid, which is crucial for easy cutting work.

31. The circle should be as small as possible to save on the reagents. However, do not touch the sections. Add two drops (approximately 100 µL) of reagents at each step.

32. Shake slides vigorously twice to remove excess water or reagents.

33. Antibodies are diluted in the previously prepared antibody-diluting solution. The following primary antibodies, dilutions, and incubation periods are used (*see* Figs. 1, 2, 3, 4, 5, and 6): anti-cytokeratin 10, 1:500, overnight at 4 °C; anti-transglutaminase, 1:100, for 60 min at room temperature; anti-ß4 integrin, 1:200, for 60 min at room temperature; anti-tryptase, 1:1,000, for 60 min at room temperature; anti-chymase, 1:500, overnight at 4 °C; and anti-BrdU, 1:100, for 60 min at room temperature.

34. Shake slides vigorously many times to remove excess water and leave the slide for some minutes to dry up the water on the slide. This allows long-term preservation of the section.

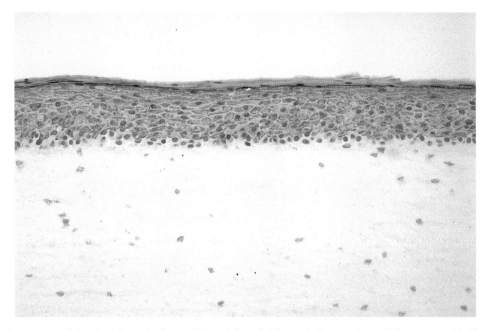

Fig. 1 Immunostaining in skin equivalents: AEC staining of skin equivalents using rabbit or mouse Ab directed against human cytokeratin 10. Skin equivalent samples were embedded in a tissue-freezing medium and frozen with liquid nitrogen. Cryostat sections of samples were air-dried on glass slides for 1 h and fixed in methanol at −20 °C for 2 min

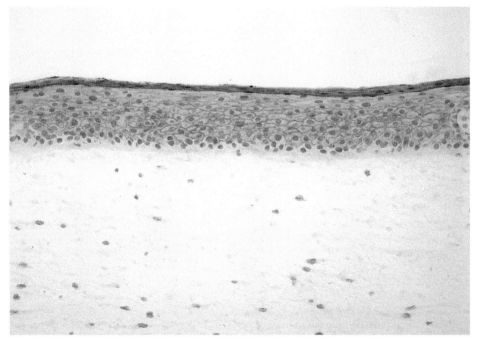

Fig. 2 Immunostaining in skin equivalents: AEC staining of skin equivalents using rabbit or mouse Ab directed against human transglutaminase. Skin equivalent samples were embedded in a tissue-freezing medium and frozen with liquid nitrogen. Cryostat sections of samples were air-dried on glass slides for 1 h and fixed in methanol at −20 °C for 2 min

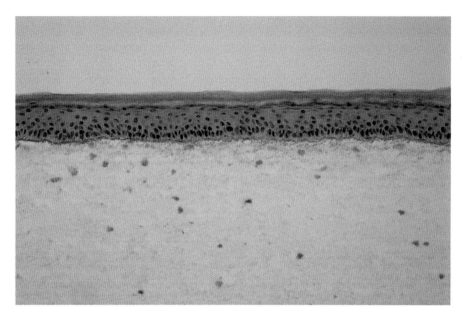

Fig. 3 Immunostaining in skin equivalents: AEC staining of skin equivalents using rabbit or mouse Ab directed against human ß4 integrin. Skin equivalent samples were embedded in a tissue-freezing medium and frozen with liquid nitrogen. Cryostat sections of samples were air-dried on glass slides for 1 h and fixed in methanol at −20 °C for 2 min

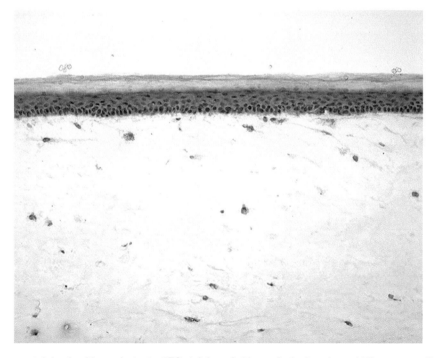

Fig. 4 Immunostaining in skin equivalents: AEC staining of skin equivalents using rabbit or mouse Ab directed against human tryptase. Skin equivalent samples were embedded in a tissue-freezing medium and frozen with liquid nitrogen. Cryostat sections of samples were air-dried on glass slides for 1 h and fixed in methanol at −20 °C for 2 min

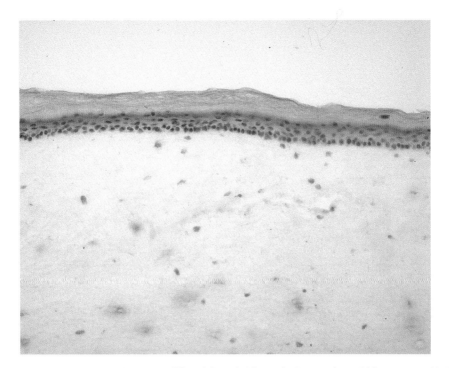

Fig. 5 Immunostaining in skin equivalents: AEC staining of skin equivalents using rabbit or mouse Ab directed against human chymase. Skin equivalent samples were embedded in a tissue-freezing medium and frozen with liquid nitrogen. Cryostat sections of samples were air-dried on glass slides for 1 h and fixed in methanol at −20 °C for 2 min

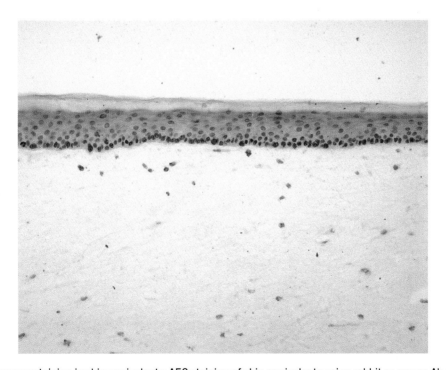

Fig. 6 Immunostaining in skin equivalents: AEC staining of skin equivalents using rabbit or mouse Ab directed against human BrdU. Skin equivalent samples were embedded in a tissue-freezing medium and frozen with liquid nitrogen. Cryostat sections of samples were air-dried on glass slides for 1 h and fixed in methanol at −20 °C for 2 min

References

1. Bell E, Ehrlich HP, Buttle DJ, Nakatsuji T (1981) Living tissue formed in vitro and accepted as skin-equivalent tissue of full thickness. Science 211:1052–1054

2. Parenteau NL, Nolte CM, Bilbo P, Rosenberg M, Wilkins LM, Johnson EW, Watson S, Mason VS, Bell E (1991) Epidermis generated in vitro: practical considerations and applications. J Cell Biochem 45:245–251

3. Fusenig NE (1994) Epithelial-mesenchymal interactions regulate keratinocyte growth and differentiation in vitro. In: Leigh IM, Lane EB, Watt FM (eds) The keratinocytes handbook. Cambridge University Press, Cambridge, pp 71–94

4. Asselineau D, Bernard BA, Bailly D, Darmon M (1989) Retinoic acid improves epidermal morphogenesis. Dev Biol 133:322–335

5. Lenoir MC, Bernard BA (1990) Architecture of reconstructed epidermis on collagen lattices varies according to the method used: a comparative study. Skin Pharmacol 3:97–106

6. Parenteau NL, Bilbo P, Nolte CJ, Mason VS, Rosenberg M (1992) The organotypical culture of human skin keratinocytes and fibroblasts to achieve form and function. Cytotechnology 9:163–171

7. Igarashi M, Irwin CR, Locke M, Mackenzie IC (2003) Construction of large area organotypical cultures of oral mucosa and skin. J Oral Pathol Med 32:422–430

8. Maas-Szabowski N, Stark HJ, Fusenig NE (2000) Keratinocyte growth regulation in defined organotypic cultures through IL-1-induced keratinocyte growth factor expression in resting fibroblasts. J Invest Dermatol 114: 1075–1084

9. Smola H, Stark HJ, Thiekotter G, Mirancea N, Krieg T, Fusenig NE (1998) Dynamics of basement membrane formation by keratinocyte–fibroblast interactions in organotypic skin culture. Exp Cell Res 239:399–410

10. Marionnet C, Pierrard C, Vioux-Chagnoleau C, Sok J, Asselineau D, Bernerd F (2006) Interactions between fibroblasts and keratinocytes in morphogenesis of dermal epidermal junction in a model of reconstructed skin. J Invest Dermatol 126:971–979

11. Ruoss SJ, Hartmann T, Caughey GH (1991) Mast cell tryptase is a mitogen for cultured fibroblasts. J Clin Invest 88:493–499

12. Nadel JA (1991) Biology of mast cell tryptase and chymase. Ann N Y Acad Sci 629:319–331

13. Algermissen B, Hermes B, Feldmann-Böddeker I, Bauer F, Henz BM (1999) Mast cell chymase and tryptase during tissue turnover—analysis on in vitro mitogenesis of fibroblasts and keratinocytes and alterations in cutaneous scars. Exp Dermatol 8:193–198

14. Grabbe J, Welker P, Dippel E, Czarnetzki BM (1994) Stem cell factor, a novel cutaneous growth factor for mast cells and melanocytes. Arch Dermatol Res 287:78–84

15. Metcalfe DD, Baram D, Mekori YA (1997) Mast cells. Physiol Rev 77:1033–1079

16. Artuc M, Hermes B, Steckelings MU, Grüzkau A, Henz BM (1999) Mast cells and their mediators in wound healing—active participants or innocent bystanders? Exp Dermatol 8:1–16

17. Henz BM, Maurer M, Lippert U, Worm M, Babina M (2001) Mast cells as initiators of immunity and host defense. Exp Dermatol 10:1–10

18. Meng H, Marchese MJ, Garlick JA, Jelaska A, Korn JH, Gailit J, Clark RA, Gruber BL (1995) Mast cells induce T-cell adhesion to human fibroblasts by regulating intercellular adhesion molecule-1 and vascular cell adhesion molecule-1 expression. J Invest Dermatol 105:789–796

19. Gruber BL, Kew RR, Jelaska A, Marchese MJ, Garlick J, Ren S, Schwartz LB, Korn JH (1997) Human mast cells activate fibroblasts. Tryptase is a fibrogenic factor stimulating collagen messenger ribonucleic acid synthesis and fibroblast chemotaxis. J Immunol 158:2310–2317

20. Gailit J, Marchese MJ, Kew RR, Gruber BL (2001) The differentiation and function of myofibroblasts is regulated by mast cell mediators. J Invest Dermatol 117:1113–1119

21. Artuc M, Steckelings UM, Grützkau A, Smorodchenko A, Henz BM (2002) A long-term coculture model for the study of mast cell-keratinocyte interactions. J Invest Dermatol 119:411–415

22. Lawrence ID, Warner JA, Cohan VL, Hubbard WC, Kagey-Sobotka A, Lichtenstein LM (1987) Purification and characterization of human skin mast cells. Evidence for human mast cell heterogeneity. J Immunol 139: 3062–3069

23. Grützkau A, Henz BM, Kirchhof L, Luger T, Artuc M (2000) alpha-Melanocyte stimulating hormone acts as a selective inducer of secretory functions in human mast cells. Biochem Biophys Res Commun 278:14–19

24. Guhl S, Artuc M, Neou A, Babina M, Zuberbier T (2011) Long-term cultured human skin mast cells are suitable for pharmacological studies of anti-allergic drugs due to high responsiveness to FcεRI cross-linking. Biosci Biotechnol Biochem 75:382–384

25. Normand J, Karasek MA (1995) A method for the isolation and serial propagation of keratinocytes, endothelial cells, and fibroblasts from a single punch biopsy of human skin. In Vitro Cell Dev Biol Anim 31:447–455

26. Stark HJ, Baur M, Breitkreutz D, Mirancea N, Fusenig NE (1999) Organotypic keratinocyte cocultures in defined medium with regular epidermal morphogenesis and differentiation. J Invest Dermatol 112:681–691

Chapter 7

The Absolute Basophil Count

Elena Borzova and Clemens A. Dahinden

Abstract

The absolute basophil count (cells/L) can be determined by manual counting of peripheral blood smears or using cell-counting chambers as well as by automated hematology analyzers and fluorescence flow cytometry. Manual basophil counting of peripheral blood smears is currently regarded as the reference method, although the limitations of this method (distribution, observer, and statistical errors) are widely recognized. Automated hematology analyzers offer an advantage of larger numbers of counted cells and high throughput but are characterized by inconsistent analytical performance for basophil enumeration. Flow cytometric enumeration of circulating basophils using panels of monoclonal antibodies is being developed as novel candidate reference method for the absolute basophil count in peripheral blood. Basophil counting using fluorescence flow cytometry is characterized by high precision and statistical superiority. Emerging innovative technologies for absolute cell counts include ImageStream technology and on-chip blood counting but their analytical performance for absolute basophil counts is yet to be established. Here, we describe various techniques for absolute basophil counting in peripheral blood including manual basophil counts in smears and hemocytometers and flow-cytometric methodologies using double-platform, bead-based, and volumetric approaches.

Key words Basophils, Absolute basophil count, Metachromatic staining, Basopenia, Basophilia, Hemocytometer, Flow cytometry, Peripheral blood smear, Leukocyte differential

1 Introduction

The absolute basophil count is defined as the number of basophils per liter of peripheral blood. Traditionally, basophil counts were presented as a percentage of white blood cells in the manual leukocyte differential. Nowadays, the absolute cell count is recommended for clinical information [1]. In research settings, absolute basophil counts can be used to determine basophil concentrations in samples used for experiments.

The basophil is a granulocyte that occurs at one of the lowest frequencies in the peripheral blood (0.5–1 % of circulating leukocytes) [2, 3]. Therefore, precise determination of the normal range and the reference intervals for circulating basophils can be challenging. Basophil numbers were reported in the range of

Bernhard F. Gibbs and Franco H. Falcone (eds.), *Basophils and Mast Cells: Methods and Protocols*, Methods in Molecular Biology, vol. 1192, DOI 10.1007/978-1-4939-1173-8_7, © Springer Science+Business Media New York 2014

20–80 cells/µL $(0.02–0.08 \times 10^9$ cells/L) using microscopic examination of peripheral blood smears and cell-counting chamber techniques [2]. Traditionally, basophil counts greater than 50 cells/µL of peripheral blood $(0.05 \times 10^9$ cells/L) were considered as basophilia, whereas basophil counts of less than 20 cells/µL $(0.02 \times 10^9$ cells/L) were regarded as basopenia [4, 5].

Current guidelines (Clinical and Laboratory Standards Institute, CLSI) [6] recommend the statistical approach for defining the reference intervals as the central 95 % distribution between lower and upper reference limits (2.5 % above and below the interval) for all tests including the absolute basophil count. Published data regarding the reference intervals for absolute basophil counts is limited. A recent study of flow cytometric enumeration of basophils reported the reference interval for absolute basophil counts of $0.014–0.087 \times 10^9$/L [7]. A cutoff of more than 290 basophils/µL of peripheral blood $(0.29 \times 10^9$ cells/L) was reported for screening for basophilia [8]. More studies are needed to establish and validate the reference intervals for peripheral blood basophils for clinical use.

Manual basophil counting using peripheral blood smears is still considered as the reference method [9]. However, the limitations of this method for cells at a frequency lower than 5 %, such as basophils, are well recognized by the current guidelines [9]. In practice, a 100- or 200-cell manual differential count is used for basophil enumeration, although a 200-cell differential count by two observers on two slides from the same blood sample is recommended for reference studies by the H20-A2 guidelines from CLSI [9]. Basophil counting using manual microscopy of peripheral blood slides is characterized by insufficient precision due to slide distributional and observer errors as well as poor statistical reliability [1, 9–11]. Optimization measures such as improving the quality of metachromatic Romanowsky dyes and the introduction of blood dispensers, automated slide makers, and automated digital microscopy for differential counting have reduced distributional and observer errors. Nevertheless, inherent statistical sampling error of manual basophil counting of peripheral blood smears prompted a strong need for an improved reference method [9, 10].

Cell-counting chambers (hemocytometers) are still widely used in laboratories. Several cell-counting chambers are currently available in research practice including the improved Neubauer modified, Fuchs-Rosenthal, Thoma chambers, etc. The protocol using Kimura stain allows basophil enumeration in peripheral blood using cell-counting chambers [12]. Recent technological advances include automated cell counting for chamber slides although this technology is yet to be applied for basophil enumeration. In general, the use of cell-counting chambers for manual basophil counts is limited by the statistical sampling error at low number of counted cells [13].

Automated basophil counts can be performed by automated hematology analyzers based on optical light scattering or electrical impedance-based technology [14]. Automated basophil counting offers the advantages of better statistical reliability due to counting a larger number of cells and higher throughput than manual microscopy. For hematology analyzers using differential cell lysis for basophil detection, the phenomenon of spurious pseudobasophilia can occur due to misclassification of plasma cells or abnormal lysis-resistant cells in some diseases including multiple myeloma and chronic leukemia [15]. In our experience, analytical performance of automated hematology analyzers for enumerating basophils appeared to be suboptimal and inconsistent in comparison with fluorescence flow cytometry [7] which is in keeping with findings of other research groups [11, 16].

Flow cytometry-based enumeration of peripheral blood basophils links multicolor immunophenotyping and absolute cell-counting technologies [17]. Several gating strategies are being evaluated for flow cytometric basophil counting [7, 11]. For example, basophil identification can be employed as a part of the monoclonal antibody panels for the five- or eight-part leukocyte differential [18, 19] or can be based on the use of basophil-specific markers for enumeration of basophil granulocytes only [7].

In flow cytometry, human basophils can be identified based on the following phenotypic characteristics: they are in the upper part of the lymphocyte scatter gate (towards the monocytes) and are CD45 medium (positive, but clearly lower than other cells in the lymphocyte gate), lin negative (CD2, CD3, CD14, CD16, CD19, CD20, CD56—however, a small fraction can be weakly positive for CD16), HLA-DR negative (only a small fraction is weakly positive), CCR3 positive, CRTH2 positive, CD123 positive (at high levels), FcεRI/IgE positive (depending on the serum IgE-level), and CD203c variable (depending on the activation state).

The markers best suited for basophil enumeration are discussed below:

CCR3: The only other cell type strongly positive for CCR3 is eosinophils which have very distinct light scatter characteristics. Although T cells can be CCR3+ in tissues, CCR3-positive T cells are extremely rare in blood even under pathological conditions. Thus, CCR3 is the only marker that can be used to robustly identify basophils by a single-color stain.

CRTH2: In addition to basophils and eosinophils, Th2-type T cells are CRTH2 positive. Thus, for the identification of basophils a CD3 stain must be included to gate out Th2 cells. Thus, the combination of T-cell markers with CRTH2 is very useful if the numbers of basophils, eosinophils, and T-cell subsets are of interest.

CD123: The only other cell type expressing IL-3 receptors at such high levels as basophils is plasmacytoid dendritic cells which are strongly positive for HLA-DR. Thus, CD123 in combination with a stain for HLA-DR is a good marker for human basophils.

FcεRI/IgE: Although used in some studies, staining of IgE or IgE receptors does not allow the unequivocal identification of basophils in individuals with low serum IgE concentrations or in patients under therapy with Xolair.

CD203c: CD203c is expressed on basophils and circulating mast cell progenitors in the peripheral blood. Basophil identification based on CD203c can be difficult because its expression varies from nearly negative to clearly positive depending on the activation state of these cells. However, the combination of CD203c with another basophil marker such as CCR3 can be useful to study in vivo basophil activation, since CD203c surface expression is enhanced by a variety of IgE-dependent and -independent stimuli.

Methods for basophil quantification by flow cytometry include single- or double-platform methodologies [17]. "Double-platform" methods allow basophil enumeration based on multiplying the percentage of basophils among leukocytes, as detected by flow cytometry, and absolute white blood cell count performed by an automated hematology analyzer [7, 20]. Absolute cell counting using microbead technology or volumetric assessment is referred to as "single-platform" method. The performance of single-platform counting techniques is characterized by lesser variation than that of a double-platform counting method [17, 20].

Flow cytometry-based absolute basophil counting offers advantages of greater precision, analysis of large number of cells, high throughput, and high specificity and, therefore, holds a promise of becoming a new candidate reference method instead of manual counting in peripheral blood smears [18]. At present, flow cytometric methods are being increasingly used for comparisons between methods for enumeration of circulating basophils [7, 11] although poor correlations were noted between absolute basophil counts derived by flow cytometry and manual microscopy [18, 19, 21]. Furthermore, disease-related changes in basophil immunophenotype (e.g., HLA-DR up-regulation) [22] may interfere with the performance of this method. More recently, imaging flow cytometry (ImageStream® technology) has emerged as an innovative approach for cell classification and identification [23] but its performance for basophil enumeration is yet to be established. Novel HematoFlow methodology (Beckman Coulter) combines the capabilities of automated hematology analyzer, flow cytometry, and Cytodiff™ staining panel for extended leukocyte differential and cellular analysis [24]. This enables the prospect of basophil counting based on combined morphological and flow cytometric parameters in the future. Future perspectives for absolute basophil counting could be linked to the development of microfluidic lab-on-a-chip technology for the complete blood cell count [25].

From a clinical perspective, abnormal basophil counts were reported in various clinical conditions including allergic diseases, chronic urticaria, and endocrine and myeloproliferative disorders [2, 4, 26]. Therefore, there is a potential for integrating absolute basophil counts in clinical decision making for screening, diagnosis, and monitoring of these diseases in the future. In clinical practice, understanding the strengths and the limitations of counting methods for peripheral blood basophils can be important for accurate interpretation of the blood test results and for an informed choice of analytical procedures for absolute basophil count. Better morphological and immunophenotypical definition of peripheral blood basophils would enhance the clinical value of basophils as biomarkers in routine clinical practice. Further advances in the knowledge of basophil biology in health and disease will contribute to the development and validation of basophil-related biomarkers for clinical use.

2 Materials

2.1 Manual Basophil Counting

2.1.1 Hemocytometer Method

1. Optical microscope with 40× objective.

2. Hemocytometer: Improved Neubauer counting chamber or modified Fuchs-Rosenthal counting chamber.

3. Thick glass cover slip.

4. 1.5 mL microcentrifuge tubes.

5. Micropipette calibrated with a maximum capacity of 200 μL.

6. Whatman Grade 41 filter paper—110 mm diameter.

7. Kimura stain [12, 27]:

   (a) Prepare a stock toluidine blue solution by dissolving 0.05 g of toluidine blue (Fluka), in 50 mL of 1.8 % NaCl solution and 11 mL 96 % ethanol. Dilute with distilled water to a final volume of 100 mL.

   (b) Prepare a stock solution (0.03 %) of light green yellowish SF (Fluka) in distilled water.

   (c) Prepare a saturated solution of saponin in 50 % ethanol with continuous stirring until orange coloration of the solution emerges [27].

   (d) 67 mM sodium phosphate buffer, pH 6.4.

   (e) Prepare Kimura stain by mixing 11 mL of 0.05 % toluidine blue solution, 0.8 mL of 0.03 % light green solution, 0.5 mL of saturated saponin solution, and 5 mL of 67 mM phosphate buffer (pH 6.4). Prepare Kimura stain freshly each week. Store at room temperature protected from the light by aluminum foil.

2.1.2 Peripheral Blood Smears

1. Absolute methanol.

2. May-Grünwald-Giemsa stain:

   (a) Prepare staining solution I: 0.3 g May-Grünwald powder in 100 mL absolute methanol and filter before use [10]. The stain should be stored in a closed container at room temperature for 24 h (do not freeze Romanowsky dyes [10]). Handle the stain with care and avoid skin contact in view of potential carcinogenicity [10].

   (b) Prepare staining solution II (Giemsa stain): Dissolve 1 g Giemsa stain powder in 66 mL glycerol and heat to 56 °C for 90–120 min. Add 66 mL of absolute methanol, mix thoroughly, and filter before use [10]. The stain should be stored in a closed container at room temperature [10]. Prepare fresh twice a day if needed.

   (c) Sörensen's buffer at pH 6.8 (see below).

3. Wright's stain [10]:

   (a) Dissolve 0.3 g of Wright's stain powder in 100 mL of methanol and filter before use. The stain should be stored tightly sealed in a closed container at a room temperature for 24 h (*see* **Note 1**). Do not freeze. Handle Wright's stain with care and avoid skin contact because of potential carcinogenicity.

   (b) Sörensen's buffer solution at pH 6.4: Dissolve 6.63 g anhydrous KH_2PO_4 and 2.56 g anhydrous Na_2HPO_4 in 1 L distilled water.

4. Frosted glass microscope slides (75×25 mm).

5. Manual staining rack or glass Coplin staining jars.

6. Light microscope with 10× and 40× objectives.

2.2 Automated Basophil Counting Using Flow Cytometry

1. Vacutainer with K_2EDTA or sodium citrate (*see* **Note 2**).

2. Directly conjugated monoclonal antibodies:

   (a) Monoclonal antibody panel 1:
   5 μL CD123-PE (BD Biosciences).
   10 μL HLA-DR-FITC (BD Biosciences).

   (b) Monoclonal antibody panel 2:
   10 μL anti-CCR3-PE (R&D).

3. Lysing Solution (BD Biosciences).

4. CellWash® (BD Biosciences).

5. CellFix® (BD Biosciences).

6. 5 mL FACS polypropylene tubes.

7. Cell-counting microbeads (for example, BD TRUCount Beads (BD Biosciences), CountBright™ Absolute Counting Beads (Invitrogen), or Cytocount™(Dako)).

8. High-performance flow cytometer (optimal for multicolor immunophenotyping).

9. Automated hematology analyzer.

3   Methods

3.1   Manual Absolute Basophil Counts in Whole Blood Stained with Kimura Stain Using Cell-Counting Chambers

1. Mix freshly drawn anticoagulated venous blood with Kimura stain in a proportion 1:10 by gentle pipetting [12]. Avoid vortexing (*see* **Note 3**).

2. Adjust a thick cover slip to the counting chamber until Newton's rings (concentric alternating dark and light ring pattern) appear.

3. Load each chamber of an improved Neubauer hemocytometer with 10 μL of diluted blood by a capillary tube or a micropipette.

4. Leave the loaded counting chamber on a bench for 1–2 min before cell counting.

5. Examine the counting chamber under the microscope. Focus the microscope on the grid of the counting chamber at low power magnification. Perform basophil count in 4–5 large squares of the counting chamber under 40× high dry objective and the blue (daylight) filter. Count cells touching upper and left borders of the counting chamber but not cells touching lower and right borders.

   To obtain basophil counts per mL using the improved Neubauer chamber, multiply average cell count per square by the dilution factor and 10^4.

3.2   Manual Absolute Basophil-Counting Procedure Using a Peripheral Blood Smear

3.2.1   Prepare a Peripheral Blood Smear

1. Mix anticoagulated blood in the tube before preparing a smear. Prepare a peripheral blood smear as quickly as possible after blood collection (preferably within 2 h) [28].

2. Use a glass capillary pipette or a blood dispenser for vacutainers to place a 2–3 mm drop of blood on a glass microscope slide approximately 1 cm from the frosted end.

3. Use another glass microscope slide as a spreader slide. Position the spreader slide at an angle of 45° in front of the drop of blood. Pull the spreader slide back towards the drop of blood at an angle of 45°. Allow the blood to spread along the edge of the spreader slide by capillary action.

4. Push the spreader slide forward at an angle around 30° with a swift smooth motion to prepare the smear (*see* **Note 4**).

5. Allow the smear to air-dry at room temperature for about 10 min. Fix the air-dried smear by flooding with absolute methanol for 2 min. Remove methanol by tilting the slide. Warning: Methanol is highly toxic even in small amounts.

6. Ensure that peripheral blood smear occupies ½–¾ of the slide length [28], is wedge shaped, and has a smooth rounded feathered end. The blood smear should not touch any slide edges and should have a sufficient area for morphological evaluation [10] where red blood cells close to each other but do not touch or overlap [29].

3.2.2 Staining a Peripheral Blood Smear with May-Grünwald-Giemsa Stain

1. Immerse the slide in May-Grünwald staining solution I (diluted with an equal volume of Sörensen's buffer, pH = 6.8) for 5 min in a Coplin jar or a staining rack.

2. Transfer the slide from a jar with May-Grünwald staining solution I to a jar with staining solution II (Giemsa stain) without washing.

3. Cover the slide with Giemsa staining solution II (diluted with 9 parts Sörensen's buffer, pH = 6.8) for 10–15 min.

4. Remove the slides from the jar and rinse the slide with Sörensen buffer (pH 6.8).

5. Wash with deionized water.

6. Place the slide into a jar with water for 2–5 min.

7. Allow the slides to air-dry in a tilted position. Do not blot dry the slide.

8. Mount the slide with a cover glass if necessary (*see* **Note 5**).

3.2.3 Staining a Peripheral Blood Smear with Wright's Stain

1. Place the slide with a fixed peripheral blood smear on the horizontal staining rack.

2. Flood the slide with Wright's stain for 2 min. Do not rinse off Wright's stain from the slide.

3. Add an equal volume of the Sörensen's buffer (pH = 6.4) to Wright's stain on the slide.

4. Mix the stain solution and the buffer gently without touching the smear on the slide and observe a metallic sheen on the surface of the staining solution mixture. Make sure that the staining solution mixture does not run off the slide.

5. Leave for 3 min.

6. Rinse the slide with deionized water for 30 s.

7. Allow the slide to air-dry in a tilted position; do not blot dry.

8. Mount the slide with a cover glass if required.

3.2.4 Evaluation of Stained Peripheral Blood Smears

1. Examine the slide at a low magnification (10× objective).

2. For optimal differential staining for Romanowsky dyes, the nuclei of white blood cells should be stained in bluish purple [29, 30].

Erythrocytes—pale to moderate pink.

Neutrophils—pale pink cytoplasm with reddish to light purple granules.

Eosinophils—blue cytoplasm with orange-red granules.

Basophils—deep purple or dark violet granules.

Lymphocytes—pale blue cytoplasm.

Monocytes—bluish grey cytoplasm.

Platelets—violet-to-purple granules in light blue cytoplasm.

3. Check the lateral edges for leukocyte distribution and basophil clumping (*see* **Note 6**).

4. Choose the examination area of the blood smear where red blood cells are close to each other and do not overlap (in at least 50 %).

5. Review the slide under higher magnification (40× objective).

6. Obtain an estimate of the white blood cell count (cells/mL) by counting the total number of leukocytes in ten 40× objective fields. For WBC estimate (WBC/mL), multiply the average number of counted WBC per field by 2,000 [31] (*see* **Note 7**).

7. Examine the smear under high oil magnification (100× objective) for WBC differentiation. Check the distribution of red blood cells of 200–250 per 100× oil immersion field [31]. Perform enumeration of at least 100 consecutive leukocytes; usually the 200 cell differential is used. (For validation studies, two 200-cell differentials on the same slide by two observers are optimal.) For differential cell counting, use a "battlement track" technique to ensure that each cell is counted only once [29] (*see* **Note 8**). Basophil counts are expressed as the percentage of the total white blood cell count.

3.3 Absolute Basophil Counts in Whole Blood Using Flow Cytometry Labeling

1. Obtain EDTA-anticoagulated venous blood.

2. Incubate 100 μL of whole peripheral blood with the combinations of monoclonal autoantibodies for 15 min at room temperature.

3. Add 5 μL CD123-PE, 10 μL HLA-DR-FITC (BD Biosciences), or 10 μL anti-CCR3-PE (R&D Systems).

4. Lyse erythrocytes with Lysing Solution® (BD Biosciences) as per the manufacturer's recommendations.

5. Wash with CELLWASH® (BD Biosciences) as per the manufacturer's specifications (*see* **Note 9**).

6. Fix the sample with CellFIX® (BD Biosciences) as per the manufacturer's recommendations if the sample analysis is delayed for 2–4 h.

7. Acquire data of 50,000 events with a flow cytometer.

8. Analyze using flow cytometric analysis software.

9. Carry out an absolute basophil count using a double-platform method, a volumetric method, or cell-counting microbeads [17] (*see* **Note 10**).

3.3.1 Double-Platform Counting Method

1. Obtain the percentage of gated basophils in the sample by flow cytometric immunophenotyping.

2. Obtain an absolute white blood cell count using an automated hematology analyzer.

3. Calculate an absolute basophil count by multiplying the percentage of gated basophils and an absolute white blood cell count and dividing by 100.

3.3.2 Single-Platform Microbead-Based Method

1. Add cell-counting microbeads (CountBright™ Absolute Counting Beads (Molecular Probes), Flowcount beads (Beckman Coulter), Flow Cytometry Absolute Count Standard™ (Bangs Laboratories, Inc.), etc.) to the sample or add the sample to the test tubes with reference fluorescent microbeads (TRUCount™ tubes, BD Biosciences) as per the manufacturer's specification. Use the same pipette and precision reverse pipetting for dispensing blood sample and cell-counting beads (*see* **Note 11**).

2. Add the beads to the sample just before data acquisition by flow cytometry. Mix carefully the sample and beads by gentle pipetting.

3. Record the known concentration of the beads.

4. Add the same amount of the beads to a control buffer sample of the same volume. Acquire the data to place a gate for a bead population in the control sample. Use this gate to obtain the bead population in the blood sample.

5. Acquire the data in the whole blood sample. Make sure that at least 1,000 events are acquired in the gate for cell-counting beads.

6. Obtain the percentage of the gated cell-counting beads in the sample. Obtain the number of events in the gate for basophils in the sample.

7. Calculate the absolute basophil count (cells/μL) in the sample by dividing the number of events in the gate for basophils by the number of bead events and multiply by the known concentration of cell-counting beads (*see* **Notes 12–14**).

3.3.3 Single-Platform Volumetric Method

Some of the flow cytometers (Accuri™ C6 (BD Biosciences), Guava™ easyCyte™ (Merck Millipore), etc.) allow a precise measurement of the sample volume and thereby volumetric cell counting.

1. Pipette the blood sample in the test tube. Use "wet tip" reverse pipetting [17] to ensure accurate pipetting. Obtain the sample volume (*see* **Note 11**).

2. Acquire the data in the sample. Obtain the number of events in the gate for basophils.

3. Calculate the absolute basophil count as a ratio of the number of events in the gate for basophils to the sample volume.

4 Notes

1. Romanowsky dyes are characterized by inherent instability and high precipitate formation [32]. On standing, certain components of Romanowsky dyes can be oxidized leading to variation in their composition including azure B content and its ratio to eosin [28, 32]. Also, minimal standing time is crucial to avoid precipitation in Romanowsky dyes and onto slides during staining [28, 32].

2. The choice of anticoagulant can be important for absolute basophil count. Dry K_2EDTA is recommended as the anticoagulant of choice for full blood cell counts by current guidelines. This solution is spray-dried by the manufacturers on the interior surface of the blood collection tubes. For liquid anticoagulants, such as K_3EDTA or sodium citrate, the dilution factor should be taken into account. Heparin is not recommended to avoid pre-analytical activation of platelets and artefacts in the staining of cells [33].

3. Basophil identification can be affected by sample-handling techniques, fixation procedures, and exposure to water-based diluents. Pre-analytical sample handling should involve gentle pipetting and avoid vortex mixing. Exposure to water-based diluents affects basophil identification by metachromatic staining and should be avoided before fixation in view of high water solubility of their granules [4]. Basophils tend to form clumps [5]; therefore, use gentle pipetting to mix the sample before data acquisition to prevent cellular aggregates.

4. In slide preparation, it is important that the drop of blood is pulled by the spreader slide rather than pushed ahead. The smear should be gradually spreading from a thicker base (closer to the frosted end of the slide) to a thinner feathered end.

5. Slide mounting with a cover glass can be considered if there is a need for a slide review by several examiners or long-term storage [10]. Slide mounting and coverslipping can protect the slides from mechanical damage or dye deterioration and reduce the biohazard when handling the slides [10].

6. In wedged slides, basophils tend to be unevenly distributed towards the feathered end of the slide [4, 10]. This may result in basophil underestimation by manual microscopy of peripheral blood smears compared to flow cytometric enumeration [10]. The use of automated slide makers may improve cell distribution on the slide [1].

7. The WBC estimate is used for internal quality control only but not for clinical use [31].

8. On microscopic examination of the peripheral blood slides, it is important to make sure that each cell is counted only once.

For this purpose, a "battlement track" technique is used [34]. Using this approach, cells in the smear area selected for the morphological examination are counted in 3–5 fields between the edges of the smear back and forth in zig-zag pattern until the necessary number of cells has been counted [34]. Following "battlement track" pattern ensures that cells distributed towards the edges of the slide will be included in the cell count, thereby accounting for distributional error [34].

9. In sample preparation for flow cytometric assays, lyse-and-wash techniques are mostly used for double-platform counting method, especially for surface markers with low-level expression [20]. Lyse-and-wash technique offers the advantage of lower fluorescence background but introduces cell losses that may affect the absolute cell count [20]. Using lyse-and-wash sample preparation leads to the loss of the original relationship between absolute cell count and the initial sample volume, thereby affecting the precision of cell count [20].

   The lyse-no-wash technique is widely used for single-platform cell-counting methods and is characterized by minimal sample manipulation [20]. Sample preparation using the lyse-no-wash technique enables absolute cell counting in relation to the initial sample volume by correcting for known dilution factors [20]. However, lyse-no-wash techniques have the drawbacks of higher background fluorescence and cell debris contamination [20]. Both techniques may have limitations due to the use of lysing solutions which may affect basophil scatter characteristics or their surface marker expression [20].

10. Flow cytometric enumeration of circulating basophils using monoclonal antibodies can be particularly helpful for patients with basophil counts at the lower reference limit. Basophil counts at the lower detection limit by manual and automated counting are characterized by increasing imprecision.

11. For single-platform methodologies, accurate pipetting should be ensured by using "wet-tip" reverse pipetting. This technique is achieved by pressing the micropipette plunger to the second stop, then placing the tip in the sample, aspirating the sample, and then dispensing the sample by pressing the plunger to the first stop [17]. Repeat this technique with the same pipette tip at least twice before dispensing the sample ("wet-tip" pipetting). Careful and regular calibration of the micropipettes is essential for precise pipetting [17].

12. In patients with allergic diseases, basophil numbers can be elevated but may rapidly decline in acute and severe clinical manifestations (asthma [12], anaphylaxis [5]). Total absence of basophils and eosinophils was reported in peripheral blood, bone marrow, and skin of a patient with chronic urticaria and vitiligo [35]. Basophil counts were also noted to be inversely

related to the severity of chronic urticaria as examined by metachromatic staining [21]. It is unknown as to whether these observations reflect a decrease in basophil counts in severe manifestations of these diseases or whether metachromatic staining is affected by basophil degranulation [16]. Therefore, flow cytometric enumeration of circulating basophils may be preferable in disorders associated with basophil degranulation. Furthermore, serial assessments of absolute basophil counts in these patients may be helpful to monitor the course of the disease.

13. Basophilia in peripheral blood should trigger further work-up to rule out hematological malignancies [36–38]. Persistent basophilia may be one of the early signs of myeloproliferative disorders [39]. In patients with myelodisplastic syndromes, the presence of basophilia (>250 cells/μL) and eosinophilia (>350 cells/μL) was shown by multivariate analysis to have a prognostic significance for reduced survival [40].

14. In clinical practice, the proportional (percentage) leukocyte differential is being replaced by absolute cell count as more informative and of greater clinical significance than the cell percentage [1, 9]. In clinical settings, the repeated differential count at the interval of less than a week on the same patient was proven not to be clinically necessary in most patients except certain clinical situations such as bleeding, severe infections, and monitoring chemotherapy [1].

References

1. Pierre RV (2002) Peripheral blood film review. The demise of the eyecount leukocyte differential. Clin Lab Med 22:279–297

2. Galli SJ, Metcalfe DD, Dvorak AM (2010) Basophils and mast cells and their disorders. In: Beutler E, Lichtman MA, Coller BS, Kipps TJ, Seligsohn U (eds) Williams' hematology, 8th edn. McGraw-Hill, New York, NY, pp 915–932

3. Falcone FH, Haas H, Gibbs BF (2000) The human basophil: a new appreciation of its role in immune responses. Blood 96:4028–4038

4. Parwaresch MR (1976) The human blood basophil. Morphology, origin, kinetics, function and pathology. Springer, New York, NY, p 235

5. Shelley WB, Parnes HM (1965) The absolute basophil count. JAMA 192:368–370

6. Horowitz GL, Altaie S, Boyd JC et al (2008) Clinical and Laboratory Standards Institute (CLSI). Defining, establishing and verifying reference intervals in the clinical Laboratory; Approved Guideline -Third Edition. CLSI document EP28-A3. Clinical and Laboratory Standards Institute, Wayne, PA

7. Ducrest S, Meier F, Tschopp C, Pavlovic R, Dahinden CA (2005) Flow cytometric analysis of basophil counts in human blood and inaccuracy of hematology analyzers. Allergy 60:1446–1450

8. Mitre E, Nutman T (2003) Lack of basophilia in human parasitic infections. Am J Trop Med Hyg 69:87–91

9. Koepke JA et al (2007) Clinical and Laboratory Standards Institute (CLSI). Reference leukocyte (WBC) differential count (proportional) and evaluation of instrument methods; Approved standard – Second edition. CLSI document H20-A2. Clinical and Laboratory Standards Institute, Wayne, PA

10. Houwen B (2002) Blood film preparation and staining procedures. Lab Hematol 6:1–7

11. Amundsen EK, Henriksson CE, Holthe MR, Urdal P (2012) Is the blood basophil count sufficiently precise, accurate and specific? Am J Clin Pathol 137:86–92

12. Kimura I, Moritani Y, Tanizaki Y (1973) Basophils in bronchial asthma with reference to reagin-type allergy. Clin Allergy 3:195–202

13. Falcone FH (2004) Basophils and immunity to parasites: an update. Rev Fr Allergol 44:14–22

14. Buttarello M, Plebani M (2008) Automated blood cell counts. State of the art. Am J Clin Pathol 130:104–116

15. Hur M, Lee YK, Lee KM et al (2004) Pseudobasophilia as an erroneous white blood cell differential count with a discrepancy between automated cell counters: report of two cases. Clin Lab Haem 26:287–290

16. Lesesve J-F, Benbih M, Lecompte T (2005) Accurate basophil counting: not an easy goal! Clin Lab Haem 27:143–144

17. Storie I (2006) Absolute cell counting. In: Guide to flow cytometry. Dako, Carpinteria, CA, pp 107–111

18. Roussel M, Davis BH, Fest T, Wood BL (2012) International Council for Standardization in Hematology (ICSH). Toward a reference method for leukocyte differential counts in blood: comparison of three flow cytometric candidate methods. Cytometry A 81A:973–982

19. Cherian S, Levin G, Lo WY et al (2010) Evaluation of an 8-colour flow cytometric reference method for white blood cell differential enumeration. Cytome B 78B:319–328

20. Brando B, Barnett D, Janossy G et al (2000) Cytofluorometric methods for assessing absolute numbers of cell subsets in blood. European Working Group on Clinical Cell Analysis. Cytometry 42:327–346

21. Grattan CE, Dawn G, Gibbs S, Francis DM (2003) Blood basophil numbers in chronic ordinary urticaria and healthy controls: diurnal variation, influence of loratadine and prednisolone and relationship to disease activity. Clin Exp Allergy 33:337–341

22. Charles N, Hardwick D, Daugas E, Illei GG, Rivera J (2010) Basophils and the T helper 2 environment can promote the development of lupus nephritis. Nat Med 16:701–707

23. Zuba-Surma EK, Mariusz ZR (2011) Analytical capabilities of the ImageStream Cytometer. Meth Cell Biol 102:207–230

24. Kim JE, Kim BR, Woo KS, Han JY (2012) Evaluation of the leukocyte differential on a new automated flow cytometry hematology analyzer. Int J Lab Hematol 34(5):547–550

25. Heikali D, Di Carlo D (2010) A niche for microfluidics in portable hematology analyzers. JALA 15:319–328

26. Denburg JA, Wilson WE, Bienenstock J (1982) Basophil production in myeloproliferative disorders: increases during acute blastic transformation of chronic myeloid leukemia. Blood 60:113–120

27. Sanz M-J, Jose PJ, Williams TJ (2000) Measurement of eosinophil accumulation in vivo.
In: Proudfoot AEI, Wells TNC, Power CA (eds) Chemokine protocols, vol 138, Methods molecular biology. Humana Press, Totowa, NJ, pp 275–283

28. Woronzoff-Dashkoff KK (2002) The Wright-Giemsa stain: secrets revealed. Clin Lab Med 22:15–23

29. Barth D (2012) Approach to peripheral blood film assessment for pathologists. Semin Diagn Pathol 29:31–48

30. Bain BJ (ed) (2007) Blood sampling and blood film preparation and examination. Blood cells: a practical guide, 4th edn. Blackwell Publishing, Carlton, VIC, pp 1–20

31. Maedel LB, Doig K (2008) Examination of the peripheral blood smear and correlation with the complete blood count. In: Rodak BF, Fritsma GA, Doig K (eds) Hematology: clinical principles and applications, 3rd edn. St. Louis, MO, Sauders Elsevier, pp 175–190

32. Horobin RW (2011) How Romanowsky stains work and why they remain valuable—including a proposed universal Romanowsky staining mechanism and a rational troubleshooting scheme. Biotech Histochem 86:36–51

33. Macey M, Azam U, McCarthy D, Webb L et al (2002) Evaluation of the anticoagulants EDTA and citrate, theophylline, adenosine and dipyridamole (CTAD) for assessing platelet activation on the ADVIA 120 hematology system. Clin Chem 48:891–899

34. Tefferi A, Hanson CA, Inwards DJ (2005) How to interpret and pursue an abnormal complete blood cell count in adults. Mayo Clin Proc 80:923–936

35. Juhlin L, Venge P (1988) Total absence of eosinophils in a patient with chronic urticaria and vitiligo. Eur J Hematol 40(4):368–370

36. George TI (2012) Malignant or benign leukocytosis. Hematol Am Soc Hematol Educ Program 2012:475–484

37. Tang G, Woods LJ, Wang SA et al (2009) Chronic basophilic leukemia: a rare form of chronic myeloproliferative neoplasm. Hum Pathol 40:1194–1199

38. Nau RC, Hoagland HC (1971) A myeloproliferative disorder manifested by persistent basophilia, granulocytic leukemia and erythroleukemic phases. Cancer 3:662–665

39. Howden B (2001) The differential cell count. Lab Hematol 7:89–100

40. Wimazal F, Germing U, Kundi M, Noesslinger T, Blum S, Geissler P, Baumgartner C, Pfeilstoecker M, Valent P (2010) Evaluation of the prognostic significance of eosinophilia and basophilia in a larger cohort of patients with myelodysplastic syndromes. Cancer 116: 2372–2381

Chapter 8

Mast Cell and Basophil Cell Lines: A Compendium

Egle Passante

Abstract

Mast cells and basophils play a crucial role during type 1 hypersensitivity reactions. However, despite efforts to elucidate their role in the pathogenesis of allergy and inflammation, our understanding of mast cell and basophil biology is still relatively scarce. The practical difficulty in obtaining a sufficient number of purified primary cells from biological samples has slowed down the process of reaching a full understanding of the physiological role of these functionally similar cell types. The establishment of several immortalized cell lines has been a useful tool to establish and perform sophisticated laboratory protocols that are impractical using primary cells. Continuous cell lines have been extensively used to investigate the allergen/IgE-mediated cell activation, to elucidate the degranulation dynamics, to investigate structural and functional properties of the high-affinity receptor (FcεRI), and to test cell-stabilizing compounds. In this chapter we review the most widely used and better characterized mast cell and basophil cell lines, highlighting their advantages and drawbacks. It must be pointed out, however, that while cell lines represent a useful in vitro tool due to their easy manipulability and reduced culture costs, they often show aberrant characteristics which are not fully representative of primary cell physiology; results obtained with such cells therefore must be interpreted with due care.

Key words Mast cells, Basophils, Cell lines, IgE receptors (FcεRI), Humanized rat basophilic leukemia cells, RBL, LAD2, HMC-1, KU812, LUVA

1 Introduction

Mast cell and basophil cell lines are increasingly used as a tool for diagnostic assays to evaluate the biological activity of allergen extracts and to assess quality control protocols and batch analysis controls of allergen preparations [1–3]. Their primary cell counterparts are key effectors in allergic diseases and inflammatory conditions such as hypersensitivity reactions, asthma, atopic dermatitis, Crohn's disease, inflammatory bowel disease, and ulcerative colitis [4–6].

Both mast cells and basophils release a large number of preformed and newly synthesized pro-inflammatory mediators following cross-linking of FcεRI-bound IgE by multivalent allergens [7]. When cross-linked by multivalent allergens, FcεRI activates an

Bernhard F. Gibbs and Franco H. Falcone (eds.), *Basophils and Mast Cells: Methods and Protocols*, Methods in Molecular Biology, vol. 1192, DOI 10.1007/978-1-4939-1173-8_8, © Springer Science+Business Media New York 2014

intracellular cascade that leads to the exocytosis of granules and the production of de novo mediators. Preformed mediators include histamine, heparin, chemotactic factors, and tryptases, while newly synthesized factors include prostaglandins, leukotrienes, and platelet-activating factors (PAF) [7]. In recent years however, several studies have highlighted that mast cell and basophil roles are not limited to the initiation of allergic responses but that they play more complex roles in adaptive and innate immune responses [8]. Both mast cells and basophils can be activated directly by pathogens through a family of pattern recognition receptors called "Toll-like receptors" (TLRs) [8, 9] Mast cells can be found in the proximity of structures at the interface of the body with the external environment (i.e., lungs, intestine, blood vessels, and nerves). These cells are the first activators of the inflammatory response, not only releasing cytokines and chemoattractants for other immune cells such as neutrophils and macrophages but also phagocytizing invading pathogens and presenting antigens to T cells [10]. The role of basophils during host defense is less well known but they are thought to sustain the inflammatory process with the release of immunoregulatory cytokines such as IL-4, IL-13, and TNF-α [11].

Mast cell and basophil research has often been hindered by practical difficulties in obtaining large amounts of homogeneous cells from biological samples. Mast cells can be obtained either by enzymatic digestion of sample tissues (*see* Chapter 3) followed by density gradient centrifugation or from circulating progenitors following in vitro differentiation (*see* Chapter 4). Basophils, on the other hand, represent less than 1 % of the white cell population and their isolation and purification consist of expensive, elaborate, and tedious multiple step protocols (*see* Chapter 2). Such purification protocols often suffer from practical pitfalls resulting in cells with low viability and purity. Furthermore, the limited yield of basophils and mast cells following such isolation procedures involves the necessity of large amounts of blood/tissue with consequent ethical and practical drawbacks. In the light of this, it is not surprising that efforts have been made to generate immortalized cell lines that could offer a practical and flexible tool to investigate several aspects of mast cell and basophil biology such as activation, signaling and survival. In the early 1970s the establishment of the first rat basophilic mast cell line (RBL-2H3) signaled a turning point providing scientists with a suitable tool to develop a solid and reliable experimental system for routine experiments and innovative protocols [12–14]. The availability of an easy-to-cultivate basophilic mast cell line allowed the development of a systematic approach to characterize fundamental aspects of mast cell/basophil molecular biology [13]. Since then, several mast cell lines have been established, all showing different physicochemical properties, expression levels of surface markers and receptors, as well as intracellular content.

It must be stressed, however, that immortalized cells, despite facilitating several practical aspects of research, show abnormalities and aberrant characteristics. Furthermore, misidentification, contamination issues, and intra-laboratory reproducibility due to different culture conditions are limitations that afflict the use of cell lines. Results obtained from such studies need therefore to be interpreted with the necessary care. This chapter provides a general overview of the development of the most commonly used mast cell and basophil lineages from their inception and it goes on to describe their major applications in experimental settings. This review is intended as a guide only and it is far from being a comprehensive description of cytochemical properties of each lineage.

2 Human Mast Cell Lines

Despite efforts to establish long-term human mast cell cultures, at present there is a limited number of immortalized lineages. For more than 10 years the only established human mast cell line was the so-called human mast cell line-1 (HMC-1) [14]. HMC-1 has been widely characterized and exploited to investigate mast cell degranulation and the anti-inflammatory properties of countless compounds but it has also been used to investigate the molecular dynamics of several intracellular pathways involved in mast cell activation and survival. More recently, Kirshenbaum and co-workers isolated two mast cell lineages (LAD-1 and LAD-2) that more closely resemble primary culture of CD34+-derived human mast cells [15]. Culturing conditions for these cells however have prohibitive costs and therefore LAD-1 and LAD-2 often are not the first choice for routine experiments. The latest entry among the human mast cell lines cohort is the recently established LUVA line. LUVA cells arose spontaneously during culture of peripheral blood CD34+ cells from a healthy donor, have been reported to degranulate after IgE receptor cross-linkage [16], and present a phenotype of fully mature mast cells. In the next sections we summarize the major features of the most exploited human cell lines.

2.1 HMC-1 and HMC-1 Sublines

The HMC-1 cell line was originally established from the peripheral blood of a patient with mast cell leukemia [15–18]. Despite the fact that their phenotype is typical of immature mast cells, HMC-1 cells show, even though at low levels, several hallmarks that characterize mastocytes [18, 19]. It has been demonstrated that HMC-1 cells express many of the typical mast cell surface antigens like CD2, CD18, CD25, CD29, CD40, and CD54; HMC-1 cells also show intracellular metachromatically staining granules containing histamine, β-tryptase, and heparin (*see* Chapter 9). On the other hand, HMC-1 cells lack functional FcεRI, α-tryptase, and chymases [17]. Another key mast cell surface marker is the so-called Kit receptor (*alias* CD117). Kit is a tyrosine kinase receptor encoded by the proto-oncogene *c-kit*.

Activation of the Kit pathway plays a vital role during mast cell differentiation, proliferation, and survival [19]. HMC-1 cells carry an isoform of Kit constitutively active due to point mutations in the intracellular domain of the receptor [20]. Such mutations consist of (a) the substitution of a valine in position 816 for an alanine (V^{816A}) and (b) the substitution of the valine in position 560 for a glycine (V^{560G}). At present, two HMC-1 sublines are available and they differ in the specific harbored CD117 mutation. In particular, HMC-1.1 line harbors both V^{560G} and V^{816A} on the juxta-membrane region and in the catalytic domain, respectively, while HMC-1.2 shows only the V^{560G} mutation. The presence of the V^{816A} mutation represents a key feature of HMC-1.1 since this mutation is often present in patients affected by adult sporadic mastocytosis and myeloproliferative disease [20–22]. HMC-1.1 and HMC-1.2 show different phenotypical characteristics such as proliferation rate and other growth characteristics. HMC-1 cells therefore can represent a useful model to better understand the effects of a constitutively active Kit on mast cell regulation, proliferation, and survival and to test the effect of Kit inhibitors. The presence of a constitutively active Kit receptor makes this cell line independent of the presence of SCF in the culture media which considerably reduces laboratory costs.

As mentioned above, HMC-1 cells lack surface expression of the high-affinity receptor FcεRI and the low-affinity FcεRII. Initial studies reported that mRNA content of the α and β chain of FcεRI is negligible while mRNA for the γ subunit is present at a high amount [17]. However, more recent evidence suggests that the FcεRIβ subunit is expressed at low levels by these cells [23, 24]. Consistently with the lack of functional FcεRI, HMC-1 cells fail to degranulate after IgE/antigen sensitization and this represents a crucial limitation to the applicability of this cell line in allergy/inflammation-related studies. The HMC-1 cell line has, however, been employed for degranulation studies following non-immunological stimulation with the calcium ionophore A23187, compound 48/80, and phorbol esters. However, the physiological meaning of such results is limited and the interpretation of these data needs to take into account that elicited pathways might not be relevant in physiological conditions, especially in the context of allergen/IgE-mediated activation.

Thus, despite its limitations HMC-1 shows undoubted advantages in that it is a relatively easy-to-cultivate cell line and a great number of homogeneous cells can be obtained in a limited time frame. Its growth is independent from the presence of growth factors and this reduces subsequent handling costs. In the light of this it is not surprising that this cell line has been widely used and has found broad applicability in laboratories worldwide. To extend the applicability of this versatile mast cell line, Xia and co-workers [24] have generated an HMC-1 subline that stably expresses the human FcεRIα subunit. This new cell line (HMCα) has been proven to bind to IgE and release cytokines (e.g., IL-8, IL-6) following antigen stimulation. However, HMCα fails to degranulate following immunological activation. The array of cytokines released from this transformed HMC-1 subline accurately reflects the panel of cytokines normally released by human mast cells during IgE/antigen challenge. The reason why HMCα cells fail to degranulate despite their ability to bind to IgE/antigen is not clear; a hypothesis might suggest that the ratio between specific forms of the FcεRI ($\alpha\gamma_2$ vs. $\alpha\beta\gamma_2$) might play a role. HMCα certainly represents a step ahead toward a more representative model of human tissue mast cells.

2.2 LAD

In 2002 Kirshenbaum and co-workers characterized two novel human mast cell lineages, namely LAD-1 and -2 [15]. These cell lines originate from bone marrow aspirates of a male patient affected by mast cell sarcoma/leukaemia and, at present, the LAD-2 cell line is available.

Unlike HMC-1, LADs do not express the activating mutation of Kit and therefore their growth is dependent on the presence of SCF in the culture medium (10 ng/ml). This characteristic makes LAD cells more similar to primary cultured mast cells. The LAD-2 cell line expresses ultrastructural features of matured mast cells such as CD4, 9, 13, 14, 22, 31, 32, 45, 64, 71, 103, 117, and 132; CXCR4 (CD184); CCR5 (CD195); and intracytoplasmic histamine, tryptase, and chymase. LAD cells also express functional FcεRI and FcγRI and they can degranulate following IgE-mediated receptor cross-linking. LAD-2 cells can be used as a tool to investigate IgE-FcεRI binding and subsequent downstream events, mast cell signaling pathways, and the effect of novel drugs. Some groups, however, have reported a decreased ability of LAD cells to release cytokines compared to other lineages and primary mast cells [25]. LAD cells represent one of the most powerful tools in mast cell research but, due to the high cost of rhSCF, LAD cells are often not the first choice as mast cell model. Additionally, LAD-2 cells also show a slow doubling time (approximately 2 weeks) which limits their applicability when large numbers of cells are required.

2.3 LUVA Cell Line

The LUVA lineage is a recently established mast cell line derived from a culture of non-transformed hematopoietic progenitor cells. LUVA cells have been extensively reviewed elsewhere [16] and therefore their main features are briefly summarized here. LUVA cells spontaneously differentiated from CD34⁺-enriched mononuclear cells from a donor with aspirin exacerbated respiratory disease but without any clonal mast cell disorder. It has been reported that LUVA cells can degranulate following FcεRI cross-linking as proved by a modest release of β-hexosaminidase [16]. Cross-linking Fc receptors also evoked the secretion of prostaglandin D_2 (PGD_2) and thromboxane A_2 (TXA_2). In addition to the expression of normal levels of FcεRI, LUVA cells also constitutively express FcγRI and FcγRII. Metachromatic intracellular granules resulted positive for tryptase, chymase, cathepsin G, and carboxypeptidase A3 (CPA3). Although LUVA cells do not show KIT mutations they can survive and proliferate in culture without the presence of SCF in the culture media; intriguingly, exogenous addition of SCF to the culture media evoked a dose-dependent increase of phosphorylation of the Kit receptor and consequent increase of cell proliferation. The LUVA cell line represents a new precious tool for future studies as it is a fully functional mast cell line without some of the aberrant characteristics that limit the applicability of other mast cell lineages.

2.4 KU812

KU812 is an immature pre-basophilic cell line obtained from a male patient affected by chronic myeloid leukemia and it shows phenotypic features of basophil precursors [26]. Characteristic of this cell line is the presence of scarce metachromatic granules containing low amounts of histamine and tryptase. KU812 cells express low levels of FcεRI and no FcεRII [27, 28]. Originally, it was reported that KU812 cells do not show surface expression of FcεRI despite the presence of mRNA transcripts for the α chain of the receptor [28–30]. However, Magnusson and co-workers [31] reported that KU812 cells do express, even though at low densities, FcεRI on their surface as proven by positive direct IgE-FITC binding. Moreover, the same authors demonstrated that IgE binds to FcεRI with high affinity and specificity toward the IgE isotype.

It has been reported that under specific conditions KU812 cells can be "directed" toward basophilic differentiation [32]. KU812 cells show the ability to spontaneously differentiate to basophil-like cells under serum-free conditions; differentiation however can be also achieved following several physiological and nonphysiological stimuli. In particular, IL-3, IL-4, IL-6, TNF-α, and hydrocortisone have been proved not only to stimulate basophil-like maturation but also enhance cell surface expression of FcεRI [28, 30, 33, 34]. Other stimuli that can induce KU812 maturation are conditioned media from the human T-cell line Mo, sodium butyrate, and dimethyl sulfoxide [35, 36]. KU812 spontaneous maturation could be due to an autocrine effect of self-produced IL-6. During differentiation it is possible to observe a morphological maturation accompanied by an increase in granulation, histamine content, and cell growth inhibition [32]. Interestingly, it has been shown that KU812 cells maintain the ability to differentiate toward other elements of the erythroid lineage. Such features, however, are lost after multiple culturing passages [28, 37]. KU812 represents the only human basophilic cell line and it has used as a model to both study cell commitment toward erythroid or basophilic differentiation and investigate antigen-dependent degranulation of basophils.

3 Rodent Cell Lines

Due to the lack of a fully mature, easy-to-cultivate human basophil or mast cell line, for many years almost the entire mast cell/basophil research landscape exploited cell lines of rodent origin. However, it must be stressed that mast cells/basophils originating from different species present important differences in their physiological properties. Therefore, between different animal species, mast cell/basophil-associated diseases show marked differences in their clinical picture and it is not a surprise if data obtained from murine cells cannot always be extrapolated to human mast cell/basophil biology. Furthermore, findings achieved with cell lines of animal origin (murine, rat, canine, equine, etc.) should always be confirmed with cells of human origin. The distinctive differences between mast cell of murine and human origin have already been extensively reviewed by Bischoff [7]. One of the major functional differences between rodent and human mast cells consists of different protease contents. Murine mast cells express several tryptases and chymases (e.g., mast cellP, mast cellP14), with different specificities, while human mast cells express just three tryptases (α, β, and γ) and one chymase [7]. Expression levels of IL-4, IL-5, and TNF also show marked differences. Responsiveness to IL-3 differs too; murine mast cell growth and survival depend on IL-3 while human mast cells respond poorly to IL-3 [38, 39]. In the next sections we summarize the major features of the most exploited rodent cell lines.

3.1 RBL Cell Lines

RBL cell lines were established following serial limited dilution of cells originating from a single rat basophilic leukemia [40, 41]. Over the years, several RBL cell lines have been created, each with different histochemical and ultrastructural features. The most widely used among the RBL cell lines is the histamine-releasing subclone RBL-2H3 obtained by Kulczycki in 1979 [40]. This cell line has been extensively reviewed elsewhere [14, 42] and here we report just a brief description of its main characteristics. RBL-2H3 cells present features of both mucosal mast cells and basophils and respond with degranulation to both immunological and non-immunological stimuli in a manner that closely resembles the degranulation dynamic of primary mast cell and basophils [13]. RBL-2H3 cells present on their surface functional FcεRI and, due to their manipulability, homogeneity and fast growth rate have been widely used for studies of IgE-mediated degranulation, to test novel mast cell stabilizers and to investigate the structural physicochemical properties of FcεRs [43, 44]. In more recent years, the use of the RBL-2H3 cell line has been extended to diagnostic and therapeutic applications following the establishment of chimeric sublines expressing human FcεRI subunits (*see* Chapter 13).

FcεRI presents a tetrameric structure composed by one α, one β, and two γ subunits (αβγ$_2$) and binds IgE with high affinity (1×10^{10} M^{-1}) [44]. The α subunit has the only function of binding the ligand through its extracellular domain. The β chain is essential for the receptor's translocation to the membrane and provides receptor stability. The β chain can also amplify the activation signal that subsequently will be transduced by the γ chain [45]. The β chain is not functionally essential and therefore a trimeric αγ$_2$ structure, despite presenting a reduced stability, is the minimum requirement for a functional Fc receptor.

Chimeric cell lines have been used as a tool to determine the biologic activity of allergen extracts. Native RBL-2H3 cells express all three subunits (α, β, γ) of the high-affinity receptor of IgE. However, rodent FcεRs do not recognize human IgE. Transfection of the RBL-2H3 cell line with human alpha/beta/gamma subunits has yielded a panel of cell lines (Table 1) that show the ability to degranulate after cross-linking IgE-bound FcεRI. Chimeric RBL cells show different levels of degranulation and different IgE-binding capacity; this might probably be due to the diverse expression levels and ratio of the subunits as well as the different surface expression of the receptors. RBL SX-38 cells express all three α, β, and γ subunits while RBL-hEIa-2B121 and RBL-30/25 cells only express the α subunit of human FcεRI. It has been shown, however, that despite the absence of the human γ subunit, the signal transduction mechanisms in RBL-hEIa-2B121 and RBL-30/25 cells are intact [48]. The differential expression of FcεRI subunits provides a reason for the different binding capacity of these cells toward human IgE, with RBL SX-38 having the highest binding capacity followed by RBL-30/25 and then RBL-hEIa-2B121 (99.9 %, 97 %, and 83 %, respectively) [3].

Like the native RBL cells, all the chimeric clones show reduced ability to bind purified IgE after approximately 2 weeks in culture. The IgE-binding capacity of these cell lines is mirrored by their ability to degranulate after allergen stimulation leading to 94 % of mediator release for RBL SX-38 followed by RBL-30/25 (84 %) and RBL-hEIa-2B121 (54 %) [3, 49]. Chimera RBL-2H3 cell lines show the same advantages of native RBL-2H3 in terms of high speed of growth, simple cell culture techniques, and affordable maintenance costs; this makes RBL cells a good research instrument. RBL chimeras have been used to ascertain the allergenicity of antigens to humans in commercialized products and diagnostic allergen preparations [50] and in assessing the activity of

Table 1
Synoptic table of the most important mast cell/basophil cell lines of human and rodent origin

Cell line	Cell type	Origin	FcεRI surface expression	FcεRI chain expressed	Kit expression	Growth factor dependence	Suggested culture conditions
HMC-1	Mast cell	Human	–	β[a], γ	+	N	IMDM + 10 % FBS + 4 mM L-glutamine + α-thioglycerol
HMC-α	Mast cell	Human	+	α[b], β, γ	+	N	
LAD-1	Mast cell	Human	+	Not known	+	Y	StemPro-34 SFM, 2 mM L-glutamine + 100 ng/ml SCF.
LAD-2	Mast cell	Human	+	α, β, γ	+	Y	
LUVA	Mast cell	Human	+	α; expression of β and γ chain not known	++	N	StemPro-34SFMat with 50 % fresh medium weekly
RBL-2H3	Mast cell/basophils	Rat	+	α, β, γ	+	N	α-MEM + 10 % FBS
RBL-hEIa-2B121	Mast cell/basophils	Rat/humanized	+	α	+	N	80 % MEM + 20 % RPMI 4 mM L-glutamine + 5 % FCS
RBL-30/25	Mast cell/basophils	Rat/humanized	+	α	+	N	
RBL SX-38	Mast cell/basophils	Rat/humanized	+	α, β, γ	+	N	
RBL-703/21	Mast cell/basophils	Rat/humanized	+	α	+	N	RPMI-1640 + 10 % FBS + 2 mM L-glutamine
IgE-binding capacity of humanized RBL cell lines: RBL SX-38 > RBL-30/25 > RBL-hEIa-2B121							
KU812	Basophils	Human	+[c]	α, β[d], γ	+	N	RPMI-1640 + 10 % FBS + 2 mM L-glutamine
LAMA-84	Basophils	Human	+	α, β	+	N	RPMI 1640 + 10 % FBS

[a]Initial study published by Nilsson and co-workers showed negligible amounts of the β subunit of FcεRI [17]; however more recent data [23, 46] have shown the presence of low amounts of FcεRIβ in HMC-1

[b]Cells stably transfected with the full-length cDNA of the IgE-binding α chain of the human Fcε [24]; HMC-α fails to show a degranulative response following immunological activation despite the ability to bind hIgE/antigen

[c]A study from Hara and co-workers reports that KU812 lacks FcεRI but cells can express it upon stimulation with IL-4 [47]

[d]The β-chain shows an unexpected low expression in KU812 clones, suggesting the possibility that both $αβγ_2$ and $αγ_2$ isoforms of the FcεRI are present

serum IgE from allergic patients [49, 51]. Chimera RBL-2H3 cells have been generated also following transfection with canine and equine FcεRI chains [41].

4   Concluding Remarks

Mast cells and basophils are key players during allergy, inflammation, as well as innate immunity [52]. Mast cell and basophil research, however, has often been impeded by the lack of readily available model systems. At present in fact, there is a limited number of mast cells and basophil cell lines and such cultures present huge variability in terms of phenotype and functionality.

Over the years, several cell lineages have been established, all bearing some but not all of the typical mast cell and/or basophil hallmarks. At present, HMC-1 cell line is the most widely used but presents the limitation of a not fully mature phenotype with lack of surface expression of the FcεRI. On the other hand, the recently established LAD-2 cell line offers an experimental system model closer to the normal mast cell physiology but the prolonged doubling time and exorbitant maintenance costs are not ideal for routine experiments. Transfection of rat basophilic leukemia cells with human FcεRI subunits has led to the generation of chimera cell lines that have been used both in research and diagnostics.

Cell lines have been proved useful to study specific molecular aspects of mast cells and basophils, clarifying their role in allergy and inflammation, acquired immunity, and other pathological conditions. However, several crucial pitfalls make this research tool inadequate for a complete understanding of molecular and physiological cell dynamics. The validity of results obtained using cultured cells is often a matter of debate as immortalized cell lines present abnormal characteristic that may not reflect primary cell physiology. Another important pitfall of the use of cell lines is the intra-laboratory reproducibility of experimental results. Therefore there is a need to standardize laboratory protocols among research groups worldwide. Information regarding experimental procedures has to be shared and made readily available among investigators in order to achieve well-defined and constant experimental conditions. This will minimize not only the intra-laboratory variation but also the costs of protocol development and optimization. Another aspect that must be considered is the potential risk of contamination and misidentification of cell lines. As a result, cell lines should only be procured from certified institutions or trusted sources. An excellent example is given by RBL cells that have been mainly regarded as mast cells despite showing a phenotype in between the one of mast cells and basophils [13]. The routine use of RBL cells to investigate mast cell behavior has produced a large amount of published material but also ambiguous and contradictory data [50].

References

1. Vogel L, Lüttkopf D, Hatahet L et al (2005) Development of a functional *in vitro* assay as a novel tool for the standardization of allergen extracts in the human system. Allergy 60: 1021–1028

2. Lin J, Renault N, Haas H et al (2007) A novel tool for the detection of allergic sensitization combining protein microarrays with human basophils. Clin Exp Allergy 37:1854–1862

3. Ladics GS, van Bilsen JHM, Brouwer HMH et al (2008) Assessment of three human FcepsilonRI-transfected RBL cell-lines for identifying IgE induced degranulation utilizing peanut-allergic patient sera and peanut protein extract. Regul Toxicol Pharmacol 51: 288–294

4. Gelbmann CM, Mestermann S, Gross V et al (1999) Strictures in Crohn's disease are characterised by an accumulation of mast cells colocalised with laminin but not with fibronectin or vitronectin. Gut 45:210–217

5. Raithel M, Winterkamp S, Pacurar A et al (2001) Release of mast cell tryptase from human colorectal mucosa in inflammatory bowel disease. Scand J Gastroenterol 36:174–179

6. Dvorak AM, Monahan RA, Osage JE et al (1980) Crohn's disease: transmission electron microscopic studies. II. Immunologic inflammatory response. Alterations of mast cells, basophils, eosinophils, and the microvasculature. Hum Pathol 11:606–619

7. Bischoff SC (2007) Role of mast cells in allergic and non-allergic immune responses: comparison of human and murine data. Nat Rev Immunol 7:93–104

8. Supajatura V, Ushio H, Nakao A et al (2002) Differential responses of mast cell Toll-like receptors 2 and 4 in allergy and innate immunity. J Clin Invest 109:1351–1359

9. Puxeddu I, Piliponsky AM, Bachelet I, Levi-Schaffer F (2003) Mast cells in allergy and beyond. Int J Biochem Cell Biol 35: 1601–1607

10. Dawicki W, Marshall JS (2007) New and emerging roles for mast cells in host defence. Curr Opin Immunol 19:31–38

11. Brunner T, Heusser CH, Dahinden CA (1993) Human peripheral blood basophils primed by interleukin 3 (IL-3) produce IL-4 in response to immunoglobulin E receptor stimulation. J Exp Med 177:605–611

12. Eccleston E, Leonard BJ, Lowe JS et al (1973) Basophilic leukaemia in the albino rat and a demonstration of the basopoietin. Nat New Biol 244:73–76

13. Passante E, Frankish N (2009) The RBL-2H3 cell line: its provenance and suitability as a model for the mast cell. Inflamm Res 58:737–745

14. Butterfield JH, Weiler D, Dewald G et al (1988) Establishment of an immature mast cell line from a patient with mast cell leukemia. Leuk Res 12:345–355

15. Kirshenbaum AS, Akin C, Wu Y et al (2003) Characterization of novel stem cell factor responsive human mast cell lines LAD 1 and 2 established from a patient with mast cell sarcoma/leukemia; activation following aggregation of FcεRI or FcγRI. Leuk Res 27: 677–682

16. Laidlaw TM, Steinke JW, Tiñana AM et al (2011) Characterization of a novel human mast cell line that responds to stem cell factor and expresses functional FcεRI. J Allergy Clin Immunol 127:815–822

17. Nilsson G, Blom T, Kusche-Gullberg M et al (1994) Phenotypic characterization of the human mast-cell line HMC-1. Scand J Immunol 39:489–498

18. Sundström M, Vliagoftis H, Karlberg P et al (2003) Functional and phenotypic studies of two variants of a human mast cell line with a distinct set of mutations in the c-kit proto-oncogene. Immunology 108:89–97

19. Edling CE, Hallberg B (2007) c-Kit-a hematopoietic cell essential receptor tyrosine kinase. Int J Biochem Cell Biol 39:1995–1998

20. Furitsu T, Tsujimura T, Tono T et al (1993) Identification of mutations in the coding sequence of the proto-oncogene c-kit in a human mast cell leukemia cell line causing ligand-independent activation of c-kit product. J Clin Invest 92:1736–1744

21. Worobec AS, Semere T, Nagata H et al (1998) Clinical correlates of the presence of the Asp816Val c-kit mutation in the peripheral blood mononuclear cells of patients with mastocytosis. Cancer 83:2120–2129

22. Longley BJ, Metcalfe DD, Tharp M et al (1999) Activating and dominant inactivating c-KIT catalytic domain mutations in distinct clinical forms of human mastocytosis. Proc Natl Acad Sci U S A 96:1609–1614

23. Cruse G, Kaur D, Leyland M et al (2010) A novel FcεRIβ-chain truncation regulates human mast cell proliferation and survival. FASEB J 24:4047–4057

24. Xia YC, Sun S, Kuek LE et al (2011) Human mast cell line-1 (HMC-1) cells transfected with FcεRIα are sensitive to IgE/antigen-mediated stimulation demonstrating selectivity towards

cytokine production. Int Immunopharmacol 11:1002–1011

25. Guhl S, Babina M, Neou A et al (2010) Mast cell lines HMC-1 and LAD2 in comparison with mature human skin mast cells-drastically reduced levels of tryptase and chymase in mast cell lines. Exp Dermatol 19:845–847

26. Kishi K (1985) A new leukemia cell line with Philadelphia chromosome characterized as basophil precursors. Leuk Res 9:381–390

27. Yamashita M, Ichikawa A, Katakura Y et al (2001) Induction of basophilic and eosinophilic differentiation in the human leukemic cell line KU812. Cytotechnology 36:179–186

28. Fukuda T, Kishi K, Ohnishi Y et al (1987) Bipotential cell differentiation of KU812: evidence of a hybrid cell line that differentiates into basophils and macrophage-like cells. Blood 70:612–619

29. Fischkoff SA, Kishi K, Benjamin WR et al (1987) Induction of differentiation of the human leukemia cell line, KU812. Leuk Res 11:1105–1113

30. Blom T, Huang R, Aveskogh M et al (1992) Phenotypic characterization of KU812, a cell line identified as an immature human basophilic leukocyte. Eur J Immunol 22:2025–2032

31. Magnusson CG, Håård J, Matsson P et al (1995) Demonstration of specific high-affinity Fc epsilon-receptors on the human basophil-like leukemia cell line KU812 by flow cytometry. Allergy 50:72–77

32. Almlöf I, Nilsson K, Johansson V, Akerblom E, Slotte H, Ahlstedt S, Matsson P (1988) Induction of Basophilic Differentiation in the Human Basophilic Cell Line KU812. Scand J Immunol 28:293–300

33. Nilsson G, Carlsson M, Jones I et al (1994) TNF-alpha and IL-6 induce differentiation in the human basophilic leukaemia cell line KU812. Immunology 81:73–78

34. Hutt-Taylor SR, Harnish D, Richardson M et al (1988) Sodium butyrate and a T lymphocyte cell line-derived differentiation factor induce basophilic differentiation of the human promyelocytic leukemia cell line HL-60. Blood 71:209–215

35. Valent P, Besemer J, Kishi K et al (1990) IL-3 promotes basophilic differentiation of KU812 cells through high affinity binding sites. J Immunol 145:1885–1889

36. Nakazawa M, Mitjavila MT, Debili N et al (1989) KU 812: a pluripotent human cell line with spontaneous erythroid terminal maturation. Blood 73:2003–2013

37. Valent P, Besemer J, Sillaber C et al (1990) Failure to detect IL-3-binding sites on human mast cells. J Immunol 145:3432–3437

38. Razin E, Ihle JN, Seldin D et al (1984) Interleukin 3: A differentiation and growth factor for the mouse mast cell that contains chondroitin sulfate E proteoglycan. J Immunol 132:1479–1486

39. Dearman RJ, Skinner RA, Deakin N, Shaw D, Kimber I (2005) Evaluation of an in vitro method for the measurement of specific IgE antibody responses: the rat basophilic leukemia (RBL) cell assay. Toxicology 206:195–205

40. Kulczycki A, Metzger H (1974) The interaction of IgE with rat basophilic leukemia cells. II Quantitative aspects of the binding reaction. J Exp Med 140:1676–1695

41. Rashid A, Sadroddiny E, Ye HT et al (2012) Review: Diagnostic and therapeutic applications of rat basophilic leukemia cells. Mol Immunol 52:224–228

42. Holowka D, Hartmann H, Kanellopoulos J et al (1980) Association of the receptor for immunoglobulin E with an endogenous polypeptide on rat basophilic leukemia cells. J Recept Res 1:41–68

43. Goetze A, Kanellopoulos J, Rice D et al (1981) Enzymatic cleavage products of the alpha subunit of the receptor for immunoglobulin E. Biochemistry 20:6341–6349

44. Kraft S, Kinet J-P (2007) New developments in FcepsilonRI regulation, function and inhibition. Nat Rev Immunol 7:365–378

45. Ra C, Jouvin MH, Kinet JP (1989) Complete structure of the mouse mast cell receptor for IgE (Fc epsilon RI) and surface expression of chimeric receptors (rat-mouse-human) on transfected cells. J Biol Chem 264:15323–15327

46. Akizawa Y (2003) Regulation of human FcepsilonRI beta chain gene expression by Oct-1. Int Immunol 15:549–556

47. Hara T, Yamada K, Tachibana H (1998) Basophilic differentiation of the human leukemia cell line KU812 upon treatment with interleukin-4. Biochem Biophys Res Commun 247:542–548

48. Gilfillan AM, Kado-Fong H, Wiggan GA et al (1992) Conservation of signal transduction mechanisms via the human Fc epsilon RI alpha after transfection into a rat mast cell line, RBL 2H3. J Immunol 149:2445–2451

49. Takagi K, Nakamura R, Teshima R et al (2003) Application of human Fc epsilon RI alpha-chain-transfected RBL-2H3 cells for estimation of active serum IgE. Biol Pharm Bull 26:252–255

50. Passante E, Ehrhardt C, Sheridan H et al (2009) RBL-2H3 cells are an imprecise model for mast cell mediator release. Inflamm Res 58:611–618

51. Hoffmann A, Jamin A, Foetisch K et al (1999) Determination of the allergenic activity of birch pollen and apple prick test solutions by mea-surement of beta-hexosaminidase release from RBL-2H3 cells. Comparison with classical methods in allergen standardization. Allergy 54:446–454

52. Galli SJ, Nakae S, Tsai M (2005) Mast cells in the development of adaptive immune responses. Nat Immunol 6:135–142

Part III

Whole Cells: Identification in Tissues, Signaling Pathways, Gene Silencing, and Reporters

Chapter 9

Detection of Mast Cells and Basophils by Immunohistochemistry

Andrew F. Walls and Cornelia Amalinei

Abstract

Staining cells or tissues with basic dyes was the mainstay of mast cell and basophil detection methods for more than a century following the first identification of these cell types using such methods. These techniques have now been largely supplanted by immunohistochemical procedures with monoclonal antibodies directed against unique constituents of these cell types. Immunohistochemistry with antibodies specific for the granule protease tryptase provides a more sensitive and discriminating means for detecting mast cells than using the classical histochemical procedures; and employing antibodies specific for products of basophils (2D7 antigen and basogranulin) has allowed detection of basophils that infiltrate into tissues. The application of immunohistochemistry to detect more than one marker in the same cell has underpinned concepts of mast cell heterogeneity based on differential expression of chymase and other proteases. The double-labelling procedures employed have also provided a means for investigating the expression of cytokines and a range of other products. Protocols are here set out that have been used for immunohistochemical detection of mast cells and basophils and their subpopulations in human tissues. Consideration is given to pitfalls to avoid and to a range of alternative approaches.

Key words Basophil, Chymase, Heterogeneity, Immunohistochemistry, Mast cell, Tryptase

1 Introduction

Mast cells were first characterized by Ehrlich in the late nineteenth century as cells with prominent cytoplasmic granules that reacted with a basic aniline dye [1]. His application of the term *Mastzellen* (well-fed cells) derived from his assumption that the intracellular material had been ingested from the local tissue. Though mast cells do indeed have phagocytic properties [2], the distinctive granules are in fact produced by the cell itself and serve as stores for a range of preformed mediators of inflammation. These include histamine, various proteases, and heparin, which can be explosively secreted in response to allergens or other stimuli. The process is accompanied by the rapid generation of new mediators including prostaglandin D_2 and leukotriene C_4, and the release of

Bernhard F. Gibbs and Franco H. Falcone (eds.), *Basophils and Mast Cells: Methods and Protocols*, Methods in Molecular Biology, vol. 1192, DOI 10.1007/978-1-4939-1173-8_9, © Springer Science+Business Media New York 2014

multiple cytokines that can be both preformed and newly generated. Methods for the identification of mast cells based on those of Ehrlich remain in use, but understanding of their constituents has led to development of immunocytochemical procedures of greater sensitivity and specificity.

Though not appreciated at the outset, the classical methods for identifying mast cells have depended on the binding of basic dyes to heparin or other proteoglycans in the granules. These procedures result also in staining of the granules of basophils, a leukocyte identified by Ehrlich in blood smears using the same aniline dyes that led to the discovery of mast cells. The most widely employed basic dyes were to become toluidine blue (which stains mast cells *metachromatically* a violet color) and Alcian blue (which stains the granules *orthochromatically* an intense blue). Other basic dyes employed in mast cell histochemistry have included safranin O, astra blue, azure A and B, and thionine, and differences in the performance of stains (possibly related to differing degrees of sulfation of proteoglycans in different granules) have led to combinations of these stains being applied in the investigation of mast cell heterogeneity (reviewed in [3]). Other approaches employed to detect mast cells have relied on the binding to proteoglycans of fluorescent dyes such as berberine sulfate or acridine orange, or avidin conjugated to enzymes or fluorescent compounds.

While the dye-based procedures are inexpensive and rapid to perform, their application may lead to an underestimation of mast cell numbers. Use of formaldehyde-based fixatives can render mast cells difficult to stain with basic dyes, particularly those of mucosal tissues in humans and rodents [4, 5]. While formaldehyde-induced loss of dye binding can be overcome to some extent by protease treatment of fixed tissues or by prolonged staining periods (generally several days required), this may be to the detriment of cell morphology and can lead to artifactual staining of other cell types [4]. A further concern with dye binding procedures is that they may fail to stain mast cells where there is extensive loss of granule contents, and unstained "phantom mast cells" have been postulated to occur in particular where there is mast cell activation [6].

The preparation of monoclonal antibodies specific for tryptase, a trypsin-like serine protease of mast cells, opened the way for methods offering important advantages in the detection of mast cells [7, 8]. Immunohistochemistry with these antibodies (*see* Fig. 1a) has now replaced the classical dye-binding techniques as the "gold standard" procedure for identifying mast cells in human tissue. This protease is largely unique to mast cells and quantities as great as 30 pg per cell may be present [9]. Basophils, the only other cell type in which tryptase has been demonstrated convincingly, have been estimated to contain less than 1 % of the amount within a mast cell [10]. Employing sensitive detection systems (e.g., with a secondary antibody and avidin-biotin complex (ABC)

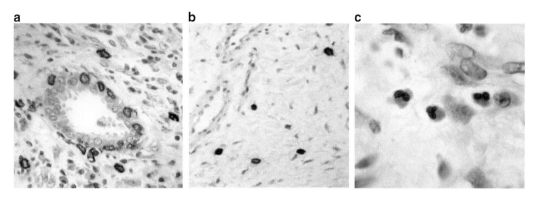

Fig. 1 (**a**) Mast cells detected using tryptase-specific monoclonal antibody AA1 in lung tissue from a case of bronchial carcinoma. Tryptase appears as *reddish brown* staining and is localized predominantly within cytoplasmic granules. The presence of extracellular immunostaining would be consistent with partial degranulation of some of the cells. (**b**) Mast cells in synovial tissue from a patient with osteoarthritis detected using a double-labelling procedure with tryptase-specific monoclonal antibody AA1 (*reddish brown* immunostaining) and chymase-specific antibody CC1 (*blue/black*). (**c**) Basophils infiltrated into lung tissue in a case of bronchial carcinoma, detected using monoclonal antibody BB1 specific for the basophil marker basogranulin. Note the lobulated nuclei (*blue* counterstain) and the presence of basogranulin in the cytoplasm (*brown*)

amplification procedures) higher signal-to-noise ratios can be achieved than with conventional basic dye procedures [8] allowing more mast cells to be detected.

Immunohistochemistry with a tryptase-specific antibody can sometimes be forgiving of poor technique, but where there is potential for loss of tryptase from the granules (either as a consequence of mast cell activation in vivo or artifactual release from tissue ex vivo, e.g., following crushing or decomposition), the use of amplification procedures and careful standardization is important. However, in most cases, mast cell degranulation in clinical disease may be partial rather than total, and tryptase will still be detected in mast cells albeit with reduced intensity. The presence of tryptase has been noted in the immediate vicinity of mast cells by immunohistochemistry (*see* Fig. 1a), occasionally as a "halo" around cells, or sometimes in discrete granules or as a "smear." Inadequate fixation can result in loss of this water-soluble protease, particularly in the case of sections of frozen tissues.

Though there is the theoretical risk that some mast cells may not be detected by immunohistochemistry with tryptase-specific antibodies on account of reduced quantities of tryptase being present following degranulation, other approaches have yet to supplant this method. A surface marker for mast cells which is not granule associated is c-kit (CD117). Immunohistochemistry with the c-kit-specific monoclonal antibody YB5.B8 can be used for the identification of mast cells [11], but this antibody has generally proved unsuitable for use with paraffin-embedded tissues. Some success has been reported using an immunohistochemical procedure with an antibody specific to histamine [12], but histamine is present also in substantial quantities in basophils and is produced by diverse other cell types including neurons, neutrophils, monocytes/macrophages, dendritic cells, and platelets [13–15].

Certain mast cell markers are restricted to a subset of these cells, and their detection by immunohistochemistry has been used to investigate heterogeneity in mast cell populations. The first such marker to be studied was chymase, a chymotryptic serine protease. On the basis of double-labelling procedures in immunohistochemistry (*see* Fig. 1b), mast cells have been categorized according to the presence of both tryptase and chymase (MC_{TC}), or of tryptase but not chymase (MC_T) [16, 17]. Relative numbers of mast cells distinguished in this way differ between anatomical sites, with MC_T cells most abundant at mucosal surfaces and cells of the MC_{TC} subset predominant in skin and the respiratory and gastrointestinal submucosa. The proportion of each subset can also be affected by disease, with cells of the MC_T population reported to be relatively sparse in the gut of AIDS patients, but present in increased numbers in the affected tissues in a range of conditions associated with inflammation or tissue remodelling (including rhinitis, conjunctivitis, scleroderma, rheumatoid arthritis, and osteoarthritis) (reviewed in [18]).

The significance of altered ratios of MC_T and MC_{TC} cells is unclear, and it remains to be determined to what extent each subset may differ in function other than that which would be conferred by the presence or the absence of chymase. On the basis of fairly limited studies, it has been suggested that another mast cell-specific protease, carboxypeptidase A3, may be restricted to the MC_{TC} subset [19] and also cathepsin G, a protease better characterized as a neutrophil product [20]. Moreover, certain inflammatory cytokines may be differentially expressed in each of the major subsets defined, at least in the respiratory tract in allergic disease (reviewed in [21]). Immunohistochemical techniques have opened the way to investigate differential expression of protein products in mast cells.

Careful optimization and standardization of procedures are crucial when applying immunohistochemical procedures for the identification and characterization of mast cell subpopulations. Published reports of relative numbers of MC_T and MC_{TC} cells detected in similar tissues have varied greatly. Some of the variation may reflect differences between subjects studied or be a consequence of sampling too small a piece of tissue. However, it seems likely that the use of different antibodies and staining protocols will have contributed to the variation observed. When double-labelling procedures are employed for tryptase and chymase, it is essential that there is effective detection of both these proteases. Different fixatives, different periods of incubation, or addition of different concentrations of primary antibodies on tissue sections can result in major differences in the proportions of MC_T and MC_{TC} subpopulations detected, and even in the appearance of cells with chymase but not tryptase MC_C [22, 23]. Immunohistochemical procedures can be effective at determining the presence within cells of specific constituents, but are less good for assessing relative amounts within each cell. The challenge is to use a limit of detection that is suitable for each study, and to adhere closely to it. Mast cells are categorized according to the presence or the absence of specific constituents by immunohistochemistry, but often it may be more appropriate to define these cells according to whether a defined constituent is abundant or present in only small amounts.

Considerations of detection sensitivity can be particularly important when applying immunohistochemistry to study mast cell subpopulations. Similar issues may arise also when seeking to distinguish mast cells from basophils and other cell types. It is generally assumed that the quantities of "mast cell proteases" present in a basophil are insufficient to be detected using standard immunohistochemical procedures; and basophils are undoubtedly less likely to be mistaken for mast cells using immunohistochemistry than using classical dye-binding techniques. However, quantities of tryptase present in the basophil can vary greatly between individuals, and by more than two orders of magnitude [24], and this issue may require reappraisal at least for tissues from some allergic individuals.

Basophil numbers in human tissues may now be determined using antibodies specific for this cell type. Monoclonal antibodies 2D7 [25] and BB1 [26] bind to proteins of unknown function that are unique to the granules of basophils, and which are secreted upon cell degranulation [27]. Antibody 2D7 binds to a protein of 72–76 kDa [25] that is produced at an early stage in basophil development from bone marrow progenitors [28], while BB1 antibody recognizes a basic protein, termed basogranulin, that is secreted as a large macromolecular complex of approximately 5,000 kDa or more [29]. Elucidation of their mediator roles could one day provide important clues as to what may be the unique contribution of basophils in disease. In the meantime, immunohistochemistry with BB1 (*see* Fig. 1c) and 2D7 can provide a valuable means for the identification of basophils in tissues.

The protocols set out below have been used successfully to detect mast cells and basophils by immunohistochemistry. As histochemical staining methods have largely been replaced by the immunohistochemical methods, they are not provided here (though protocols for staining by dye binding are available elsewhere [30]). Mast cell and basophil markers are here described only for human cells. While the basic immunohistochemical procedures outlined may be suitable for use with cells and tissues from nonhuman species, such is the extent of mast cell heterogeneity between species that markers used in man may be inappropriate even if suitable antibodies were available for the nonhuman homologue. There are species-related differences not only in the distribution of mast cell proteases but also in the types of protease. Thus, for example, multiple chymases (with quite different patterns of expression) have been characterized in several species of small mammal, but there is just one chymase in man (reviewed in [18]). Simple categorization into MC_T and MC_{TC} populations is unlikely to be possible for many nonhuman species.

The techniques described are intended not as blueprints to be followed rigidly, but as guides that may be helpful when developing suitable methods for a specific system being studied. It is important to validate and optimize methods for each source of material. Suggestions are made for antibodies to employ, for the preparation of some widely employed fixatives and reagents; and there is a list of basic equipment. The primary approach for which details are provided involves fixation and processing tissues in paraffin wax, though methods are indicated also for preparing and fixing cyto-centrifuge preparations. Loss of antigenicity often occurs during fixation, and a heat-induced epitope retrieval procedure is described for use following de-waxing and rehydration of tissue sections. Protocols are provided for immunohistochemistry with one primary antibody or with two different antibodies. Pitfalls to avoid, and possible alternative materials and strategies for immunohisto-chemistry, are suggested in Subheading 4 to the methods.

2   Materials

2.1   Antibodies

Monoclonal antibodies specific for mast cell tryptase (e.g., AA1), chymase (e.g., CC1), or basophils (e.g., BB1), or to an irrelevant antigen as a control (e.g., specific for *Aspergillus niger* glucose oxidase, X0931).

Biotinylated antiserum to the primary antibody (e.g., goat anti-mouse immunoglobulins).

2.2   Fixatives, Tissue Processing, and Slide Preparation

See **Note 1**.

1. 10 % Neutral buffered formalin: 100 mL 40 % formaldehyde stock is diluted with 900 mL distilled water, and 4 g of sodium dihydrogen orthophosphate and 6.5 g of disodium hydrogen orthophosphate (anhydrous) are added and dissolved. The pH is adjusted to 7.0–7.6.

2. Aldehyde-based fixatives:
   Glutaraldehyde.
   Paraformaldehyde: A solution of 2.26 % sodium dihydrogen orthophosphate (41.5 mL) is added to 2.52 % sodium hydroxide (8.5 mL) and heated to 60–80 °C in a covered container. Paraformaldehyde (2 g) is added, and the mixture is

stirred until it becomes clear. This is filtered, cooled, and adjusted to pH 7.2–7.4. This fixative should be freshly prepared on each occasion.

3. Mercuric chloride fixatives (B5 fixative): A stock B5 solution is made with 60 g mercuric chloride, and 12.5 g sodium acetate dissolved in 1 L of distilled water. A working solution is prepared immediately before use by mixing 90 mL of the stock B5 solution with 10 % neutral buffered formalin as prepared above.

Zenker's fixative: Prepared by dissolving 25 g potassium dichromate and 50 g mercuric chloride in 950 mL distilled water and adding 50 mL glacial acetic acid. The solution should be mixed overnight to ensure solubilization of mercuric chloride crystals.

4. Alcohol fixatives: Carnoy's fluid: A mixture of 60 mL absolute ethanol, 30 mL chloroform, and 10 mL glacial acetic acid. Methacarn: A mixture of 60 mL absolute methanol, 30 mL chloroform, and 10 mL glacial acetic acid.

5. Susa fixative: A stock solution is prepared with 4.5 g mercuric chloride, 2 g trichloroacetic acid, and 0.5 g sodium chloride dissolved in 80 mL distilled water. To this is added a mixture of 20 mL 40 % formaldehyde and 4 mL glacial acetic acid.

6. Acetone.

7. Methanol.

8. Absolute alcohol.

9. Histoclear II (or other xylene substitute).

10. Poly-L-lysine.

2.3 Reagents for Antigen Retrieval and Immunohistochemistry

1. Antigen retrieval solution: 0.01 M sodium citrate buffer, pH 6.0. Prepare stock solutions of 0.1 M citric acid solution (by dissolving 21 g of citric acid, monohydrate 1 L of distilled water), and 0.1 M sodium citrate solution (by dissolving 29.4 g trisodium citrate dihydrate in 1 L of distilled water). A working solution is prepared by adding 9 mL of 0.1 M citric acid and 41 mL of 0.1 M sodium citrate to 450 mL of distilled water and adjusting the pH to 6.0.

2. Peroxidase-blocking solution: 0.5 % hydrogen peroxide, 0.1 % sodium azide in methanol (*see* **Note 2**).

3. Nonspecific protein-binding blocking buffer:
For use with hydrogen peroxide reporting enzyme: 1 % fraction V bovine serum albumin in phosphate-buffered saline (PBS-albumin).

For use with alkaline phosphatase reporting enzyme (as in double-labelling immunohistochemistry protocol):

1% fraction V bovine serum albumin in Tris-buffered saline (TBS-albumin).

4. Wash buffer:

For use with hydrogen peroxide: Phosphate-buffered saline (PBS), pH 7.4 (*see* **Note 3**).

For use with alkaline phosphatase: Tris-buffered saline, pH 8.0.

5. ExtrAvidin®-peroxidase conjugate or ExtrAvidin®-alkaline phosphatase conjugate (*see* **Note 4**).

6. Substrates:

For horseradish peroxidase: A stock solution is prepared with 10 mg/mL 3-amino 9-ethylcarbazole (AEC) in dimethylformamide (*see* **Note 5**). This can be stored in the dark for up to 1 week at 4 °C. The AEC substrate for applying to sections comprises 1 mL AEC stock, 19 mL 0.1 M acetate buffer, pH 5.0, and 3.3 μL 30 % hydrogen peroxide. This should be filtered immediately before use. *See* **Note 6**.

For alkaline phosphatase: Prepare stock solutions of (1) 50 mg/mL 5-bromo-4-chloro-3-indolyl phosphate (*p-toluidine* salt; BCIP) in dimethylformamide (BCIP stock), (2) 75 mg/mL *p*-nitrotetrazolium blue (NBT) in 70 % dimethylformamide (BCIP stock), and (3) 0.1 M glycine, 1 mM magnesium chloride, and 1 mM zinc chloride, pH 10.4 (alkaline phosphatase buffer). These can be stored at 4 °C. Prior to use, prepare the alkaline phosphatase substrate solution by adding 75 μL BCIP stock and 100 μL NBT stock to 20 mL alkaline phosphatase buffer; and 0.25 mg/mL levamisole should be added (to block most endogenous alkaline phosphatases).

7. Counterstain: Mayer's hemalum. Filter each time before use.

2.4 Equipment

1. Glass microscope slides.

2. Microtome for cutting tissue sections.

3. Delimiting pen.

4. Access to automated tissue-processing equipment is useful where there is high throughput of samples.

5. Water bath.

6. Microwave (if employed for fixation or for unmasking antigens prior to immunohistochemistry).

7. Slide tray which holds the slides above a pool of tap water. A close-fitting lid for the tray allows a humidified atmosphere to be maintained and prevents sections from drying out during immunohistochemistry.

8. Staining trough and slide racks.

9. Hemocytometer.

10. Cytocentrifuge.

3   Methods

3.1   Fixation and Processing of Tissues

1. Carefully cut tissues into pieces small enough to allow good penetration of the fixative (generally 1 cm³ or less). *See* **Note 7**.

2. Fix specimens as soon as possible to preserve tissue architecture by incubating in 10 % neutral buffered formalin for 6–24 h (*see* **Note 8**).

3. Decant the fixative and dispose according to local regulations. Add PBS and mix gently on a spiral or a rotary mixer at 4 °C for 1–2 h to wash out the fixative.

4. At intervals of an hour or more, dehydrate the specimens through a series of graded alcohols, incubating progressively with 70 % ethanol, 90 % ethanol, and 100 % ethanol (twice) with gentle mixing at 4 °C.

5. Embed the tissues in paraffin wax (*see* **Note 9**).

6. Cut into 4–6 µm sections (*see* **Note 10**) and float them in a tank of water.

7. Pick up cut sections from the water tank onto slides coated with poly-L-lysine (to provide an adherent surface). *See* **Note 11**.

8. Maintain at 58 °C in a drying oven (with thermostat) for better adherence of tissue to the slides (*see* **Note 12**).

3.2   Preparation and Fixation of Cytocentrifuge Preparations

1. Establish the number of cells in suspension using a hemocytometer, and then adjust to 10^6 cells per mL using a physiological buffer.

2. Assemble slides in cytocentrifuge according to the manufacturer's instructions, then load 100 µL of cell solution per slide, and centrifuge for 5 min at 500 rpm ($28 \times g$).

3. Remove the slides, taking care not to smear the cells when removing the filter cards. Allow the cells to air-dry, and then fix in methanol or acetone for 1 min. *See* **Note 12**.

3.3   De-waxing and Rehydration of Tissue Sections

1. Immerse slides with tissue sections in a trough of xylene and heat in the oven at 58 °C, for 45 min.

2. Incubate twice in Histoclear II (or other proprietary, less toxic substitute for xylene) at room temperature for 10 min each time.

3. Incubate three times in 100 % ethanol for 10 min each time.

4. Incubate in 96 % ethanol for 10 min.

5. Incubate in 80 % ethanol for 10 min.

6. Incubate in 70 % ethanol for 10 min.

7. Rinse in distilled water twice each for 10 min.

8. It may be helpful to use a delimiting pen to draw a circle around the specimen on the slide (*see* **Note 13**). The trace is water repellent and should help to prevent reagents added from running off the slide. *See* **Note 14**.

3.4 Heat-Induced Epitope Retrieval

(*See* **Note 15**.)

1. Transfer slides to a heat-proof vessel containing the sodium citrate buffer antigen retrieval solution—buffer solution and heat in a water bath at 97–99 °C for 20–30 min (*see* **Note 16**). If necessary, add more solution during this process to prevent the tissue sections from drying out.

2. While still submerged, allow slides to cool at room temperature for an additional 30–40 min.

3. Wash in distilled water for 5 min at room temperature, and proceed to immunohistochemistry.

3.5 Immunohisto-chemistry with a Single Primary Antibody

(*See* **Note 17**.)

1. With the slides placed flat in a humid environment (e.g., in slide tray), add the peroxidase-blocking solution for 5 min (to inhibit endogenous peroxidase activity).

2. Discard the peroxidase-blocking solution and wash with distilled water for 5 min.

3. Block nonspecific protein-binding sites by adding the protein-blocking solution for 10 min.

4. Discard the protein-blocking solution and wipe around sections with a piece of tissue.

5. Apply 100 μL primary antibody at a preestablished working dilution (*see* **Note 18**) in PBS-albumin to the section, and incubate overnight at 4 °C (*see* **Note 19**).

6. Wash the slides three times with wash buffer, for 10 min each wash.

7. Wipe around the sections and apply 100 μL of biotinylated secondary antibody for 30 min, at room temperature.

8. Wash the slides as described in **step 6**.

9. Wipe around the sections and apply 100 μL ExtrAvidin®-peroxidase diluted 1/20 in PBS-albumin. Incubate the slides for 30 min at room temperature.

10. Wash the slides as described in **step 6**, and while sections are being washed, prepare the AEC substrate solution.

11. Apply the AEC substrate solution for 3–4 min or until a reddish brown color develops (checking briefly under the microscope if necessary). In practice this means starting to collect slides in a rack after 2 min as staining can continue with the slides in a vertical position. *See* **Note 6**.

12. Wash slides in a trough of running tap water for 5 min, avoiding excessive turbulence that could result in detachment of sections. Rinse briefly in distilled water.

13. Counterstain in Mayer's hemalum for 3 min, and then wash as described in **step 12**.

14. When the sections have dried completely, mount a cover slip using aqueous mounting medium (*see* **Note 20**).

3.6 Double-Labelling Immunohisto-chemistry for MC$_T$ and MC$_{TC}$ Subpopulations

(*See* **Note 21**.)

1. With the slides in a humid environment, add the peroxidase-blocking solution for 5 min (as in Subheading 3.5; *see* **Note 22**).

2. Discard the peroxidase-blocking solution and wash with distilled water for 5 min.

3. Block nonspecific protein-binding sites by adding the protein-blocking solution for 10 min.

4. Discard the protein-blocking solution and wipe around sections with a piece of tissue.

5. Apply 100 μL primary antibodies at preestablished working dilutions (*see* **Note 18**) in TBS-albumin to the section, and incubate for 3 h (*see* **Note 19**). The antibodies added should comprise (1) peroxidase-conjugated anti-tryptase antibody, (2) biotinylated anti-chymase antibody, and (3) both peroxidase-conjugated anti-tryptase antibody and biotinylated anti-chymase antibody added together. Appropriate negative control antibodies (of the same isotype and quantity as each of the other antibodies) should also be included.

6. Wash the slides three times with wash buffer, for 10 min each wash, and meanwhile prepare the AEC substrate solution.

7. Apply the AEC substrate solution for 5 min. A reddish brown color should develop.

8. Wash the slides as described in **step 6**.

9. Wipe around the sections and apply 1/20 ExtrAvidin®-alkaline phosphatase in TBS-albumin for 1 h.

10. Wash the slides as described in **step 6**, and while sections are being washed, prepare the BCIP/NBT substrate solution.

11. Apply the BCIP/NBT substrate solution for 10 min.

12. Wash slides in a trough of running tap water for 5 min avoiding excessive turbulence. Rinse briefly in distilled water.

13. Counterstain in Mayer's hemalum for 3 min, and then wash as described in **step 12**.

14. When the sections have dried completely, mount a cover slip using aqueous mounting medium. Using this protocol, there should be reddish brown immunostaining for tryptase and blue/black for chymase (almost invariably co-localized with the reddish brown color).

4 Notes

1. There are hazards associated with the constituents of many fixatives, and their preparation and use should be carried out in a well-ventilated area with personal protective equipment (PPE). Formaldehyde, paraformaldehyde, and mercuric chloride have irritant and corrosive effects on the eye and skin. Mercuric chloride is corrosive to metals. It should not be brought in contact with any metal object, and waste should not be poured down the drain.

2. Sodium azide is highly toxic, so PPE should be worn.

3. PBS may be adequate as a wash buffer in many situations, but where there is heavy background staining, there may be a need for a more extensive washing protocol, and to add a suitable detergent, e.g., Tween 20® (Polysorbate 20) or increase the salt concentration of the wash buffer. A protocol that has been used in mast cell identification [30] has involved sequential washing with three separate wash buffers comprising:
Buffer A: 0.4 M NaCl, 50 mM Tris, 0.05 % Tween 20, pH 8.5.
Buffer B: 0.15 M NaCl, 50 mM Tris, 0.05 % Tween 20, pH 8.5.
Buffer C: 50 mM Tris, 0.1 % Tween 20, pH 8.5.
   As phosphate ions inhibit alkaline phosphatase activity, a TBS rather than a PBS-based wash buffer should be used where this is the reporter enzyme employed (as in the double-labelling protocol here).

4. The protocols described involve an avidin-biotin complex (ABC) amplification step which relies on the high affinity of avidin for biotin. ExtrAvidin®, a modified form of avidin that retains affinity for biotin, is associated with less nonspecific binding at neutral pH, and its use is described here. Modified forms of avidin from other suppliers include NeutrAvidin®; and the bacterially derived streptavidin has also been employed in immunohistochemistry.
   The principle of the ABC staining method is that a biotinylated secondary antibody is allowed to bind to the primary antibody once it has bound to the target antigen in tissue. This is in turn incubated with a mixture of biotinylated reporter enzyme (horseradish peroxidase or alkaline peroxidase) and free ExtrAvidin®. As avidin is tetravalent, a complex is formed that allows many more molecules of the reporter enzyme to be attached (via biotin) to the secondary antibody than would be possible by simply conjugating the enzyme directly to the immunoglobulin.
   Various reporter enzymes are available, though the methods described here are restricted to horseradish peroxidase and to alkaline phosphatase (whose use is described in the

double-labelling protocol). The techniques set out could be adapted also to use fluorescent reporters, which may be particularly suitable where several different primary antibodies are employed on the same section, though the staining pattern can be short-lived (unlike with enzyme reporters). An alternative to avidin-biotin complex amplification of signal is the labelled avidin-biotin (LAB) staining method (or LSAB where streptavidin is used instead of avidin) in which the enzyme reporter is conjugated directly to avidin (or streptavidin) molecules. Further amplification could be obtained by the use of a tertiary antibody directed against the reporter enzyme (peroxidase anti-peroxidase or phosphatase anti-phosphatase (PAP) method), though such a sensitive approach is unlikely to be required for mast cell or basophil identification in most situations.

5. When using dimethylformamide in preparing the substrate, avoid polystyrene vessels because these are attacked by the solvent. Avoid bright lights with AEC, and wear PPE.

6. A commonly used alternative substrate (to AEC) for horseradish peroxidase is 3,3'-diaminobenzidine (DAB) diluted 1:20 in substrate buffer, pH 7.5. DAB solution has to be prepared within 30 min before developing the reaction (being photosensitive, strong light should be avoided when handling it). If using DAB as substrate, washing and counterstaining should proceed as described for AEC, though thereafter, there should be dehydration in graded alcohols and clarification in Histoclear II (or other xylene substitutes), before mounting a cover slip using a synthetic organic medium (e.g., DPX).

7. Prolonged fixation in formalin-based fixatives is likely to lead to antigens being masked so that they are not recognized by the primary antibody in immunohistochemistry. Careful optimization of the antigen retrieval stage may be required in such cases.

8. A number of other commonly employed fixatives are listed above, but selection of the most appropriate for each type of tissue is beyond the scope of this chapter. Fixatives differ in their suitability for different types of tissues, and vary in their speed of penetration and in the degree of structural alterations they induce in the tissues (shrinkage, hardness rendering cutting difficult, masking of antigens, etc.).

   Tissue imprints, blood smears, cell cultures, and purified cells can be fixed with acetone (5 s, and then 10 min and then rehydrated in buffer) or 10 % neutral buffered formalin (as for tissue). Cells can also be centrifuged into a pellet (or cells resuspended in gelatine), and the pellet (or cells in gelatine) processed for histology as described for tissue specimens. Microwave treatment can be used for fixation of fresh cells or frozen tissues by heating, or can be used to speed fixation by heating tissues in fixative.

9. A temperature higher than 60 °C should be avoided during processing of tissues in wax as this can result in loss of antigenicity.

10. In general, sections should be cut thinly, as when more than 5 μm thick there are likely to be multiple layers of cells present rendering interpretation more difficult.

11. Clean slides should be soaked in a 10 % solution of poly-L-lysine for 10 min, and then air-dried with the use of a fan or a drying oven (40 °C), prior to storage or use.
    When picking sections up onto the slides, it is important that sections are flat and that they adhere to the slides without forming ridges; otherwise they may be torn off during processing.

12. Sectioned tissue on slides or cytocentrifuge preparations can be wrapped in aluminum foil and stored at 4 °C for up to 2 weeks before performing immunohistochemistry.

13. Drawing around the section with a delimiting pen is not universally practised and it may be sufficient (and less work) to simply rely on surface tension to maintain small volumes of liquid on top of the section in subsequent steps. In this case, more care may be required in wiping around the tissue sections at later stages when the surface of the slide has become wet.

14. After de-waxing and rehydration, sections can be stored for a short period with buffer to prevent drying out, but it is preferable to proceed directly to the next stage (antigen retrieval or immunohistochemistry) as soon as possible.

15. An antigen retrieval step may not be necessary for some fixatives, but is often required where there has been prolonged incubation of the tissue with formalin. Masking of the epitope so that it does not bind to primary antibody can be a consequence of formalin-induced cross-linking of peptides either within or adjacent to the epitope. This can be associated with conformational changes or alterations in charge at the epitope, such that the antibody no longer binds or fails to penetrate to the epitope.

    Though a single technique is described here, a range of antigen retrieval methods are available, and for some tissues, fixation methods, and antibodies employed, it may be necessary to try more than one for best results, as well as varying conditions for each. Heat-induced epitope retrieval is thought to reverse some of the peptide cross-linkages that occur during fixation, and allow restoration of secondary or tertiary structure at the epitope. Protease-induced epitope retrieval methods are also widely employed and involve addition of proteinase K, trypsin, pepsin, or other proteases to cleave peptides that may be masking the epitope. Protease-based methods require careful titration to avoid loss of tissue morphology or degradation of the epitope of interest with prolonged incubation with protease or too high a concentration.

16. Heat-induced epitope retrieval can be performed also using microwave ovens, pressure cookers, vegetable steamers, and autoclaves. Microwave protocols can involve 5-min periods of heat with the antigen retrieval buffer added directly to the slide, followed by replacement of the buffer.

17. Sodium azide inhibits horseradish peroxidase activity, and so should not be used as a preservative in buffers employed for immunohistochemistry with the method described using this enzyme for detection of antibody binding.

18. Antibodies should be titrated before using for the first time. As a rough guide, concentrations of monoclonal antibodies of around 1 µg/mL generally give good results, but the optimum concentration can differ between tissues processed in different ways as well as between different batches of antibody. If the type of tissue of interest is in short supply, an alternative that is more readily available can be used in antibody titration, ideally processed in exactly the same way. Staining patterns for serial dilutions of antibody should be carefully compared and a concentration of antibody selected that gives a clear signal and minimal background staining.

    Appropriate control antibodies should be employed as well as the antibody of interest. Ideally these should include a negative control antibody in the staining run, and buffer-only controls. Anti-tryptase antibody AA1 can be suitable as a positive control antibody in many situations (even where mast cells are not the principal cell of interest) as it gives a strong signal and will detect mast cells clearly in most human tissues. Detection of basophils in tissues can be more problematic, as they can be sparse or absent altogether. Confirmation that the technique for immunohistochemistry is working appropriately in such situations can be provided by including sections of tissues in which basophil infiltration has been demonstrated previously, or of a pellet of basophils or buffy coat cells that has been processed using similar histological procedures (greater volumes of such material can be produced by embedding the cells in gelatine prior to processing).

19. Incubation periods employed in immunohistochemistry are generally chosen to correspond to a point *after* the antibody-antigen reaction has achieved equilibrium. As such there is generally scope for shortening incubation periods to speed up the staining process if required, or to fit the procedure into the working day. Thus for example, instead of incubating the primary antibody overnight at 4 °C, it may be acceptable for this incubation period

to be reduced to 90 min at room temperature [30], or for a shorter period. However, once a protocol has been established in a study it should be followed consistently to minimize variation in results.

20. A xylene-based mountant such as DPX should not be used with AEC as it will solubilize the stain (though it is appropriate with other substrates such as DAB; *see* **Note 6**).

21. The protocol here is for detection of tryptase and chymase in mast cells, but it could equally well be adapted for use with pairs of antibodies specific for other markers (e.g., to localize a cell product to mast cells or basophils, or to determine the location of either of these cells in relation to other cells or structures). In order that the binding of two different primary antibodies can be visualized simultaneously, it is necessary to use different reporting enzymes for each, and to select chromogenic substrates which will yield contrasting colors. The present method employs a biotinylated antibody specific for chymase (for which the signal is amplified by avidin-biotin complex formation with alkaline phosphatase), and an antibody specific for tryptase that is labelled with horseradish peroxidase. Using this protocol, the amplification step should be for the antibody that gives the weaker signal (either on account of the properties of the antibody or the quantity of antigen available to bind). In the present case, chymase is less abundant in mast cells than tryptase [9]. It is crucial that care is exercised to get the correct balance of staining of the two target proteins, and it should be ensured that antigen retrieval steps if applied are appropriate for both antigens being studied. As with all immunohistochemistry, antibody concentrations should be titrated and incubation times selected carefully (*see* **Note 18**).

22. As alkaline phosphatase is inhibited by phosphate ions, PBS should not be employed as buffer or in washing steps in this protocol (*see* **Note 3**).

Acknowledgements

Special thanks to Professor Marius Raica from the Department of Histology of "Victor Babes" University of Medicine and Pharmacy Timisoara, Romania, and to Dr Mark Buckley, formerly of the Immunopharmacology Group, University of Southampton, UK, for fruitful discussions on immunohistochemical technique. Dr Anne-Marie Skitt and Dr Mark Buckley helped with provision of photographs. Financial support from the Medical Research Council, the National Institute for Health Research and Asthma, UK, is gratefully acknowledged.

References

1. Ehrlich P (1879) Contributions to the theory and practice of histological staining. In: Himmelweit F (ed) The collected papers of Paul Ehrlich. Pergamon Press, New York, NY, pp 65–68

2. Wesolowski J, Caldwell V, Paumet F (2012) A novel function for SNAP29 (Synaptosomal-Associated Protein of 29 kDa) in mast cell phagocytosis. PLoS One 7(11):e49886

3. Heard BE (1986) Histochemical aspects of the staining of mast cells with particular reference to heterogeneity and quantification. In: Kay AB (ed) Asthma, clinical pharmacology and therapeutic progress. Blackwell, Oxford, pp 286–294

4. Walls AF, Roberts JA, Godfrey RC, Church MK, Holgate ST (1990) Histochemical heterogeneity of human mast cells: disease-related differences in mast cell subsets recovered by bronchoalveolar lavage. Int Arch Allergy Appl Immunol 92:233–241

5. Wingren U, Enerback L (1983) Mucosal mast cells of the rat intestine: a re-evaluation of fixation and staining properties, with special reference to protein blocking and solubility of the granular glycosaminoglycan. Histochem J 15:571–582

6. Claman HN, Choi KL, Sujansky W, Vatter AE (1986) Mast cell "disappearance" in chronic murine graft-vs-host disease (GVHD) – ultrastructural demonstration of "phantom mast cells". J Immunol 137:2009–2013

7. Craig SS, DeBlois G, Schwartz LB (1986) Mast cells in human keloid, small intestine, and lung by an immunoperoxidase technique using a murine monoclonal antibody against tryptase. Am J Pathol 124:427–435

8. Walls AF, Jones DB, Williams JH, Church MK, Holgate ST (1990) Immunohistochemical identification of mast cells in formaldehyde-fixed tissue using monoclonal antibodies specific for tryptase. J Pathol 162:119–126

9. Schwartz LB, Irani A-MA, Roller K, Castells MC, Schechter NM (1987) Quantitation of histamine, tryptase and chymase in dispersed human T and TC mast cells. J Immunol 138:2611–2615

10. Castells MC, Irani AM, Schwartz LB (1987) Evaluation of human peripheral blood leukocytes for mast cell tryptase. J Immunol 138:2184–2189

11. Mayrhofer G, Gadd SJ, Spargo LD, Ashman LK (1987) Specificity of a mouse monoclonal antibody raised against acute myeloid leukaemia cells for mast cells in human mucosal and connective tissues. Immunol Cell Biol 65:241–250

12. Johansson O, Virtanen M, Hilliges M, Yang Q (1994) Histamine immunohistochemistry is superior to the conventional heparin-based routine staining methodology for investigations of human skin mast cells. Histochem J 26:424–430

13. Xu X, Zhang D, Zhang H, Wolters PJ, Killeen NP, Sullivan BM, Locksley RM, Lowell CA, Caughey GH (2006) Neutrophil histamine contributes to inflammation in mycoplasma pneumonia. J Exp Med 203:2907–2917

14. Oh C, Suzuki S, Nakashima I, Yamashita K, Nakano K (1988) Histamine synthesis by non-mast cells through mitogen-dependent induction of histidine decarboxylase. Immunology 65:143–148

15. Alcañiz L, Vega A, Chacón P, El Bekay R, Ventura I, Aroca R, Blanca M, Bergstralh DT, Monteseirín J (2013) Histamine production by human neutrophils. FASEB J 27:2902–2910

16. Irani A-MA, Bradford TR, Kepley CL, Schechter NM, Schwartz LB (1989) Detection of MCT and MCTC types of human mast cells by immunohistochemistry using new monoclonal anti-tryptase and anti-chymase antibodies. J Histochem Cytochem 37:1509–1515

17. Buckley MG, McEuen AR, Walls AF (1999) The detection of mast cell subpopulations in formalin-fixed human tissues using a new monoclonal antibody specific for chymase. J Pathol 189:138–143

18. Walls AF (2000) The roles of neutral proteases in asthma and rhinitis. In: Busse WW, Holgate ST (eds) Asthma and rhinitis, 2nd edn. Blackwell, Boston, MA, pp 968–998

19. Irani A-MA, Bradford TR, Schwartz LB (1991) Human mast cell carboxypeptidase. Selective localization to MCTC cells. J Immunol 147:247–253

20. Schechter NM, Irani AM, Sprows JL, Abernethy J, Wintroub B, Schwartz LB (1990) Identification of a cathepsin G-like proteinase in the MCTC type of human mast cell. J Immunol 145:2652–2661

21. Bradding P, Walls AF, Holgate ST (2006) The role of the mast cell in the pathophysiology of asthma. J Allergy Clin Immunol 117:1277–1284

22. KleinJan A, Godthelp T, Blom HM, Fokkens WJ (1996) Fixation with Carnoy's fluid reduces the number of chymase-positive mast cells: not all chymase-positive mast cells are also positive for tryptase. Allergy 51:614–620

23. Beil WJ, Schulz M, McEuen AR, Buckley MG, Walls AF (1997) Number, fixation properties, dye-binding and protease expression of duodenal mast cells: comparisons between healthy subjects and patients with gastritis or Crohn's disease. Histochem J 29:759–773

24. Foster B, Schwartz LB, Devouassoux G, Metcalfe DD, Prussin C (2002) Characterization of mast-cell tryptase-expressing peripheral blood cells as basophils. J Allergy Clin Immunol 109:287–293

25. Kepley CL, Craig SS, Schwartz LB (1995) Identification and partial characterization of a unique marker for human basophils. J Immunol 154:6548–6555

26. McEuen AR, Buckley MG, Compton SJ, Walls AF (1999) Development and characterization of a monoclonal antibody specific for human basophils and the identification of a unique secretory product of basophil activation. Lab Invest 79:27–38

27. Mochizuki A, McEuen AR, Buckley MG, Walls AF (2003) The release of basogranulin in response to IgE-dependent and IgE-independent stimuli: validity of basogranulin measurement as an indicator of basophil activation. J Allergy Clin Immunol 112:102–108

28. Kepley CL, Pfeiffer JR, Schwartz LB, Wilson BS, Oliver JM (1998) The identification and characterization of umbilical cord blood-derived human basophils. J Leuk Biol 64:474–483

29. McEuen AR, Calafat J, Compton SJ, Easom NJ, Buckley MG, Knol EF, Walls AF (2001) Mass, charge, and subcellular localization of a unique secretory product identified by the basophil-specific antibody BB1. J Allergy Clin Immunol 107:842–848

30. Buckley MG, Walls AF (2008) Identification of mast cells and mast cell subpopulations. In: Jones MG, Lympany P (eds) Allergy methods and protocols, vol 138, Methods in molecular medicine. Humana, Totowa, NJ, pp 285–297

Chapter 10

Measuring Histamine and Cytokine Release from Basophils and Mast Cells

Bettina M. Jensen, Sidsel Falkencrone, and Per S. Skov

Abstract

Basophils and mast cells are known for their capability to release both preformed and newly synthesized inflammatory mediators. In this chapter we describe how to stimulate and detect histamine released from basophils in whole blood, purified basophils, in vitro cultured mast cells, and in situ skin mast cells. We also give an example of an activation protocol for basophil and mast cell cytokine release and discuss approaches for cytokine detection.

Key words Basophils, Mast cells, Histamine, Cytokines

---

1 Introduction

Basophils and mast cells are granulocytes, the former usually residing in the blood, and the latter in other tissues, which play an important role in inflammatory responses. Mast cells have long been known to be one of the "troublemakers" of allergic reactions (characterized by the presence of allergen-specific IgE) due to the expression of high-affinity IgE receptors (FcɛRI) which, when cross-linked, causes mast cells to degranulate. Even though basophils also express FcɛRI they seem to have a more secondary role in the allergic reaction. Nevertheless, both basophils and mast cells can produce a large repertoire of inflammatory mediators when activated via FcɛRI. The IgE-mediated activation of basophils and mast cells is, however, not the only way to stimulate these cells to degranulation. Other well-known triggers of activation are complement components, TLR ligands, and neurogenic factors (primarily for mast cells). In addition formyl-methionyl-leucyl-phenylalanine (fMLP) is a well-known basophil activator [1–3] whereas compound 48/80 has been used as a mast cell activator [4–6].

Bernhard F. Gibbs and Franco H. Falcone (eds.), *Basophils and Mast Cells: Methods and Protocols*, Methods in Molecular Biology, vol. 1192, DOI 10.1007/978-1-4939-1173-8_10, © Springer Science+Business Media New York 2014

In the following we describe some of the main mediators released by basophils and mast cells, primarily after cross-linking of FcεRI, and give examples of methods to detect these mediators.

1.1 Histamine

Histamine is a biogenic amine derived from the decarboxylation of the amino acid histidine, a reaction catalyzed by the enzyme L-histidine decarboxylase. Histamine is found pre-stored in the granules within basophils and mast cells and can therefore quickly be released after stimulation. Activation caused by cross-linking of FcεRI will result in histamine release [7]. However, non-IgE-mediated stimuli such as complement 3a and 5a, substance P, fMLP, or compound 48/80 can also result in histamine release. Activation through TLRs can also result in histamine release but only from certain phenotypes of mast cells [8–12].

1.2 Cytokines

In contrast to histamine, cytokines belong to the group of newly generated mediators meaning that basophils and mast cells in general do not contain large amounts of pre-stored cytokines. Nevertheless, TNFα might be found in resting mast cells [13].

As is the case for histamine release, cross-linking of FcεRI will result in cytokine release from both basophils and mast cells but the range and amount of cytokines released from the two cell types are not identical. Mast cells appear to release a broader range of cytokines when compared to basophils and, depending on the mast cell phenotype, the following cytokines have been associated with FcεRI stimulation: IL-1β, IL-5, IL-6, IL-8, IL-10, IL-13, IFNα, GM-CSF, TNFα, and VEGF [7, 14]. The major cytokines released from basophils after FcεRI stimulation are IL-4, IL-13, and VEGF but new cytokines are still reported such as TNFα [15].

TLRs have been described to activate both basophils and mast cells to release cytokines [8–11].

2 Materials

2.1 Histamine Release and Detection

1. 96-well glass fiber coated plates (RLA 210) and HR-Test Reagent kit HISTAREADER (RLA700) (RefLab, Member of R-Biopharm Group).
2. PIPES buffer: 3.02 g PIPES sodium salt, 19.05 g $CH_3COONa \cdot 3H_2O$, 0.491 g CH_3COOK, 0.088 g $CaCl_2 \cdot 2H_2O$, 0.224 g $MgCl_2 \cdot 6H_2O$, distilled water up to 1 L, adjust pH to 7.4 with 1 M Trizma-base.
3. Histamine release buffer (HR-buffer): PIPES + 0.5 % human serum albumin.
4. Distilled water with a conductivity of <20 μS/cm.
5. Reagents for maximal histamine release: Phorbol 12-myristate 13-acetate (PMA) (1 μg/mL final concentration) and ionomycin (5 μg/mL final concentration).

6. Incubator at 37 °C.

7. Microdialysis fibers: Assemble dialysis fibers by threading single-dialysis fibers from a hemodialysator (model GFE 18; Gambro Dialysaten AG, Hechingen, Germany) with a 0.1 mm stainless steel guidewire (Sandvik A/S) and glue this to nylon tubing.

8. Cannulas (23G).

9. Syringes (1 mL).

10. Catheter connector 20–24 G (B. Braun Medical, Melsungen, Germany).

11. Micro-injection pumps (CMA/100; CMA/Microdialysis, Stockholm, Sweden).

12. High-sensitivity fluorometer.

2.2 Cytokine Release and Detection

1. Basophil culture medium: RPMI 1640, penicillin/streptomycin (100 U/mL/100 µg/mL), L-glutamine (1 mM), human AB serum (5 % v/v).

2. 48-well cell culture plate.

3. CO_2 incubator.

3   Methods

3.1 Histamine Release and Detection

Stimulation of basophils and mast cells to release histamine varies depending on the cell source and therefore different techniques are described below. However, the method to detect histamine is the same and the one described in this chapter is dependent on glass fiber-coated plates and fluorometric detection. Other protocols for histamine detection, like histamine ELISAs, can also be used according to the manufacturer's guidelines, but they are not described here.

All the reagents used for cell activation are made up 2× the final concentration (e.g., if cells will be stimulated with 100 ng/mL anti-IgE make solutions of 200 ng/mL anti-IgE). Avoid concentrations above 1 mg/mL since such solutions might cause unspecific binding to the glass fibers. A typical anti-IgE titration curve could range from 1 ng/mL to 1 µg/mL (*see* **Note 1**). Do not include fetal bovine serum in the buffer since it contains diamine oxidase which degrades histamine.

In order to express the results as % histamine release, one can include a stimulation of the cells using a solution of phorbol 12-myristate 13-acetate (PMA) (1 µg/mL final concentration) and ionomycin (5 µg/mL final concentration) in order to obtain a "maximal" histamine release.

It is also possible to lyse the cells and thereby estimate the total histamine content. This can be done by lysing 100 µL cell suspension with 30 μL 7 % HClO$_4$ (vortex after adding the HClO$_4$) for 5 min at room temperature followed by neutralization with 100 μL PIPES buffer.

3.1.1 Histamine Reaction in Whole Blood

1. Heparinized blood (use within 24 h after venipuncture) is centrifuged (600 ×*g*, 10 min, 20 °C).

2. Mark the level of the total volume (blood cells and plasma) and remove the plasma (*see* **Note 2**).

3. Reconstitute the plasma volume with PIPES buffer (add buffer up to the marked level) and mix the blood by inverting the tube. This is now termed "washed blood."

4. Use a 96-well glass fiber-coated plate (*see* Fig. 1). Add 50 μL PIPES buffer to the first column (includes a histamine standard) and rows A and B (these are kept for background values) on the plate. Add 50 μL stimulant of interest to the other wells. Add 50 μL washed blood to all wells (also the first column and rows A and B).

5. Immediately after adding the washed blood to the plate, cover it with a lid (do not cover it by tape) and incubate at 37 °C for 1 h. During this time, stimulated basophils will release histamine which will then bind to the glass fibers present in the plate. The histamine release can sometimes be improved by adding IL-3 to the blood (*see* **Note 3**); however, not all blood donors have responding basophils (*see* **Note 4**).

6. After incubation the blood cells are removed by washing the plate; add 100 μL distilled water (conductivity <20 μS/cm) to

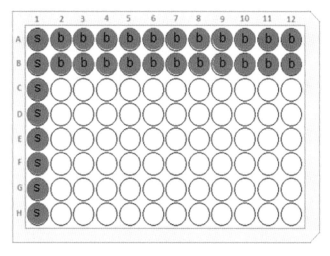

Fig. 1 Design of a glass fiber-coated plate. *Grey wells* are for buffer (*s* histamine standard, *b* blanks). *White wells* are for samples

the wells, aspirate by inverting plate over a sink, add 200 μL distilled water, and aspirate again by inverting the plate over a sink (*see* **Note 5**).

7. Repeat this two more times and finish by taping the plate semidry on paper (*see* **Note 6**).

8. The plate can now either be stored (upside down and protected from light) for 1 month or used immediately for histamine detection according to Subheading 3.1.4.

3.1.2 Histamine Reaction with Purified Basophils

In order to obtain pure basophils it is preferable to use a negative selection protocol since positive selection may cause activation of the cells, leaving them desensitized and thereby unable to release histamine during the experiment.

1. Centrifuge the purified basophils and resuspend in HR buffer to a concentration of 100,000 cells/mL.

2. Prepare reagents in HR buffer and add 50 μL to a v-shaped 96-well plate.

3. Add 50 μL cell suspension to the plate, cover it with a lid (do not cover it by tape), and incubate at 37 °C for 1 h. During this time stimulated basophils will release histamine.

4. Reconstitute a glass fiber-coated 96-well plate by adding 25 μL PIPES buffer to all wells.

5. Centrifuge the cell plate (10 min, $300 \times g$, 4 °C, acc 5, brake 3) and transfer 25 μL supernatant to wells designed for samples in the reconstituted glass fiber-coated plate.

6. Add HR buffer to the first lane (histamine standard) and to the blanks (A2-A12, B2-B12) (*see* Fig. 1).

7. Cover the glass fiber plate with a lid and incubate for 30 min at 37 °C.

8. Wash the plate with distilled water; add 150 μL distilled water (conductivity <20 μS/cm) to the wells, aspirate by inverting plate over a sink, add 200 μL distilled water, and aspirate again by inverting plate over a sink.

9. Repeat this two more times and finish by taping the plate semidry on paper. An ELISA plate washer can also be used for the washing procedure as described in **Note 5**.

10. The plate can now either be stored (upside down and protected from light) for 1 month or used right away for histamine detection according to Subheading 3.1.4.

3.1.3 Histamine Reaction with In Vitro Cultured Human Mast Cells

Stem cell-derived human mast cells (*see* Chapter 4) do not have IgE bound to their high-affinity IgE receptors and therefore need to be sensitized if IgE-dependent histamine release is to be studied. IgE sensitization can be performed by culturing the cells overnight with 100 ng/mL–1 μg/mL human IgE.

1. Centrifuge the human mast cells and resuspend in HR buffer to a concentration of 100,000 cells/mL.

2. Prepare reagents in HR buffer and add 50 μL to a v-shaped 96-well plate.

3. Add 50 μL cell suspension to the plate, cover it with a lid (do not cover it by tape), and incubate at 37 °C for 1 h. During this time stimulated mast cells will release histamine.

4. Assay histamine release as described earlier (Subheading 3.1.2, steps **4–10**).

3.1.4 Histamine Reaction with In Situ Mast Cells

Microdialysis is a minimally invasive sampling technique used for continuous measurement of substances in the extracellular fluid of virtually any tissue. It has traditionally been used to assess neurotransmitters and hormones in neuroscience and to measure exogenous compounds (e.g., pharmaceuticals) to investigate distribution within the body [16–18]. Microdialysis is, however, also a highly relevant technique when applied to the skin for investigation of the various functions of tissue-residing mast cells. While human primary tissue-residing mast cells can be isolated, it is not clear as to what degree tissue dispersion and subsequent isolation with digestive enzymes affect mast cell functions [19]. Microdialysis in the skin can be performed in vivo in humans and experimental animals [20–22] but can also be used to investigate mast cell functions in excised skin since these mast cells remain responsive several hours after the skin is removed (unpublished data).

1. Introduce 23G cannulas into the upper dermis at a length of 1 cm and a depth of 0.7 mm.

2. Introduce microdialysis fibers into the skin by threading the fiber through the 23G guide cannula and remove the cannula to leave the fiber in the skin (*see* **Note 7**).

3. Connect the inlet of each dialysis fiber to individual syringes mounted in micro-injection pumps (CMA/100; CMA/ Microdialysis, Stockholm, Sweden).

4. Perfuse the fibers in parallel at a rate of 3.0 μL/min with NaCl or PIPES buffer (*see* **Note 8**).

5. Challenge the skin sites above the fibers by injecting 50 μL buffer/activator intradermally.

6. After challenge, collect eluates from the microdialysis fibers for 30 min and analyze for histamine according to Subheading 3.1.1, steps **2–5**.

3.1.5 Histamine Detection

1. Allow the HR-Test Reagent Kit HISTAREADER to reach room temperature (20–25 °C) before use.

2. Prepare coupling reagent by transferring 1 OPA disc to the bottle containing 10 mL diluent for coupling reaction (sufficient for one plate).

3. Leave the reaction mix for 45 min (avoid light). Invert the bottle gently before use. The disc will *not* dissolve.

4. In order to remove blood compounds that still might be present add 150 μL wash solution to the plates. Incubate the plate for 30 min at 37 °C.

5. Aspirate the wash buffer by inverting plate over a sink and then rinse the plate three times; add 200 μL distilled water and aspirate again by inverting the plate over a sink.

6. Repeat this two more times and finish by taping the plate on highly absorbent paper towel until it is free of any residual water.

7. Add 75 μL coupling reagent to all used wells and leave plate for exactly 10 min.

8. Stop the reaction by adding 75 μL stop solution into the wells.

9. Read the plate using a highly sensitive fluorometer within the same day. *See* **Note 9** for calculation of % histamine release.

3.2 Cytokine Release and Detection

Cytokine secretion experiments are often more time consuming than histamine release since many cytokines need to be produced before the cells can release them. However, the secretion rate can be different which is why studies have to be designed according to the specific cytokine of interest. Please note that, if anti-IgE-mediated cytokine release is to be studied in in vitro generated human mast cells, it is necessary to sensitize the cells with IgE before activation (*see* Subheading 3.1.3). All the reagents used for cell activation are made up to 10× the final concentration (if cells will be stimulated with 100 ng/mL anti-IgE make solutions of 1,000 ng/mL anti-IgE). The volume of the cell samples depends on the following analysis but cultures of 200 μL should be sufficient for most cytokine analysis and it is the volume used in the description below.

3.2.1 Cytokine Release with Purified Basophils or In Vitro-Cultured Human Mast Cells

1. Centrifuge the purified basophils or in vitro-cultured human mast cells ($300 \times g$, 10 min, room temp.).

2. Resuspend in basophil or mast cell culture media, respectively, to a cell density of 1.11×10^6 cells/mL. This will result in a final density of 10^6 cells/mL in the cell sample. The culture medium for basophils is given in Subheading 2; for human mast cells the choice of culture medium depends on the culture protocol used (*see* Chapter 4).

3. Use a 48-well cell culture plate and add 20 μL of stimulant or medium to the wells. Add 180 μL cell suspension and place the culture plate in the CO_2 incubator (37 °C) for a time point relevant for the specific cytokine of interest (which can vary from 4 to 24 h).

4. After incubation, transfer the cell suspension to 0.5 mL tubes and centrifuge ($300 \times g$, 10 min, 4 °C). Save the supernatant (containing released cytokines) and continue with cytokine detection or store the supernatant at –80 °C until further analysis. Avoid freeze/thaw cycles (*see* **Note 10**).

3.2.2 Cytokine Detection

Quantification of cytokines can be performed in several ways and many commercial ELISA kits and multiplex technologies are available. Most of these kits are ready-to-use assays and accompanied by a clear protocol from the manufacturer.

The ELISA assays are typically offered as ready-coated 96-well plates with prepared reagents for a quick and convenient way to determine one cytokine per sample. Several companies also offer ELISA assays as kits consisting of a standard, HRP-streptavidin, and capture and detection antibodies. These kits require more preparation time and method optimization but once established can be a more economic and customizable assay when measuring larger quantities of samples. The ELISA method does not require specific laboratory equipment except from a plate reader and the procedure takes only between 1 and 2 days depending on the ELISA kit. The detection limit is generally good (down to 10–100 pg/mL) but since only a single cytokine can be measured per ELISA, you will need many cells in order to generate enough material for several cytokine tests.

The multiplex technology has added a new dimension to the cytokine detection. Several cytokines can now be measured in the same sample using a bead-antibody-fluorometric based platform and it appears that only the number of cytokines in the catalogue sets the limit of cytokines which can be detected in one sample. In comparison to the ELISA, most multiplex assay can be run in a 96-well plate format but the cytokine detection requires a special flow cytometer which some laboratories might not have. On the other hand, the detection limit is quite good (down to few pg/mL) and sometimes lower compared with an ELISA. Unfortunately, there might be variations between multiplex assays since differences in reproducibility and absolute quantities of detected cytokines have been reported [23–25].

4 Notes

1. The histamine release curve is bell shaped. Therefore, it is important to find the right concentration—too low or too high a concentration will result in no or very little histamine release.

2. Be careful not to disturb the white blood cell layer on top of the red blood cells (leave 2 mm plasma above the cell layer).

3. IL-3 will often improve the basophil histamine release. Concentrations from 10 pg/mL to 1 ng/mL have been used to potentiate the anti-IgE mediated histamine release. Higher concentrations might cause histamine release by IL-3 alone.

4. 10–20 % of the population has non-releasing basophils [26]. This term is used when basophils do not release histamine when stimulated with anti-IgE. However, other stimuli, like fMLP, will activate these cells to release histamine [27].

5. An ELISA plate washer can also be used for the washing procedure. You must be able to adjust the nozzles for dispensing and aspiration so that they are 2–3 mm above the fiber matrix. Run three cycles with distilled water (conductivity <20 µS/cm). It is very important that the ELISA plate washer is clean of regular ELISA wash buffers. Salt solutions will disturb the histamine binding.

6. No blood should be visible in the plate. If so, repeat one more wash cycle or, if the blood is at the side of the well, remove it with cotton swabs without disturbing the fiber matrix.

7. Microdialysis fibers can be assembled but require specially made guidewire for stability.

8. Allow a recovery phase of 10 min before initiation of the experiments to wash out any histamine released due to insertion trauma from the cannula. Physiological saline can be used for perfusion; alternatively use PIPES buffer which is a buffer adjusted to give optimal histamine release.

9. Expression of % histamine release: The glass fiber plate contains blank wells and wells with 50 ng histamine which is used for calculating the histamine concentration in the unknown sample:

$$ng/mL\ histamine\ in\ sample = (Sample_{FU} - Blank_{FU})/(50\ ng_{FU} - Blank_{FU})$$

where $Blank_{FU}$ is the mean fluorescence intensity of the blank wells (A1-D1) and $50\ ng_{FU}$ is the mean fluorescence intensity of the wells containing 50 ng histamine (well E1-H1). $Sample_{FU}$ is the fluorescence intensity of the sample. The % histamine release (of maximal release) can be calculated from the PMA/ionomycin results:

$$\%\ Histamine\ release = (histamine\ in\ sample/histamine\ in\ PMA/ionomycin) \times 100\%$$

10. When measuring mediator release from both mast cells and basophils please be aware that the supernatants may contain large amounts of proteases that can degrade the cytokines present. If possible, keep your supernatants at –80 °C until measuring and avoid freeze-thaw cycles for the best possible outcome.

References

1. Ishizaka T, Dvorak AM, Conrad DH, Niebyl JR, Marquette JP, Ishizaka K (1985) Morphologic and immunologic characterization of human basophils developed in cultures of cord blood mononuclear cells. J Immunol 134:532–540

2. Nolte H, Spjeldnaes N, Kruse A, Windelborg B (1990) Histamine release from gut mast cells from patients with inflammatory bowel diseases. Gut 31:791–794

3. Okayama Y, Church MK (1992) IL-3 primes and evokes histamine release from human basophils but not mast cells. Int Arch Allergy Immunol 99:343–345

4. Hate KR, Schneider R (1966) The difference in behaviour of basophil leucocytes and mast cells towards compound 48/80. Br J Pharmacol Chemother 28:282–288

5. Lowman MA, Rees PH, Benyon RC, Church MK (1988) Human mast cell heterogeneity: histamine release from mast cells dispersed from skin, lung, adenoids, tonsils, and colon in response to IgE-dependent and nonimmunologic stimuli. J Allergy Clin Immunol 81: 590–597

6. Oskeritzian CA, Zhao W, Min HK, Xia HZ, Pozez A, Kiev J, Schwartz LB (2005) Surface CD88 functionally distinguishes the MCTC from the MCT type of human lung mast cell. J Allergy Clin Immunol 115:1162–1168

7. Galli SJ, Nakae S, Tsai M (2005) Mast cells in the development of adaptive immune responses. Nat Immunol 6:135–142

8. Sumbayev VV, Yasinska I, Oniku AE, Streatfield CL, Gibbs BF (2012) Involvement of hypoxia-inducible factor-1 in the inflammatory responses of human LAD2 mast cells and basophils. PLoS One 7:e34259

9. McCurdy JD, Olynych TJ, Maher LH, Marshall JS (2003) Cutting edge: distinct Toll-like receptor 2 activators selectively induce different classes of mediator production from human mast cells. J Immunol 170:1625–1629

10. Varadaradjalou S, Feger F, Thieblemont N, Hamouda NB, Pleau JM, Dy M, Arock M (2003) Toll-like receptor 2 (TLR2) and TLR4 differentially activate human mast cells. Eur J Immunol 33:899–906

11. Kulka M, Alexopoulou L, Flavell RA, Metcalfe DD (2004) Activation of mast cells by double-stranded RNA: evidence for activation through Toll-like receptor 3. J Allergy Clin Immunol 114:174–182

12. Supajatura V, Ushio H, Nakao A, Akira S, Okumura K, Ra C, Ogawa H (2002) Differential responses of mast cell Toll-like receptors 2 and 4 in allergy and innate immunity. J Clin Invest 109:1351–1359

13. Zhang B, Alysandratos KD, Angelidou A, Asadi S, Sismanopoulos N, Delivanis DA, Weng Z, Miniati A, Vasiadi M, Katsarou-Katsari A, Miao B, Leeman SE, Kalogeromitros D, Theoharides TC (2011) Human mast cell degranulation and preformed TNF secretion require mitochondrial translocation to exocytosis sites: relevance to atopic dermatitis. J Allergy Clin Immunol 127:1522–1531

14. Galli SJ, Tsai M (2012) IgE and mast cells in allergic disease. Nat Med 4:693–704

15. Falkencrone S, Poulsen LK, Bindslev-Jensen C, Woetmann A, Odum N, Poulsen BC, Blom L, Jensen BM, Gibbs BF, Yasinska IM, Sumbayev VV, Skov PS (2013) IgE-mediated basophil tumour necrosis factor alpha induces matrix metalloproteinase-9 from monocytes. Allergy 68:614–620

16. Blakeley J, Portnow J (2010) Microdialysis for assessing intratumoral drug disposition in brain cancers: a tool for rational drug development. Expert Opin Drug Metab Toxicol 6: 1477–1491

17. Boddu SH, Gunda S, Earla R, Mitra AK (2010) Ocular microdialysis: a continuous sampling technique to study pharmacokinetics and pharmacodynamics in the eye. Bioanalysis 2:487–507

18. Plock N, Kloft C (2005) Microdialysis–theoretical background and recent implementation in applied life-sciences. Eur J Pharm Sci 25: 1–24

19. Kulka M, Metcalfe DD (2010) Isolation of tissue mast cells. *Curr Protoc Immunol* Chapter 7:Unit 7.25

20. Brazis P, Barandica L, Garcia F, Clough GF, Church MK, Puigdemont A (2006) Dermal microdialysis in the dog: in vivo assessment of the effect of cyclosporin A on cutaneous histamine and prostaglandin D2 release. Vet Dermatol 17:169–174

21. Groth L, Jorgensen A, Serup J (1998) Cutaneous microdialysis in the rat: insertion trauma and effect of anaesthesia studied by laser Doppler perfusion imaging and histamine release. Skin Pharmacol Appl Skin Physiol 11: 125–132

22. Petersen LJ, Church MK, Skov PS (1997) Histamine is released in the wheal but not the flare following challenge of human skin in vivo: a microdialysis study. Clin Exp Allergy 27: 284–295

23. Berthoud TK, Manaca MN, Quelhas D, Aguilar R, Guinovart C, Puyol L, Barbosa A, Alonso PL, Dobaño C (2011) Comparison of commercial kits to measure cytokine responses to Plasmodium falciparum by multiplex microsphere suspension array technology. Malar J 10:1–9

24. Breen EC, Reynolds SM, Cox C, Jacobson LP, Magpantay L, Mulder CB, Dibben O, Margolick JB, Bream JH, Sambrano E, Martínez-Maza O, Sinclair E, Borrow P, Landay AL, Rinaldo CR, Norris PJ (2011) Multisite comparison of high-sensitivity multiplex cytokine assays. Clin Vaccine Immunol 18:1229–1242

25. Moncunill G, Aponte JJ, Nhabomba AJ, Dobaño C (2013) Performance of multiplex commercial kits to quantify cytokine and chemokine responses in culture supernatants from Plasmodium falciparum stimulations. PLoS One 8:1–10

26. Kepley CL, Youssef L, Andrews RP, Wilson BS, Oliver JM (1999) Syk deficiency in nonreleaser basophils. J Allergy Clin Immunol 104:279–284

27. Knol EF, Mul FP, Kuijpers TW, Verhoeven AJ, Roos D (1992) Intracellular events in anti-IgE nonreleasing human basophils. J Allergy Clin Immunol 90:92–103

Chapter 11

Flow Cytometric Allergy Diagnosis: Basophil Activation Techniques

Chris H. Bridts, Vito Sabato, Christel Mertens, Margo M. Hagendorens, Luc S. De Clerck, and Didier G. Ebo

Abstract

The basis of flow cytometric allergy diagnosis is quantification of changes in expression of basophilic surface membrane markers (Ebo et al., Clin Exp Allergy 34: 332–339, 2004). Upon encountering specific allergens recognized by surface receptor FcεRI-bound IgE, basophils not only secrete and generate quantifiable bioactive mediators but also up-regulate the expression of different markers (e.g., CD63, CD203c) which can be detected by multicolor flow cytometry using specific monoclonal antibodies (Ebo et al., Cytometry B Clin Cytom 74: 201–210, 2008). Here, we describe two flow cytometry-based protocols which allow detection of surface marker activation (Method 1) and changes in intragranular histamine (Method 2), both reflecting different facets of basophil activation.

Key words Basophil activation tests, CD203c, CD63, HistaFlow

1 Introduction

Basophil activation assays have predominantly focused on histamine and leukotriene release assays. However, time-consuming procedures were needed to isolate cells, to incubate with activators, and to quantify (sometimes labile) mediators. Two decades ago, the discovery of the markers CD63 (a.k.a. gp53) and subsequently CD203c (a.k.a. ENPP-3) facilitated the development of a novel technique to analyze and quantify allergen-specific in vitro activation of basophils: the so-called basophil activation test (BAT) [2]. Briefly, the BAT relies on a flow cytometric identification and quantification of various specific activation markers on the surface membrane or activated proteins inside the cells. These changes can be detected and quantified on a single-cell level using specific monoclonal antibodies coupled to fluorochromes. Practically, basophils are identified by specific markers such as CCR3/CD3 [3], CD123/HLA-DR [4], or IgE/CD203c [5]. Of these markers, only CD203c is lineage specific. Subsequently, after activation with

Bernhard F. Gibbs and Franco H. Falcone (eds.), *Basophils and Mast Cells: Methods and Protocols*, Methods in Molecular Biology, vol. 1192, DOI 10.1007/978-1-4939-1173-8_11, © Springer Science+Business Media New York 2014

an allergen, the upregulation or the appearance of specific surface activation markers, such as CD63 and/or CD203c, can be measured. Activation of basophils can also be quantified by means of intracellular molecules, such as phosphorylation of MAPK (p38MAPK) [6, 7] or STAT5 (pSTAT5) [8]. At present, BAT has proven to be a rapid and reliable diagnostic method that allows the diagnosis of allergy to various allergens like food (including pollen-related food allergies), natural rubber latex, hymenoptera venom, and certain drugs. In addition, the technique has proven to be useful in non-IgE-mediated reactions, such as in drug hypersensitivity as well as in the detection of IgG anti-FcεRI or anti-IgE autoantibodies in chronic autoimmune urticaria.

Finally, it was recently shown that intracellular histamine and its release by in vitro-activated basophils can successfully be analyzed by multicolor flow cytometry (HistaFlow) [9] applying an enzyme-affinity fluorochrome method, based on the affinity of the histaminase diamine oxidase for its substrate [10]. We developed a flow cytometric technique (HistaFlow) which enables the measurement of histamine release by individual basophils in combination with cell membrane markers. Conjugating diamine oxidase to fluorochromes together with phenotyping activated basophils, histamine content, and release can be quantified in whole blood with standardized flow cytometry techniques.

2 Materials

All solutions must be prepared with sterile ultrapure water. We use a Millipore Milli Q System and water purification is performed with the use of a reversed osmosis system followed by ultra-purification to attain 18 MΩ at room temperature.

2.1 Blood Sample

10 mL peripheral heparinized blood is obtained and immediately brought to the laboratory. Incubation and analysis must be completed within 8 h (see **Note 1**).

2.2 Reagents

1. Interleukin-3 (IL-3)
   IL-3 is sometimes used to preactivate ("prime") basophils. It must be noted that IL-3 can upregulate CD203c.

   (a) Stock solution: 10 μg IL-3 in 10 mL water, divide per 100 μL in sterile tubes. Store at –20 °C.

   (b) Storage solution: Dilute 100 μL stock solution in 5 mL BAT buffer and divide per 500 μL. Store at –20 °C.

   (c) Working solution: Dilute storage solution with an equal volume of buffer; prepare daily before use. The final concentration is 10 ng/mL.

2. BAT buffer

   (a) A BAT buffer is prepared under STERILE conditions just before use.

   (b) Dilute 1.9 mL Hanks' balanced salt solution 10× concentrated (HBSS with Ca^{2+} and Mg^{2+}) with 17 mL H_2O.

   (c) Add 0.6 mL 7.5 % $NaHCO_3$.

   (d) Add 0.4 mL 1 M Hepes.

   (e) Adjust pH to 7.4.

3. Lysis solution
   Lysis solution (BD Biosciences) is diluted 1:10 with water and stored at room temperature.

4. Phosphate-buffered saline (PBS 1×)

   (a) PBS (10× concentrated without Ca^{2+} or Mg^2) is diluted with water to obtain an isotonic PBS (1×) buffer. Adjust pH to 7.4.

5. PBS-EDTA
   Dissolve 10 mmol/L Na_2EDTA in PBS (1×). Adjust pH to 7.4.

6. PBS-NaN_3
   Dissolve 0.5 g/L NaN_3 in PBS (1×). Adjust pH to 7.4. Store at room temperature.

7. PBS-0.1 % BSA
   Mix 50 mL PBS with 0.66 mL BSA (albumin bovine fraction V 7.5 %); pH should be 7.4.

8. Anti-human IgE Alexa Fluor©488 (aIgE)
   Since anti-IgE (Sigma-Aldrich, Clone GE-1) is currently not available conjugated with an Alexa Fluor©488 Dye, this antibody is labeled in house using the procedure by the manufacturer Life Technologies described in Subheading 3 below.

9. CD63-PE or CD63-FITC
   Anti-CD63-PE or anti-CD63-FITC (BD Biosciences) must be stored at 2–8 °C in the dark. This antibody is ready to use (*see* **Note 2**).

10. Anti-CD123-PE/anti-HLAdr-PERCP/anti-CD63-FITC
    All antibodies available commercially ready to use (BD BioSciences) (*see* **Note 2**).

11. Mouse anti-human IgE (mHu-antiIgE)

    (a) This antibody (BD Biosciences, clone G7-18) is used as a positive control to stimulate basophils. Stock solution: 0.5 mg/mL in BAT buffer.

    (b) Working solution: Between 1 and 10 µg/mL in BAT buffer.

12. CD203c-APC
    Anti human CD203c (clone NP4D6) labeled with APC (BD Biosciences or BioLegend), ready to use (*see* **Note 2**).

13. Allergens
    Allergens can be protein extracts, recombinant proteins, or drugs. They must be water soluble and used in concentrations which are not toxic for basophils (*see* **Note 3**).

14. DAO-PE or DAO-V500 (BD Biosciences)

    (a) Diamine oxidase or histaminase (Sigma-Aldrich) has been conjugated with phycoerythrine or Horizon V500 at the laboratories of BD Biosciences.

    (b) Prepare a working solution 1:1 (DAO-PE) or 1:20 (DAO-V500) in PBS/EDTA. Every new batch has to be titrated and measured with a flow cytometer in order to find the optimal staining concentration for intracellular histamine.

15. Lysis/fixing solution (BD Biosciences)

    (a) BD Phosflow Lyse/Fix buffer (5× concentrate: BD Biosciences) is used to lyse and fix whole blood for use with intracellular staining techniques. Store at room temperature.

    (b) Dilute 1:5 just before use in H_2O.

16. PBS-TX100
    Working solution is 0.1 % Triton X-100 in PBS: Add 0.1 mL pure Triton X-100 (Sigma-Aldrich) to 100 mL PBS (1×). Store at room temperature.

17. Calibration particles
    Rainbow Calibration Particles six peaks or eight peaks (BD Biosciences). Store undiluted at 4 °C in the dark. Mix well before use. Dilute 3–5 drops in 1 mL buffer. Use immediately.

3   Methods

3.1   Flow Cytometric Basophil Activation Technique: Membrane Markers (Method 1)

All procedures are carried out at room temperature, in a laminar air-flow cabinet when necessary, unless otherwise specified (*see* **Note 7**).

3.1.1   Alexa Fluor© 405 Labeling of Mouse Monoclonal Anti-human IgE

1. Labeling procedure: Mouse monoclonal anti-human IgE (clone GE-1) is diluted in $NaHCO_3$ (0.1 mol/L in H_2O, pH 8.3) at a concentration of 5 mg/mL.

2. Alexa Fluor 488 carboxylic acid, succinimidyl ester, and triethylammonium salt (Life Technologies, Molecular Probes) can be stored at –20 °C for a maximum of 3 months. When dissolved in DMSO, the solution becomes unstable. A working solution is made fresh by dissolving 1 mg in 0.1 mL DMSO.

3. Mix 2 mL anti-IgE in $NaHCO_3$ slowly with 0.1 mL Alexa Fluor© 488 working solution for 1 h at room temperature in the dark. Mix regularly.

4. Dialyze overnight with PBS at 4 °C.

5. Add NaN_3 until a final concentration of 0.05 % is reached. Store at 2–8 °C.

6. Working solution: 1:50 in PBS-NaN_3. Store at 2–8 °C. The working solution has to be titrated every time a new batch is made (*see* also **Note 2**).

3.1.2 Preparation of Positive and Negative Controls (Exclusion of Non-responders)

1. Incubate 100 μL blood with 100 μL negative (BAT buffer) or positive control (anti-IgE) during 20 min at 37 °C.

2. Using the procedure described below, stain with aIgE-AF488 and CD203c-APC (*see* **Note 4**) or CD123/HLA-Dr and CD203c-APC (*see* **Note 4**).

3. When basophils do not react one can decide to stimulate with two concentrations of the allergen to exclude non-reactivity to anti-IgE (*see* **Note 5**).

3.1.3 Allergen Procedure

1. All blood samples, buffers, and allergens are prewarmed without mixing for 15 min at 37 °C in warm water bath (WWB) (*see* **Note 6**).

2. Prepare incubation tubes and add 100 μL allergen solution to the allergen tubes. Dilutions depend on the allergen used (*see* **Note 3**). Use BAT buffer as a negative control or for FMO evaluation (*see* **Note 2**).

3. Add anti-IgE as positive control to a positive control tube. Add 100 μL BAT buffer to a negative control tube.

4. Add to all tubes 100 μL prewarmed whole blood.

5. Incubate during 20 min at 37 °C in WWB.

6. Stop reaction by adding 1 mL PBS-EDTA.

7. Spin at $200 \times g$ for 10 min at 4 °C without setting on the brake of the centrifuge. Remove supernatant.

8. Add 20 μL aIgE-AF488 and 10 μL anti-CD63-PE (or in case at 10 μL CD123/HLADr/CD63). Add 5 μL aCD203c-APC.

9. Incubate on ice for 20 min in the dark.

10. Add 2 mL lysis solution and incubate at room temperature for 20 min.

11. Spin for 10 min at $250 \times g$ at room temperature. Remove supernatant.

12. Add 2 mL PBS and spin again for 10 min $250 \times g$ at room temperature. Remove supernatant.

13. Add 300 μL PBS-NaN_3. The tubes are now ready to measure with a flow cytometer.

152   Chris H. Bridts et al.

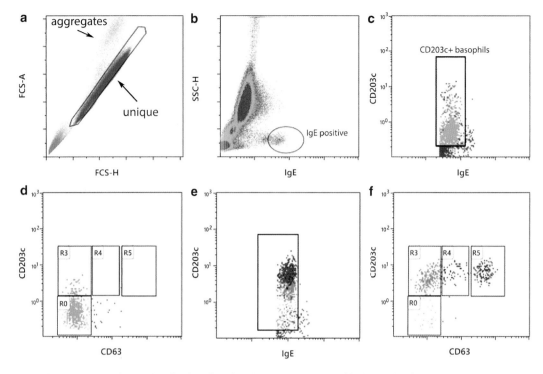

Fig. 1 Basophil selection and activation. Panel **a**: Aggregates are avoided by selecting unique cells based on FCS (forward scatter) area and FCS height plot. Plot **b**: IgE high positive cells are gated out. Panel **c**: Gated cells are IgE$^+$ and CD203$^+$ (without stimulation). Panel **d**: Activated basophils in control setting: R0 are CD203c$^+$CD63$^-$, R3 are CD203c^{hi+}CD63$^-$, R4 are CD203c^{hi+} CD63^{low+}, R5 are CD203c^{hi+}CD63hi$^+$. Panels **e** and **f** are equal to **c** and **d** but after activation with anti-IgE as a positive control

14. Count at least 500 basophils which are defined as aIgE$^+$ and CD203c$^+$.

15. Store data in an FCS-formatted file, which can be analyzed with flow cytometric software.

16. Define CD203c^{hi+}CD63$^-$ basophils and CD203c^{hi+}CD63^{hi+} as activate basophil populations (*see* Fig. 1).

17. Expression as %CD203c^{hi+}CD63$^-$ or %CD203c^{hi+}CD63^{hi+} basophils by subtracting % positive control or allergen with % negative control.

3.2 HistaFlow: Basophil Activation Technique with Intracellular Staining of Histamine (Method 2)

All procedures are carried out at room temperature, in a laminar airflow cabinet when necessary, or unless otherwise specified. The procedure is identical as in Method 1 (except volumes) until **step 9**.

3.2.1 Preparation of Positive and Negative Controls (Exclusion of Non-responders)

1. Incubate 200 µL of blood with 200 µL negative (BAT buffer) or positive control (anti-IgE) for 20 min at 37 °C.

2. Using the procedure described below, stain with aIgE-AF488 and CD203c-APC (*see* **Note 4**)

3. When basophils do not respond one can decide to stimulate with two concentrations of the allergen to exclude non-reactivity to anti-IgE (*see* **Note 5**).

3.2.2 Allergen Procedure

1. All blood samples, buffers, and allergens are prewarmed without mixing for 15 min at 37 °C in warm water bath (WWB) (*see* **Note 6**).

2. Prepare incubation tubes and add 200 µL allergen solution to the allergen tubes. Dilutions depend on the allergen used (*see* **Note 3**). Use BAT buffer as a negative control or for FMO evaluation (*see* **Note 2**).

3. Add anti-IgE as positive control to a positive control tube. Add 100 µL BAT buffer to a negative control tube.

4. Add to all tubes 100 µL prewarmed whole blood.

5. Incubate during 20 min at 37 °C in WWB.

6. Stop reaction on ice and add 1 mL PBS-EDTA.

7. Spin at $500 \times g$ for 10 min at 4 °C without setting on the brake of the centrifuge. Remove supernatant.

8. Add 20 µL anti-IgE-AF405, 10 µL anti-CD63-FITC, and 5 µL anti-CD203c-APC.

9. Incubate at 4 °C for 20 min in the dark.

10. Add 2 mL Phosflow Lyse/Fix work solution and incubate at 37 °C in WWB for 20 min.

11. Spin for 10 min at $500 \times g$ at room temperature. Remove supernatant.

12. Add 2 mL 0.1 % PBS-TX100 and spin again for 10 min $500 \times g$ at room temperature. Remove supernatant.

13. Add 100 µL 0.1 % PBS-TX100 and 10–40 µL (depending on titration) DAO-V500.

14. Stain for 45 min at 37 °C in WWB. Mix several times during stain procedure.

15. Add 2 mL PBS and spin at $500 \times g$ for 10 min at room temperature. Remove supernatant.

16. Add 300 µL PBS-NaN$_3$.

17. The tubes are now ready to be measured with a flow cytometer.

18. Count at least 1,000 basophils, defined as aIgE$^+$ and CD203c$^+$.

19. Store data in an FCS-formatted file, which can be analyzed with flow cytometric software.

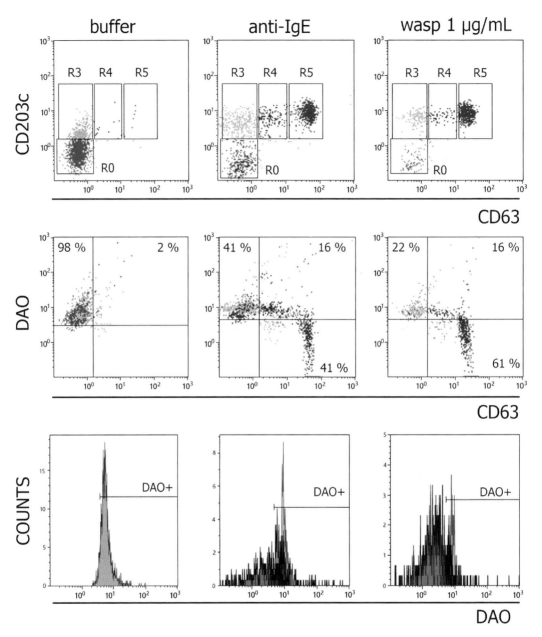

Fig. 2 HistaFlow analysis: Basophils are selected as described in Fig. 1. See also legend Fig. 1 for R0–R5 defini-tion. The *left* column displays results of buffer (negative control), the *second* column shows results of positive control, and the *right* column displays results of activation with wasp antigen in a wasp allergic patient. DAO results (histamine content) show histamine release in 61 % of the basophils after activation with wasp antigen

20. Define CD203c^{hi+}CD63$^-$ basophils and CD203c^{hi+}CD63^{hi+} as activated basophil populations. Define histamine content using the compensation setting described below. This setting must be unique for every sample. Figure 2 shows an example of HistaFlow analysis of basophils stimulated with wasp venom in a wasp allergic patient.

Table 1
Compensation method

Tube	1	2	3	4
Type	CD63–DAO–	CD63–DAO+	CD63++DAO+	CD63++DAO–
Explanation	Negative cells	DAO+ cells without activation	DAO+ and *intracellular* CD63+ staining *WITHOUT* stimulation	DAO and CD63 staining *WITH* stimulation
Incubation/activation procedure (*see* Method 2)				
Whole blood	200 µL	200 µL	200 µL	200 µL
BAT buffer	200 µL	200 µL	200 µL	–
mHu-antiIgE (pos. control)	–	–	–	200 µL
Incubation (*see* Method 2)				
Membrane-staining procedure				
CD63	None	None	None	none
IgE/CD203c	20 µL/10 µL	20 µL/10 µL	20 µL/10 µL	20 µL/10 µL
Lyse/fix (*see* Method 2)				
Wash with PBS_0.1 % TritonX				
Intracellular staining procedure (*see* Method 2)				
PBS-TX100	100 µL	100 µL	100 µL	100 µL
CD63	–	–	10 µL	10 µL
DAO	–	10 µL	10 µL	10 µL
Population by correct compensation (*see* Fig. 4)	*Grey cell in gate C* (no staining for DAO and CD63)	*Green cells in gate D* (DAO+ staining alone)	*Blue cells in gate E* (all basophils are positive for DAO and CD63; note that there is no CD203c upregulation)	*Red cells in gate F* (histamine-releasing cells)

3.3 Compensation Procedure

A functional assay like the HistaFlow technique needs an optimal flow cytometric compensation setting which is not always necessary when measuring populations, as long as the populations can be differentiated. In the case of histamine release, we must be aware that not all basophils release the same amount of histamine; hence different populations can (and must) be observed.

One could also explain this by comparing it with taking a picture with a digital camera. You need a correct exposure to see all the details. To do so, one needs a correct exposure time or shutter speed (=PMT setting in flow cytometry) and a correct aperture (=compensation setting in flow cytometry).

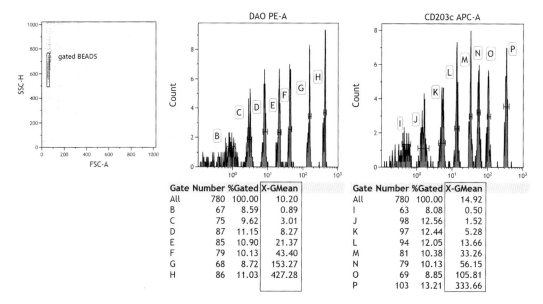

Fig. 3 Selection of standardized beads (*left*) and calculation of geometric mean of eight different intensities (*middle*: PE, *right*: APC). Results are shown in column X_Gmean

Gate Number	%Gated	X-GMean
All	780	100.00	10.20
B	67	8.59	0.89
C	75	9.62	3.01
D	87	11.15	8.27
E	85	10.90	21.37
F	79	10.13	43.40
G	68	8.72	153.27
H	86	11.03	427.28

Gate Number	%Gated	X-GMean
All	780	100.00	14.92
I	63	8.08	0.50
J	98	12.56	1.52
K	97	12.44	5.28
L	94	12.05	13.66
M	81	10.38	33.26
N	79	10.13	56.15
O	69	8.85	105.81
P	103	13.21	333.66

This is in fact what we do by combining the data of the four tubes in the compensation setting of the HistaFlow technique (*see* Table 1).

The first tube is without staining for DAO/CD63. These are the histamine-negative basophils. The second tube is DAO staining alone. These are the DAO (or histamine)-positive basophils.

The third tube is special: DAO as well as CD63 staining AFTER fixation and WITHOUT stimulation: this will give us the optimal staining for all populations.

The fourth tube is DAO and CD63 after activation (just like a positive control): This tube gives us the possibility to optimize the compensation setting (under an optimal PMT setting). By fine-tuning one will easily observe the different population releasing basophil populations.

After staining each tube separately, we can mix them to find out the optimal setting or one can measure every tube individually and, using software, add all the data in one data file. Afterwards we measure all tubes of the same patient with this setting.

Ensure that you repeat this for every donor due to potential differences in histamine content.

3.4 Calibration Procedure

1. Measure working solution of diluted beads with the identical flow cytometric settings as for the HistaFlow analysis (*see* Fig. 3).

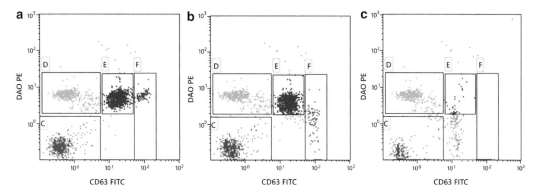

Fig. 4 Correct compensation setting. Basophils were selected as CD203⁺antIgE⁺. Panel **a** shows undercompensation, Panel **b** is correctly compensated, and Panel **c** is overcompensated

2. Make a calibration graph (lin-log) with the use of the channel number and the median fluorescence intensity (MFI) as described by the manufacturer (*see* Fig. 4).

3. Use this calibration curve to calculate the MFI of the histamine-containing cell population.

4   Notes

1. Although different BAT techniques are described using EDTA or even citrate-treated blood, the best results are obtained with heparinized blood as basophil activation is very calcium dependent and using chelators or calcium-binding products can have deleterious effect on test results. Anti-histamines, which target the histamine receptors, have no influence on basophil activation tests in contrast to corticosteroids and immune-suppressive drugs.

2. All antibodies can be used labeled with different fluorochromes. Be aware that correct titration is necessary. This can be done by using different dilutions of the antibody and, using the correct flow cytometric settings, looking for the optimal resolution in comparison with an FMO (fluorescence minus one) measurement as a control.

3. Allergens can be protein extracts, recombinant proteins, or drugs. They must be water soluble and used in concentrations which are not toxic for basophils. To test toxicity, incubate basophils with different concentrations of the allergen or mouse anti human-IgE (positive control) for 20 min at 37 °C and measure viability using propidium iodide or Live/Dead viability/ Cytotoxicity Kit for mammalian cells (e.g., Life Technologies). Do not use preparations for skin testing. These solutions contain preservatives or sometimes modified proteins which can inhibit

basophil activation in vitro. Be aware that food allergens are very difficult to standardize. The optimal concentration of an allergen to stimulate basophils must be determined in a dose–response curve experiment including about ten well-defined patients positive to the antigen and ten controls negative to the allergen. Because such a response can result in a bell-shaped curve, in routine practice at least two concentrations have to be used to define a positive result.

4. Basophils can be differentiated with different markers. Basophils are IL-3 receptor (CD123) positive and HLA-DR negative (monocytes and dendritic cells are HLA-DR positive and also CD123 positive). Because CD203c is the only lineage marker known until now for basophils (mast cells are also positive, but they do not circulate in the blood), we prefer to define basophils as CD203c$^+$/IgE$^+$. Nevertheless the CD203c density in resting basophils can be too low to differentiate cells.

5. In about 5–10 % of the patients, basophils do not respond to a positive control, be it anti-IgE, fMLP, or anti-Fc εRI. In such a case one can decide to stimulate with the allergen. Nevertheless if the allergen also gives a negative response, the procedure has to be stopped because it could be a false-negative response (the so-called non-responder). Results will be inconclusive.

6. Basophil activation results in an immediate response (1 min) that lasts for about 20–30 min at maximum response. To obtain highly reproducible results, all solutions are best pre-warmed to 37 °C.

7. Wear gloves, lab coat, and safety glasses while handling all human blood products. Dispose of all pipettes, etc. into bagged waste collection bins. Wipe work surfaces with disinfectant before and after running tests.

References

1. Ebo DG, Hagendorens MM, Bridts CH, Schuerwegh AJ, De Clerck LS, Stevens WJ (2004) In vitro allergy diagnosis: should we follow the flow? Clin Exp Allergy 34:332–339

2. Ebo DG, Bridts CH, Hagendorens MM, Aerts NE, De Clerck LS, Stevens WJ (2008) Basophil activation test by flow cytometry: present and future applications in allergology. Cytometry B Clin Cytom 74:201–210

3. Hausmann OV, Gentinetta T, Bridts CH, Ebo DG (2009) The basophil activation test in immediate-type drug allergy. Immunol Allergy Clin North Am 29:555–566

4. Ebo DG, Bridts CH, Hagendorens MM, Mertens CH, De Clerck LS, Stevens WJ (2006) Flow-assisted diagnostic management of anaphylaxis from rocuronium bromide. Allergy 61:935–939

5. Sabato V, Verweij MM, Bridts CH, Levi-Schaffer F, Gibbs BF, De Clerck LS et al (2012) CD300a is expressed on human basophils and seems to inhibit IgE/FcepsilonRI-dependent anaphylactic degranulation. Cytometry B Clin Cytom 82:132–138

6. Ebo DG, Dombrecht EJ, Bridts CH, Aerts NE, De Clerck LS, Stevens WJ (2007) Combined analysis of intracellular signalling and immunophenotype of human peripheral blood basophils by flow cytometry: a proof of concept. Clin Exp Allergy 37:1668–1675

7. Verweij MM, De Knop KJ, Bridts CH, De Clerck LS, Stevens WJ, Ebo DG (2010) P38 mitogen-activated protein kinase signal transduction in the diagnosis and follow up of immunotherapy of wasp venom allergy. Cytometry B Clin Cytom 78:302–307

8. Verweij MM, Sabato V, Nullens S, Bridts CH, De Clerck LS, Stevens WJ et al (2012) STAT5 in human basophils: IL-3 is required for its FcepsilonRI-mediated phosphorylation. Cytometry B Clin Cytom 82:101–106

9. Ebo DG, Bridts CH, Mertens CH, Hagendorens MM, Stevens WJ, De Clerck LS (2012) Analyzing histamine release by flow cytometry (HistaFlow): a novel instrument to study the degranulation patterns of basophils. J Immunol Methods 375:30–38

10. Nullens S, Sabato V, Faber M, Leysen J, Bridts CH, De Clerck LS et al (2013) Basophilic histamine content and release during venom immunotherapy: insights by flow cytometry. Cytometry B Clin Cytom 84:173–178

Chapter 12

Microscopy Assays for Evaluation of Mast Cell Migration and Chemotaxis

Monika Bambousková, Zuzana Hájková, Pavel Dráber, and Petr Dráber

Abstract

A better understanding of the molecular mechanisms leading to mast cell migration and chemotaxis is the long-term goal in mast cell research and is essential for comprehension of mast cell function in health and disease. Various techniques have been developed in recent decades for in vitro and in vivo assessment of mast cell motility and chemotaxis. In this chapter three microscopy assays facilitating real-time quantification of mast cell chemotaxis and migration are described, focusing on individual cell tracking and data analysis.

Key words Mast cells, Cell migration, Chemotaxis, Chemokine, Chemoattractant

1 Introduction

Mast cells are best known for their role in mediating allergic diseases [1]. Recent studies have highlighted their important functions in the innate immunity contributing to protection against bacterial infection, angiogenesis, and autoimmunity [2, 3]. Under pathological conditions, mast cells are involved in immediate hypersensitivity, chronic allergic reactions, asthma, and other inflammatory diseases [4]. As highly effective sentinel cells they are localized close to blood vessels in common sites of potential infection, such as skin, airways, and the gastrointestinal tract. Chemoattractant-directed migration of mature mast cells or their progenitors might be one of the key mechanisms responsible for local accumulation of these cells under physiological or pathological conditions [5]. Chemotactic mechanisms can be therefore potentially targeted by therapeutic interventions.

$CD13^+/CD34^+/CD117$ (c-Kit)$^+$ mast cell progenitors arise in bone marrow where they start their differentiation under the influence of chemokines and growth factors [6]. During this process they leave bone marrow and migrate into bloodstream to reach

Bernhard F. Gibbs and Franco H. Falcone (eds.), *Basophils and Mast Cells: Methods and Protocols*, Methods in Molecular Biology, vol. 1192, DOI 10.1007/978-1-4939-1173-8_12, © Springer Science+Business Media New York 2014

various body sites. The key signal for mast cell homing and recruitment into peripheral tissues is provided by interaction of the stem cell factor (SCF) with its receptor, the c-Kit [7]. In rodents another critical factor, interleukin-3 (IL-3), which binds to its surface receptor is involved [8]. In peripheral tissues mast cell progenitors mature and terminally differentiate under the influence of the local environment. Two predominant phenotypes of mature mast cells, the connective tissue and the mucosal mast cells, differ by the expression of various secretory granule proteins [9] (*see* Chapter 9). Migration of mast cell progenitors to the site of their residency is directed by various chemokines which bind to chemokine receptors [10]. The expression pattern of these molecules is different in progenitors and mature mast cells and differences are also observed between particular mast cell subtypes [11]. Several other chemotactic ligands affecting mast cell migration have been identified; these include sphingosine-1-phosphate [12], arachidonic acid metabolites as leukotriene B4 [13], and prostaglandin E_2 (PGE_2) [14, 15], as well as antigen, recognized by IgE anchored to the high-affinity IgE receptor (FcεRI) [16, 17]. In target tissues mast cells participate actively in immune responses against various pathogens by releasing a broad spectrum of mediators, either stored in secretory granules or rapidly synthesized after cell triggering. Mediators produced by mast cells include leukotrienes, prostaglandins, cytokines, and chemokines (*see* Chapter 10), which in turn can recruit other immune cells to sites of inflammation [18, 19]. Importantly, mature mast cells in sensitized individuals exposed to allergens produce mediators that attract mast cell-committed progenitors to the place of pathogen entry [13]. In healthy tissues the number of mast cells is stable and can be regulated by proliferation, migration, and mast cell survival. On the other hand, inflamed tissues show an increased number of mast cells, and their enhanced accumulation is characteristic for a number of pathological states [20, 21].

Numerous methods have been developed for studies on mast cell migration and chemotaxis towards various chemoattractants. Most of the in vitro studies utilized various modifications of Boyden's chamber system where cells migrate through pores (usually 5 or 8 µm) of polycarbonate membrane towards increasing concentrations of chemoattractants [22]. These techniques are well established for quantification of chemotactic responses [13, 15, 23]. However, they do not allow recording the movement of individual cells at selected time intervals and analyzing cell trajectories. Therefore, new methods have been developed for analysis of chemotaxis using real-time imaging. The gradient of chemoattractant is usually created by arranging special chambers in various settings [24]. Alternatively, a gradient is produced by embedding chemoattractants in porous materials such as agarose [25–27]. Using a microscope equipped with a camera and proper software, the images are processed with image analysis software capable of obtaining coordinates of individual trajectories. They are then used for calculation of cell movement parameters (e.g., directionality, achieved distance, velocity) [24, 28, 29]. Since primary mast cells are non-adherent, the 2D or the 3D tracking of their movement encounters some difficulties. To overcome these problems, mast cells are attached to the surface with some natural adhesive compounds, such as fibronectin. Furthermore, cell attachment has to be preserved during the whole experiment to prevent any artificial movement of cells during analysis. These techniques resulted in the development of new methods for analysis of migration and chemotaxis of non-adherent mast cells. In this chapter we describe several experimental settings for real-time analysis of cell motility or directed chemotaxis optimized for non-adherent mast cells. The techniques utilize commercially available migration chambers or simple homemade devices.

2 Materials

2.1 Chemicals

1. Fibronectin from bovine plasma for cell cultures.

2. Recombinant murine IL-3.

3. Recombinant murine SCF: Stock solution containing 1 mg/mL of SCF in H_2O is aliquoted to avoid repeated freeze-thaw cycles.

4. Agarose.

5. Collagen I (3.1 mg/mL).

6. PGE_2 (1 mM stock solution is prepared in DMSO).

2.2 Buffers and Media

1. HEPES solution (1 M).

2. RPMI-1640.

3. Minimum essential medium (MEM) nonessential amino acids.

4. 10× concentrated MEM Eagle with Hanks' salts (H-MEM).

5. Migration medium (MM): RPMI-1640, 0.1 % BSA (w/v), 20 mM HEPES, pH 7.4.

6. StemPro-34® serum-free medium.

2.3 Mast Cells

1. Bone marrow from femurs and tibias of 6–10-week-old mice is used as a source of mast cell precursors. The cells are cultured in RPMI-1640 supplemented with 20 mM HEPES, pH 7.5, 100 U/mL penicillin, 100 μg/mL streptomycin, 100 μM MEM nonessential amino acids, 1 mM sodium pyruvate, 41 μM 2-mercaptoethanol, 10 % (v/v) fetal calf serum, IL-3 (20 ng/mL), and SCF (15 ng/mL). After 5–7 weeks, most of the cultured cells (up to 95 %) express FcεRI and c-Kit, markers of mast cells. Such bone marrow-derived mast cells (BMMCs)

have been extensively used in studies on cell signaling since they closely resemble normal mast cells in respect to their requirement of IL-3 and SCF for optimal growth and their ability to respond to various physiological stimuli, and particularly because they can be isolated from mouse strains deficient in genes which are possibly involved in a variety of signaling pathways.

2. A particular cell line derived from mouse BMMCs (BMMCL) has been isolated by Hibbs [30]. These cells are cultured in complete RPMI-1640 supplemented as described above but without SCF and with recombinant IL-3 replaced by 10 % (v/v) WEHI-3 cell supernatant. These cells can be recovered after freezing in 10 % (v/v) DMSO and storage at –70 °C or liquid nitrogen. BMMCL can be used instead of BMMCs for their easier culturing and fast growth. Further, they react in almost the same way as BMMCs to a variety of treatments [31].

3. The human mast cell line (LUVA) was originally obtained by growing CD34+-enriched mononuclear cells derived from the peripheral blood of a human donor [32] (*see* Subheading 2.3 in Chapter 8). LUVA cells are maintained in StemPro-34 serum-free medium in the absence of any exogenously added cytokines. Although they have the morphology of mast cells, after several passages in vitro they lose surface expression of FcεRI (our own unpublished data).

2.4 Other Materials

1. Test tubes and 1.5 mL Eppendorf tubes.

2. 96-Well black optical bottom plates, suitable for microscopy.

3. Bevelled pipette tips for filling ports on μ-Slide.

4. Slant tweezers for plug handling.

5. Cell culture dishes 40×11 mm.

6. Glass beads (2 mm diameter).

7. μ-Slide Chemotaxis[3D] chambers containing μ-Slide[3D] for evaluation of cell chemotaxis in three samples, a cultivation lid, and 18 plugs (Ibidi).

2.5 Equipment

1. Laminar flow box.

2. CO_2 incubator.

3. Inverted microscope equipped with 10× bright-field objective, camera for time-lapse video recording, motorized stage, and CO_2- and temperature-regulated chamber.

4. Automated microscopy system equipped with 10× and 20× bright-field objectives, camera for recording time-lapse video, motorized stage, CO_2- and temperature-regulated chamber, and platform for 96-well plates.

5. Milli-Q water purification system or equivalent.

2.6 Software	1. MetaMorph Offline (Version 7.7.9.0; Molecular Devices). 2. ImageJ (Version 1.46; National Institutes of Health) with Chemotaxis and Migration Tool plug-in (Version 1.01; Ibidi).

3   Methods

For quantitative studies of mast cell migration and chemotaxis by microscopy, three assays are presented: simple motility assay, chemotaxis measured in μ-Slide chemotaxis chamber, and chemotaxis analyzed in homemade chamber with chemoattractants embedded in agarose cone.

3.1   Motility Assay

This technique is used to determine the general ability of mast cells to move. It is useful when cells of different properties are investigated or if activity of selected drugs on cell movement is tested. The method allows measurement in 96-well plate format. Mast cells are allowed to attach to fibronectin-coated surfaces and are treated with an activator such as PGE_2. The velocities of cell movement and/or the distances reached from the start point are automatically determined (*see* Fig. 1). However, no information on directionality of migration is provided.

All solutions intended for handling live cells and the microscope heating chamber should be pre-warmed to 37 °C.

1. Prepare fibronectin-coated 96-well optical bottom plate by adding 50 μL of fibronectin (50 μg/mL) in PBS into each well of the plate and incubate for 14–16 h at 4 °C (*see* **Note 1**).

2. Grow BMMCs at concentration 2×10^6/mL without SCF and IL-3 for 12–16 h before experiment (*see* **Note 2**).

3. Wash the cells twice with MM, resuspend in MM, and adjust the concentration to 5×10^5/mL.

4. Wash the fibronectin-coated surfaces briefly with PBS and pipet 100 μL of cell suspension into each well.

5. Allow the cells to attach for 30 min at 37 °C and then gently wash the wells once with warm MM (*see* **Note 3**).

6. Add carefully 100 μL of MM or activator (e.g., PGE_2) diluted in MM into each well (*see* **Note 4**).

7. Monitor the cell motility on automated microscopy system with 10× or 20× objective and define the number of examined sites per well and their XYZ positions. Take time-lapse images for 1–2 h at 1-min intervals (*see* **Note 5**).

8. Analyze the data using the procedure described in Subheading 3.4.

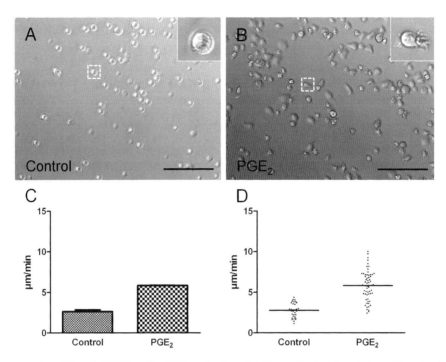

Fig. 1 Increased motility of BMMCs after PGE$_2$ activation. (**a**) Non-activated (control) or (**b**) activated (PGE$_2$) BMMCs, attached to fibronectin-coated surface, were monitored with automated microscopy system with 20× objective. Time-lapse images were taken for 60 min at a frequency of 1.27 min/frame. Representative cells are magnified and shown in *inserts* (**a**, **b**; *right upper corners*). (**c**) Individual trajectories of 30–50 cells were processed and the average velocity ± SD was calculated from duplicates in one representative experiment. (**d**) Distribution of velocities of individual cells is presented with vertical scatterplot; average values of all analyzed cells are also shown. Bars in (**a**) and (**b**) = 100 μm

3.2 Mast Cell Chemotaxis in μ-Slide Chemotaxis³ᴰ Chambers

The μ-Slide Chemotaxis³ᴰ chambers make it possible to study directed migration of non-adherent cells towards the chemoattractant. Each μ-Slide³ᴰ contains three identical chambers for parallel monitoring of samples. Cells are kept in a chamber using 3D collagen I gel. The unique working arrangement of μ-Slide³ᴰ enables to create the required chemoattractant gradient. Mast cell movement is monitored by time-lapse microscopy followed by data analysis (*see* Subheadings 3.4 and 3.5).

All procedures with μ-Slide Chemotaxis³ᴰ chambers are performed in a laminar flow box to maintain sterility.

1. One day before the experiment, place the culture medium for BMMCs, BMMCL, or LUVA cells, sterile H$_2$O for tissue culture, and the μ-Slide³ᴰ (*see* Fig. 2a) into incubator for gas equilibration. Aqueous solutions should be transferred into semi-closed test tubes, while the μ-Slide³ᴰ should stay packaged to maintain sterility (*see* **Note 6**).

2. Prepare a mast cell suspension at a concentration of 9×10^6 cells/mL in proper equilibrated culture medium (*see* **Note 7**).

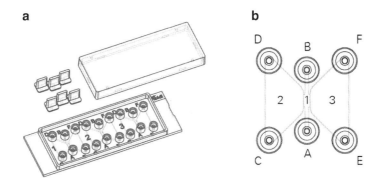

Fig. 2 Components of µ-Slide Chemotaxis[3D] and configuration of a chamber for evaluation of cell motility in one tested sample. (**a**) µ-Slide Chemotaxis[3D] contains a slide with chambers for simultaneous evaluation of three samples (areas *1–3*), six plugs, and a lid. (**b**) Chamber configuration. *1*, channel (observation area); *2*, left reservoir; *3*, right reservoir; *A–F*, filling ports

3. Mix 6 µL of 10× H-MEM, 21.9 µL of sterile H_2O for tissue culture, 2.1 µL of 7.5 % (w/v) $NaHCO_3$, and 15 µL of proper culture medium in a sterile Eppendorf tube (premix; total volume 45 µL). Pipet 30 µL of collagen I into a second Eppendorf tube (*see* **Note 8**).

4. Using tweezers close the filling ports C, D, E, and F (*see* Fig. 2b) with the plugs in the µ-Slide[3D]. Prepare a humid chamber by placing moistened tissue into a sterile 10 cm Petri dish.

5. Pipet 45 µL of the premix into Eppendorf tube containing 30 µL of collagen I and immediately add 15 µL of cell suspension. Mix well, but carefully with a 100 µL pipette (*see* **Note 9**).

6. Apply 6 µL of the mixture to the top of filling port A (use bevelled pipette tip). Immediately after loading aspirate the air from the opposite port B to fill the channel (*see* #1 in Fig. 2b) homogenously with the mixture (*see* **Note 10**). Repeat this step in all three chambers.

7. Remove all plugs from the slide and close filling ports A and B with plugs (filling ports A and B will stay closed till the end of the experiment). Insert the slide into the humid chamber and put into CO_2 incubator for 30–40 min (*see* **Note 11**).

8. Meanwhile dilute chemoattractant (SCF or PGE_2) stocks 1:5,000 in proper culture medium to obtain 200 ng/mL SCF or 0.2 µM PGE_2, respectively. Prepare 40 µL of the chemoattractants for one chamber (*see* **Note 12**).

9. After collagen polymerization, fill the reservoirs (*see* #2 and #3 in Fig. 2b). First, close reservoir #2 with plugs (close filling ports C and D) and directly pipet 65 µL of chemoattractant-free medium through one of the two opened filling ports (E or F). Then remove plugs from filling ports C and D and

close filling ports E and F. Fill reservoir #2 with 65 μL of chemoattractant-free medium. Repeat this step twice to fill reservoirs in all three chambers.

10. To create the chemoattractant gradient, apply 15 μL of 2× concentrated chemoattractant (e.g., SCF or PGE$_2$) to the top of the filling port C and immediately aspirate 15 μL of the medium from the filling port D. This time press the pipette tip directly inside the port. Repeating this step again leads to filling of 30 μL of 2× concentrated chemoattractant into the reservoir. Close all filling ports. An equilibrium gradient of chemoattractant is created during 1–2 h (*see* **Note 13**).

11. Monitor cell chemotaxis with an inverted microscope immediately after chemoattractants are added. Define XYZ positions of channels (observation areas) of all three chambers. Take time-lapse images for 7–10 h at 2-min intervals with the intensity of 71 and exposure time 6 ms. Autofocus can be used during the time-lapse (*see* **Note 14**).

12. Analyze the data using the procedure described in Subheading 3.4.

Further information about this method is available online (*see* **Note 15**).

3.3 Chemotaxis in Homemade Chambers

This method allows characterizing directional movement of cells towards chemoattractant embedded in an agarose cone. After attachment of cells to a fibronectin-coated surface, chemoattractant embedded in an agarose cone is added. Movement of cells starts after an initial 15-min period of sensing the chemoattractant. As a relatively simple and cheap alternative to commercial systems this method can be used for observation of cell behavior and changes in morphology during chemotaxis.

1. Prepare a fibronectin-coated culture dish by adding 1 mL of fibronectin (50 μg/mL) in PBS and incubate it for 12–16 h at 4 °C (*see* **Note 1**).

2. Grow BMMCs at concentration 2×10^6/mL without SCF and IL-3 for 12–16 h (*see* **Note 2**).

3. For preparation of the agarose cone with embedded chemoattractant dissolve 1 % (w/v) agarose in PBS by short heating at 80 °C followed by slow chilling to approximately 40 °C. Keep the agarose solution at the same temperature and dilute PGE$_2$ in agarose solution to final 1 μM concentration. Dispense 15 μL aliquots of this solution to the bottom of 1.5 mL Eppendorf tubes (tubes should be pre-warmed to 40 °C). Immediately insert a glass bead into the agarose solution at the bottom of each tube (*see* Fig. 3a). The glass bead acts as a weight and will help stabilize the cone at the same position in culture dish during the test. Prepare control cones without chemoattractant in the same way. Let the agarose solidify in

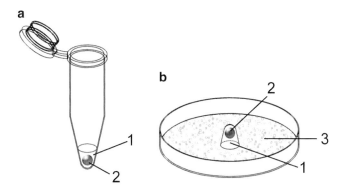

Fig. 3 Agarose cone with embedded chemoattractant. (**a**) Agarose cone with embedded chemoattractant and glass bead in Eppendorf tube; (**b**) position of agarose cone in a culture dish with cells and medium; *1.* Chemoattractant in 1 % agarose; *2.* glass bead; *3.* cell layer

the tubes at 4 °C for at least 15 min and keep it so until use (*see* **Note 16**).

4. Wash the cells with MM and adjust their concentration to 5×10^5/mL.

5. Wash the fibronectin-coated dish with 1 mL of PBS before attaching the cells.

6. Dispense 2 mL aliquots of cell suspension (1×10^6 cells) into each dish and incubate undisturbed for 30 min at 37 °C.

7. Gently wash the dish with 1 mL of MM and add 5 mL of new MM.

8. Fix the dish in a proper position in microscope. Carefully remove the agarose cone containing the glass bead from the Eppendorf tube using tweezers and place it slowly in the middle of the dish with the flat bottom facing down the cell layer (*see* Fig. 3b). Cover the dish with a lid.

9. Find the edge of the agarose cone in the field of view of the inverted microscope with a 10× objective (*see* Fig. 4a) and monitor the cells in time-lapse images for 2–3 h at 1-min intervals (*see* Fig. 4b).

10. Analyze the data as described in Subheading 3.4 (*see* Fig. 4c and d). Start the analysis at frame 60 and end with frames 120–180 (*see* **Note 17**).

3.4 Tracking Cells   Automatic tracking using a MetaMorph program with optimized parameters for mast cells is described in the following section. However, there are also other options to track cells in bright-field time-lapse movies (*see* **Note 18**).

[*Italic font style is used for buttons, option buttons, and headlines. Underlined text refers to dialog boxes.*]

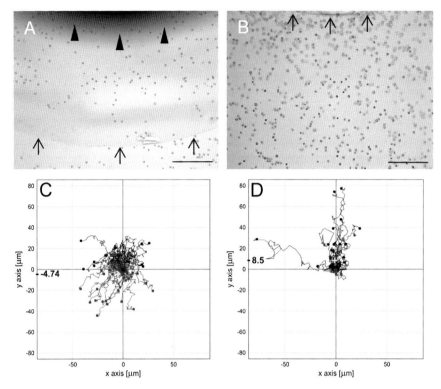

Fig. 4 Mast cell chemotaxis towards PGE$_2$ embedded in an agarose cone. (**a**) The edge of agarose cone is marked by *arrows* and the glass bead by *triangles*. (**b**) BMMCs were attached to fibronectin-coated surface, and the agarose cone with embedded PGE$_2$ was inserted into the dish containing the cells. The cone edge is indicated by *arrows*. The image was captured 15 min after insertion of the cone (when the first changes in cell morphology were observed in the vicinity of agarose cone). Images were taken with an inverted microscope equipped with a 10× objective. (**c, d**) Representative images from a single experiment showing migration trajectory graphs expressing directionality of BMMC movement. Chemotaxis towards PGE$_2$ is reflected by a shift of a center of cell mass in *x*-axis (*crosses*). Bars = 250 μm

1. Open time-lapse sequence in the MetaMorph program. Choose *Threshold → Threshold Image*. Mark off *Inclusive* and use the slider to adjust the threshold so that only the cells of interest are marked (*see* Fig. 5a) (*see* **Note 19**).

2. Select *Apps → Track Objects* and set the following parameters in <u>Track Objects dialog box</u>:

   (a) In *Source for images* mark off *Stack*.

   (b) Using *Search Options* button open <u>Search Options dialog box</u> and in *Algorithm* set *Threshold Results*. Then choose what the program should do in *If object not found* (e.g., *Select position*). Also set *Delay* (e.g., 0 s/object) and *Object size match requirement* (*as* %) (e.g., 35).

   (c) Set other parameters in <u>Track Objects Interval Options</u>, <u>Track Overlay Options</u>, and <u>Origin Options dialog boxes</u> by

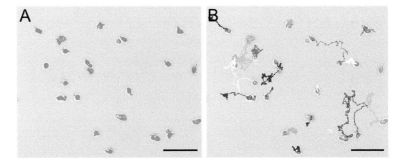

Fig. 5 Analysis of cell migration with MetaMorph. (**a**) Representative thresholded image of time-lapse sequence. (**b**) Trajectories of individual cells. Chemotaxis of BMMCs towards 100 µM PGE$_2$ loaded into the left reservoir of µ-Slide Chemotaxis^{3D} chamber. Images were taken with an inverted microscope with a 10× objective. Bars = 100 µm

choosing *Set Interval*, *Set Overlay*, and *Set Origin* buttons, respectively.

(d) Choose *Track* to select tracked cells.

3. Select Objects dialog box appears. To choose objects to be tracked hold down the [Ctrl] and click on each object using the left mouse button. Adjust the size of the search regions (*see* **Note 20**). Then choose *OK* and object tracking will proceed automatically.

4. It is recommended to follow tracking during whole analysis. In case MetaMorph tracks in a wrong way (e.g., skips to another cell) press [Esc] to stop tracking. The Tracking dialog box will open. If necessary press the *Step Back* to return the analysis to the last correctly tracked plane. Then do a correction by hand (move the search region to the correct position using left mouse button), and continue in the analysis by choosing *Update Position And Continue* in Tracking dialog box. In such cases it can be worth marking off *Continue one step and pause* in Tracking dialog box.

5. If MetaMorph loses an object during the tracking, it proceeds according to the previous selection in the *If object not found* options in Search Options dialog box. In case *Select position* is marked off, it is necessary to do the correction by hand as described in **step 4**.

6. After the tracking is finished, all trajectories of individually tracked cells are marked in the time-lapse movie (*see* Fig. 5b) and Track Objects dialog box appears again.

(a) Select *Open Log*, and define where the data should be saved and a blank Excel file opens. Thereafter choose *Log Data* to save all the data from tracking. Sometimes it is easier to track only several cells at one time and each time log newly tracked data to the same Excel document.

3.5 Presenting Chemotaxis Data

Chemotaxis is analyzed by means of Chemotaxis and Migration Tool. This is a free software for ImageJ that can be downloaded at http://ibidi.com/software/chemotaxis_and_migration_tool/.

[*Italic font style is used for buttons, check boxes, and headlines. Underlined text refers to bookmarks.*]

1. Download and open Chemotaxis and Migration Tool in the ImageJ. Import the data table from MetaMorph by choosing *Import Data* in Import dataset bookmark (*see* **Note 21**).

2. Choose which cell tracks from the data table will be analyzed by filling in the *Number of slices*. Only specified tracks with exact number or within entered range of slices will be used. Then choose *Add dataset*, and mark off *Selected Dataset* in the main panel (*see* **Note 22**).

3. Calibrate the software in Settings bookmark. XY coordinates from MetaMorph are in pixels; it is therefore necessary to define the size of one pixel in *X/Y Calibration*. Also fill in *Time interval* that was used during time-lapse monitoring. Afterwards choose *Apply settings* in the main panel.

4. To analyze only selected time intervals from imported time-lapse choose *Open restrictions* in the main panel, mark off *Split dataset* check box, and fill in required slices (*see* **Note 23**). Then choose *Apply settings* in the main panel.

5. Now the tool is prepared to plot graphs and diagrams and export various statistic values. One can plot Chemotaxis Plot in Plot feature bookmark → *Plot graph* (*see* Figs. 4c, d and 6a, b). Sector feature and Diagram feature bookmarks allow plotting other graphs (e.g., Rose diagram; *see* Fig. 6c, d). Statistic feature bookmark provides statistic values that can be used for further statistical analysis.

4   Notes

1. Alternatively, fibronectin-coated surface can be prepared by 1-h incubation at 37 °C.

2. Starvation of BMMCs for IL-3 should not exceed 14–16 h. In case of suboptimal results, overnight culturing with a small amount of IL-3 can be optionally tested.

3. Removal of fibronectin-unbound cells is an important step and should be carried out with maximal caution to avoid any washing out or damaging of fibronectin-attached cell layer.

4. Best results are achieved with PGE_2 concentrations between 50 and 100 nM.

5. The length of time intervals depends on the number of monitored sites. If many sites are being examined, it is advisable to

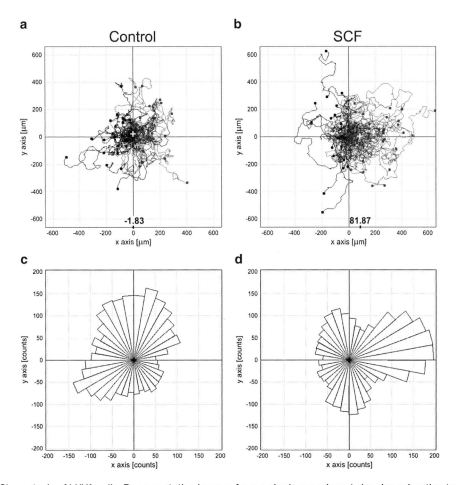

Fig. 6 Chemotaxis of LUVA cells. Representative images from a single experiment showing migration trajectory graphs (**a**, **b**) and rose diagrams expressing direction tendencies of LUVA cells (**c**, **d**). Cells without (**a**, **c**; control) and with 100 ng/mL SCF in the right reservoir (**b**, **d**; SCF). Chemotaxis of LUVA cells towards SCF is reflected by a shift of the center of cell mass in *x*-axis (*crosses* in **a**, **b**). LUVA cells in collagen I matrix were monitored for 10 h in an inverted microscope equipped with a 10× objective

choose as short time interval as possible. Cells become most active after the initial 15 min. An optimal time interval for subsequent analysis can be defined for individual experiments.

6. Equilibration prevents formation of air bubbles during loading of the μ-Slide[3D]. Packaged μ-Slide[3D] enables gas equilibration. Do not equilibrate collagen I.

7. Cell suspension will be consequently diluted into final concentration of 1.5×10^6 cells/mL. Cell concentration could vary according to individual experimental preferences—more cells for obtaining extensive statistic data, and less cells for easier cell tracking (cells are isolated and trajectories do not interfere).

8. This amount corresponds to collagen I concentration 1 mg/mL.

9. Mix well, but avoid generating bubbles. Polymerization starts approximately 5 min after mixing collagen I with premix.

10. Do not inject the mixture directly; rather maintain a small gap between the tip and the filling port A. Insert then the pipette tip directly into the filling port B and aspirate until the gel level reaches the pipette tip. Both ports should be filled but not overfilled.

11. Cell concentration and morphology should be checked with a microscope. The remaining gelation mixture in the Eppendorf tube helps determine the moment when the process of polymerization is completed.

12. To generate chemoattractant gradient, only half of the reservoir will be filled. Therefore, to achieve the desired final concentration, double the chemoattractant concentration.

13. Reservoirs must be filled, but not overfilled. This will prevent unwanted medium fluxes.

14. For later easier cell tracking it is better to contrast the cells against the background rather than perfectly focus the cells themselves.

15. Further information about working with μ-Slide Chemotaxis[3D] chambers can be found on the Ibidi website, http://ibidi.com/applications/chemotaxis/u-slide-chemotaxis-3d/.

16. Manipulation with viscous agarose solution might be facilitated if pipette tips with cut off narrow ends are used. Low-melting-point agarose with gelling point around or below 40 °C is not recommended.

17. Do not include data obtained during the first 60 min into analysis because of possible irregularities caused by addition of agarose cone.

18. Cells can be also tracked with Manual Tracking plug-in for ImageJ, which is freely available. Furthermore, several commercially available platforms offer automated cell tracking online (e.g., Wimasis Image Analysis, http://www.wimasis.com/Products/chemotaxis-assay.html).

19. If the time-lapse displays dark borders or periphery, it is advisable to cut it off from the time-lapse sequence. The goal is to get as many marked cells as possible without marked background. Cells that are not properly marked are not tracked easily. On the other hand, too much background signal slows down the tracking process. It is possible to modify the threshold during automated tracking.

20. For this type of tracking it is best to use search regions of the size similar to that occupied by the cell.

21. Data loaded from MetaMorph must be in the same order and format as those from the Manual Tracking from ImageJ. It is therefore necessary to alter the .xlsx file from MetaMorph.

The first column should contain numbers of each tracked slice (from 1 to the very last line). The second column should indicate the number of tracks (Track no.). The third column should show the number of each slice in every track (Slice no.). Two other columns indicate X and Y coordinates. Save data table as .txt file.

22. This tool enables to work with more imported datasets at one time.

23. This option enables to analyze cell chemotaxis from the same time after adding the chemoattractant in every experiment.

Acknowledgements

This work was supported in part by Grants P302-14-09807S, P305-14-00703S, 301/09/1826, P302/10/1759, P302/12/G101, and P302/12/1673 from the Czech Science Foundation, project LD13015 and LD12073 from the Ministry of Education, Youth and Sport of the Czech Republic. We also acknowledge support of the COST Action BM1007 Mast Cells and Basophils—Targets for Innovative Therapies as well as Institutional support RVO 68378050. M.B. and Z.H. were supported in part by the Faculty of Science, Charles University, Prague.

References

1. Galli SJ, Tsai M, Piliponsky AM (2008) The development of allergic inflammation. Nature 454:445–454

2. Abraham SN, St. John AL (2010) Mast cell-orchestrated immunity to pathogens. Nat Rev Immunol 10:440–452

3. Maltby S, Khazaie K, McNagny KM (2009) Mast cells in tumor growth: angiogenesis, tissue remodelling and immune-modulation. Biochim Biophys Acta 1796:19–26

4. Galli SJ, Tsai M (2012) IgE and mast cells in allergic disease. Nat Med 18:693–704

5. Halova I, Draberova L, Draber P (2012) Mast cell chemotaxis - chemoattractants and signaling pathways. Front Immunol 3:119

6. Kirshenbaum AS, Metcalfe DD (2006) Growth of human mast cells from bone marrow and peripheral blood-derived CD34+ pluripotent progenitor cells. Methods Mol Biol 315:105–112

7. Ashman LK (1999) The biology of stem cell factor and its receptor c-Kit. Int J Biochem Cell Biol 31:1037–1051

8. Lantz CS, Boesiger J, Song CH, Mach N, Kobayashi T, Mulligan RC, Nawa Y, Dranoff G, Galli SJ (1998) Role for interleukin-3 in mast-cell and basophil development and in immunity to parasites. Nature 392:90–93

9. Welle M (1997) Development, significance, and heterogeneity of mast cells with particular regard to the mast cell-specific proteases chymase and tryptase. J Leukoc Biol 61:233–245

10. Taub D, Dastych J, Inamura N, Upton J, Kelvin D, Metcalfe D, Oppenheim J (1995) Bone marrow-derived murine mast cells migrate, but do not degranulate, in response to chemokines. J Immunol 154:2393–2402

11. Okayama Y, Kawakami T (2006) Development, migration, and survival of mast cells. Immunol Res 34:97–115

12. Jolly PS, Bektas M, Olivera A, Gonzalez-Espinosa C, Proia RL, Rivera J, Milstien S, Spiegel S (2004) Transactivation of sphingosine-1-phosphate receptors by FcεRI triggering is required for normal mast cell degranulation and chemotaxis. J Exp Med 199:959–970

13. Weller CL, Collington SJ, Brown JK, Miller HRP, Al-Kashi A, Clark P, Jose PJ, Hartnell A, Williams TJ (2005) Leukotriene B4, an activation product of mast cells, is a chemoattractant for their progenitors. J Exp Med 201:1961–1971

14. Weller CL, Collington SJ, Hartnell A, Conroy DM, Kaise T, Barker JE, Wilson MS, Taylor GW, Jose PJ, Williams TJ (2007) Chemotactic action of prostaglandin E2 on mouse mast cells acting via the PGE_2 receptor 3. Proc Natl Acad Sci 104:11712–11717

15. Kuehn HS, Jung M-Y, Beaven MA, Metcalfe DD, Gilfillan AM (2011) Prostaglandin E2 activates and utilizes mTORC2 as a central signaling locus for the regulation of mast cell chemotaxis and mediator release. J Biol Chem 286:391–402

16. Ishizuka T, Okajima F, Ishiwara M, Iizuka K, Ichimonji I, Kawata T, Tsukagoshi H, Dobashi K, Nakazawa T, Mori M (2001) Sensitized mast cells migrate toward the antigen: a response regulated by p38 mitogen-activated protein kinase and Rho-associated coiled-coil-forming protein kinase. J Immunol 167:2298–2304

17. Kitaura J, Kinoshita T, Matsumoto M, Chung S, Kawakami Y, Leitges M, Wu D, Lowell CA, Kawakami T (2005) IgE- and IgE + Ag-mediated mast cell migration in an autocrine/paracrine fashion. Blood 105:3222–3229

18. Echtenacher B, Mannel DN, Hultner L (1996) Critical protective role of mast cells in a model of acute septic peritonitis. Nature 381:75–77

19. Malaviya R, Ikeda T, Ross E, Abraham SN (1996) Mast cell modulation of neutrophil influx and bacterial clearance at sites of infection through TNF-α. Nature 381:77–80

20. Brightling CE, Bradding P, Symon FA, Holgate ST, Wardlaw AJ, Pavord ID (2002) Mast-cell infiltration of airway smooth muscle in asthma. N Engl J Med 346:1699–1705

21. Quintás-Cardama A, Jain N, Verstovsek S (2011) Advances and controversies in the diagnosis, pathogenesis, and treatment of systemic mastocytosis. Cancer 117:5439–5449

22. Boyden S (1962) The chemotactic effect of mixtures of antibody and antigen on polymorphonuclear leucocytes. J Exp Med 115: 453–466

23. Hálová I, Dráberová L, Bambousková M, Machyna M, Stegurová L, Smrž D, Dráber P (2013) Crosstalk between tetraspanin CD9 and transmembrane adaptor protein non-T cell activation linker (NTAL) in mast cell activation and chemotaxis. J Biol Chem 288:9801–9814

24. Lee J, Veatch SL, Baird B, Holowka D (2012) Molecular mechanisms of spontaneous and directed mast cell motility. J Leukoc Biol 92: 1029–1041

25. Heit B, Kubes P (2003) Measuring chemotaxis and chemokinesis: the under-agarose cell migration assay. Sci STKE 2003:pl5

26. Wiggins HL, Rappoport JZ (2010) An agarose spot assay for chemotactic invasion. Biotechniques 48:121–124

27. Poole TJ, Zetter BR (1983) Stimulation of rat peritoneal mast cell migration by tumor-derived peptides. Cancer Res 43:5857–5861

28. Kuiper JWP, Sun C, Magalhães MA, Glogauer M (2011) Rac regulates PtdInsP3 signaling and the chemotactic compass through a redox-mediated feedback loop. Blood 118:6164–6171

29. Zengel P, Nguyen-Hoang A, Schildhammer C, Zantl R, Kahl V, Horn E (2011) μ-Slide chemotaxis: a new chamber for long-term chemotaxis studies. BMC Cell Biol 12:21

30. Hibbs ML, Tarlinton DM, Armes J, Grail D, Hodgson G, Maglitto R, Stacker SA, Dunn AR (1995) Multiple defects in the immune system of Lyn-deficient mice, culminating in autoimmune disease. Cell 83:301–311

31. Hájková Z, Bugajev V, Dráberová E, Vinopal S, Dráberová L, Janáček J, Dráber P, Dráber P (2011) STIM1-directed reorganization of microtubules in activated mast cells. J Immunol 186:913–923

32. Laidlaw TM, Steinke JW, Tinana AM, Feng C, Xing W, Lam BK, Paruchuri S, Boyce JA, Borish L (2011) Characterization of a novel human mast cell line that responds to stem cell factor and expresses functional FcεRI. J Allergy Clin Immunol 127:815–822

Chapter 13

Use of Humanized Rat Basophil Leukemia (RBL) Reporter Systems for Detection of Allergen-Specific IgE Sensitization in Human Serum

Daniel Wan, Xiaowei Wang, Ryosuke Nakamura, Marcos J.C. Alcocer, and Franco H. Falcone

Abstract

Determination of allergen-specific IgE levels in human blood samples is an important diagnostic technology for assessment of allergic sensitization. The presence of specific IgE in human serum samples can be measured by sensitizing humanized rat basophil leukemia (RBL) cell lines with diluted serum and measuring cellular activation after challenge with the suspected allergens. This has been traditionally performed by measuring the levels of β-hexosaminidase released upon RBL degranulation. Here, we describe the use of two recently developed humanized RBL reporter cell lines which offer higher sensitivity and are amenable to high-throughput-scale experiments.

Key words Reporter system, Luciferase, DsRed, RBL, IgE, Allergy, RS-ATL8, NFAT-DsRed

1 Introduction

Immunoglobulin E (IgE) is the antibody isotype which is at the center of the pathology of allergic disease. Many of its effects are mediated via the tetrameric high-affinity IgE receptor FcεRI. Because of the key role of IgE, diagnosis of type I allergy has been traditionally focused on measuring the levels of allergen-specific and total IgE in serum or plasma of allergic individuals. This is routinely performed in vitro by measuring IgE binding to solid-phase bound allergens and detection via enzymatically labelled secondary antibodies and fluorescent substrates, using devices available in automated or semiautomated formats from various companies [1]. More recently, new methods have taken advantage of protein array technology (ISAC: ImmunoSolid phase Allergen Chip) [2], allowing simultaneous testing of more than 100 allergens using a small blood sample. Methods based on allergen-specific IgE measurements have high sensitivity, but their clinical relevance is not always

Bernhard F. Gibbs and Franco H. Falcone (eds.), *Basophils and Mast Cells: Methods and Protocols*, Methods in Molecular Biology, vol. 1192, DOI 10.1007/978-1-4939-1173-8_13, © Springer Science+Business Media New York 2014

clear, as they report the ability of IgE to bind allergen but not to induce an allergic reaction. As a result, IgE tests are frequently accompanied by clinically more relevant skin prick tests (SPTs), and a detailed medical history. However SPTs also have a range of disadvantages since the use of certain medications can interfere with the test results resulting in some patients being excluded from this type of test. The residual hazard also requires these tests to be carried out in specialized units. Another more recent type of allergy test is based on the assessment of basophil activation in whole blood (basophil activation tests, BAT) using flow cytometry. These tests work by monitoring the upregulation of CD63 and/or CD203c on the surface of basophils after incubation of heparinized whole blood with the suspected allergen (see Chapter 11). There is currently no widely accepted standard protocol for BATs, and these tests need to be performed within a day after blood sampling (whereas serum samples can be stored). As a result, this test is still not widely used clinically, but only performed in specialized, research-active laboratories.

Another technique has been available for about two decades but, due to its perceived limitations, has not found a widespread use. This is the use of humanized rat basophilic leukemia (RBL) cells for monitoring of specific allergen sensitization in patient serum. The RBL cell lines need to be humanized with at least the human α chain of FcεRI [3], as human IgE does not bind to the rodent IgE receptor [4]. A critical issue with this cell line has been the cytotoxicity of certain human sera for the rat cells, requiring high dilutions and resulting in insufficient sensitization and subsequently negative tests. However, a new generation of reporter cell lines is now replacing the previous humanized RBL cell lines taking advantage of sensitive reporter genes such as luciferase or fluorescent proteins. This enables detection of allergen-specific IgE even when using serum dilutions as high as 1:100 [5, 6]. In this chapter, we describe the use of two such humanized RBL reporter systems, RS-ATL8 and NFAT-DsRed, for detection of allergen-specific IgE in human serum samples. Both methods pave the way for high-throughput measurements, and the latter can also be used in conjunction with allergen arrays [7].

2 Materials

All reagents and supplies should be sterile. Follow local waste disposal regulations.

2.1 Reagents

1. RBL medium: Minimum essential medium (MEM), 10 % v/v heat-inactivated fetal bovine serum, 100 U/mL penicillin, 100 μg/mL streptomycin, 2 mM L-glutamine (if not already present in MEM). Store at 4 °C.

2. RS-ATL8 and NFAT-DsRed reporter cell lines, available from the authors through a Material Transfer Agreement (MTA).

3. G418 sulfate (Geneticin).

4. Blasticidin S (for NFAT-DsRed cells).

5. Hygromycin B (for RS-ATL8 cells).

6. DPBS without Ca^{2+} or Mg^{2+}.

7. Trypsin–EDTA or cell scrapers.

8. Patient sera.

9. Allergens.

10. Anti-human IgE.

11. Lysis buffer: 1 % v/v Triton X-100 in DPBS (for fluorescence assay). Store at 4 °C.

12. ONE-Glo Luciferase Assay System (Promega), for luminescence assay. Follow local regulations regarding the handling of suspected carcinogens. Prepare and store as described by the manufacturer. Warm to room temperature before use.

2.2 Supplies

1. Graduated pipettes and pipette tips.

2. 25 cm^2/75 cm^2 cell culture flasks.

3. 50 mL centrifuge tubes.

4. Clear 96-well plates.

5. Black 96-well plates (for fluorescence assay).

6. White 96-well plates (for luminescence assay).

2.3 Equipment

1. Pipettors for graduated pipettes/tips.

2. Water bath.

3. Class II microbiological safety cabinet.

4. Cell culture incubator: Humidified incubator set to 37 °C and 5 % CO_2.

5. Heat block.

6. Hemocytometer.

7. Centrifuge capable of holding 50 mL tubes.

8. Plate reader for fluorescence or luminescence.

3 Methods

3.1 General Cell Culture

Work in a class II microbiological safety cabinet using sterile techniques.

1. If starting from frozen stocks, partially defrost a vial of cells by warming in hand, and then add 1 mL pre-warmed RBL medium to fully defrost.

2. Transfer cells to a 25 cm² flask containing 8 mL RBL medium, and place in a cell culture incubator overnight.

3. When the cells are confluent in the 25 cm² flask (this may take several days, depending on the viability of frozen cells), transfer cells to a 75 cm² flask by detaching adherent cells using trypsin–EDTA (*see* **steps 1–9** of Subheading 3.3 below).

4. Maintain cells in 10 mL RBL medium supplemented with 1 mg/mL G418 sulfate and 20 μg/mL blasticidin S (NFAT-DsRed) or 500 μg/mL G418 sulfate and 200 μg/mL hygromycin B (RS-ATL8), in a 75 cm² flask, in the cell culture incubator.

5. Passage cells when confluent using trypsin–EDTA (*see* **steps 1–10** below). Replacing the flask with 20 % cells will result in confluence after 3 days. Replace with 10 % of cells for confluence (*see* **Note 1**) after 4 days (refresh the medium after 2 or 3 days). Top up the level of liquid in the flask to 10 mL.

6. Freeze stocks of cells in larger batches, i.e., from several flasks. Centrifuge cells at $300 \times g$ for 5 min, and resuspend in RBL medium with 10 % v/v DMSO to obtain a cell concentration of 5×10^6 cells/mL. Work quickly since DMSO is toxic to cells at room temperature. Aliquot 1 mL cells/cryovial, transferring cryovials to a Mr. Frosty™ (Nalgene) container filled with isopropanol, and place in a –80 °C for several hours or overnight. After freezing, transfer the cryovials to a liquid nitrogen Dewar flask for long-term storage. Defrost a vial to check the viability of the batch.

3.2 Treatment of Serum Before Sensitization (Optional)

1. If necessary, heat human serum in an Eppendorf tube at 56 °C for 5 min (*see* **Note 2**) on a heat block and then place it on ice.

3.3 Sensitization

Cells are sensitized for 16–20 h by incubating them in RBL medium with the desired dilution of previously heat-inactivated serum (*see* **Note 3**).

1. Pre-warm RBL medium to 37 °C in a water bath.

2. Remove medium from 75 cm² flask of confluent cells (*see* **Note 4**).

3. To the flask, add 10 mL DPBS without Ca²⁺ or Mg²⁺ (*see* **Note 5**).

4. Tilt the flask to wash the cells with DPBS.

5. Discard the DPBS in the flask.

6. Add 2 mL trypsin–EDTA to the flask.

7. Tilt the flask to ensure that the cells are exposed to the trypsin–EDTA solution.

8. Incubate the flask for 5–15 min at 37 °C in a cell culture incubator, until clumps of cells are visibly detached (*see* **Note 6**).

9. Add 8 mL pre-warmed RBL medium to the flask and resuspend the cell suspension (*see* **Note 7**).

10. Transfer the cells to a 50 mL tube. Some cells can be left behind in the flask for passaging (*see* Subheading 3.1).

11. Count a sample of cells in a hemocytometer and calculate the total cell number.

12. Pellet the cells by centrifuging at $300 \times g$ for 5 min.

13. Resuspend the cells to a concentration of 1×10^6 cells/mL using RBL medium.

14. Sensitize cells using appropriate concentration of serum (*see* **Note 2**).

15. Pipette 50 μL cells/well of a 96-well plate.

16. Incubate the plate overnight in the cell culture incubator.

3.4 Stimulation

1. Check the plate under a light microscope to see if the cells are in healthy state.

2. Prepare appropriate dilutions of allergens or other stimuli in RBL medium. Optimal concentrations may vary for each allergen and will need to be determined experimentally. Use an appropriate amount of anti-human IgE as a positive control (*see* **Note 8**).

3. Remove the medium from the cells in the 96-well plate.

4. Add 50 μL stimuli to appropriate wells of the plate. Do this quickly so that the cells do not dry out when the medium is removed. Smaller steps, e.g., 3–6 wells at a time, can be done instead.

5. Incubate the plate in the cell culture incubator for 24 h (fluorescence assay with NFAT-DsRed) or 3 h (luciferase assay with RS-ATL8).

3.5 Measurement of Activation

3.5.1 Fluorescence Assay with NFAT-DsRed

1. Wash the cells once with 50 μL DPBS, remove DPBS, and add 100 μL 1 % Triton X-100 in DPBS to lyse the cells.

2. Tap the plate gently to mix, then transfer the lysate in each well to a black 96-well plate, and measure fluorescence in a plate reader (*see* Fig. 1).

3.5.2 Luciferase Assay (EXiLE Test, See Note 9)

1. Allow the luciferase assay reagent and cells to come to room temperature before mixing. The assay is temperature sensitive and this method allows more reproducible results.

2. Add 50 μL ONE-Glo Luciferase Assay Substrate (Promega) directly to stimulated cells (no need to remove medium containing stimulus).

3. Transfer the 100 μL mixture in each well to a white 96-well plate, and measure luminescence in a plate reader (*see* **Notes 10–12**).

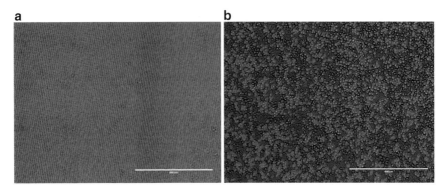

Fig. 1 Fluorescence microscopy image of NFAT-DsRed reporter cell line sensitized with monoclonal IgE without stimulation (**a**) and 24 h after stimulation with anti-IgE antibody (**b**). Note that not all cells appear to have been activated by this treatment and that the intensity of fluorescence varies between individual cells

4   Notes

1. A 1/20 split (5 % cells) is not recommended for routine passaging as this can cause "colonies" to form and unhealthy cells in the middle of the cell clusters.

2. Human sera are frequently cytotoxic for RBL cells (*see* Fig. 2). This is in part due to the presence of activated complement, which is traditionally inactivated by heating at 56 °C for 30 min. This prolonged treatment however also induces irreversible conformational changes in IgE molecules, ablating its ability to bind to FcεRI. A shorter heat inactivation will be sufficient to inactivate complement while preserving the integrity of IgE. We have had good results with this protocol, even with 20 % serum concentration (1:5). Not all sera, however, require heat inactivation. In most cases, a 1:50 or a 1:100 dilution will be sufficient to remove cytotoxicity without any heat treatment. Thus the heat treatment is described as optional.

3. We routinely start the sensitization protocol at 3 pm, and the stimulation at 9 am the following day.

4. Once fully confluent, a 75 cm² flask contains enough cells to fill two 96-well plates.

5. Cell scrapers can be used to detach the cells instead of trypsin–EDTA. Simply refresh RBL medium and scrape the cells. There is no need for a DPBS wash.

6. You can speed up the detachment process by repeatedly knocking the bottom of the flask with your knuckles, holding it tight with the other hand. Be careful, however, as the use of too much force can split the flask.

7. Make sure that any visible clumps are broken up, by pipetting up and down. We routinely use a 5 mL serological pipette for

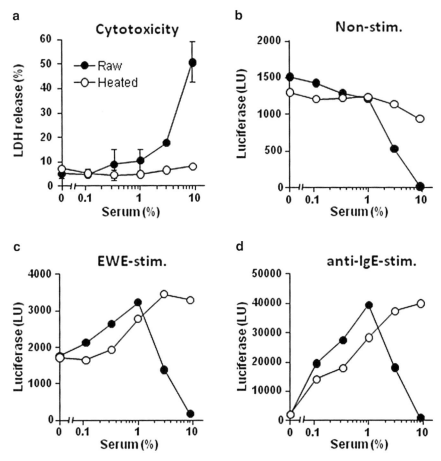

Fig. 2 Cytotoxicity of human serum on the RS-ATL8 cells. A serum sample of an egg white allergic patient (7 years, male, total IgE 1388 IU/mL egg white sIgE 12.8 U$_A$/mL) was heated at 56 °C for 30 min. The RS-ATL8 cells were sensitized overnight with the serum at various concentrations. (**a**) Cytotoxicity of the sera on the cells as revealed by LDH release assay. EXiLE response after 3-h treatment of (**b**) control medium, (**c**) egg white extract (EWE), and (**d**) anti-human IgE

this purpose, as these have a narrower tapered end. Make sure that you do not create bubbles when pipetting up and down by always leaving some medium in the pipette when expelling the liquid and not taking up any air when aspirating it.

8. The optimal amount of anti-IgE will depend on the type (species, clonality, affinity, etc.) used and needs to be determined empirically. Optimum concentrations can range between 100 ng/mL and 2 μg/mL which therefore need to be determined by testing the anti-IgE antibody over a wide range of concentrations (e.g., at least five orders or magnitude). This should result in a bell-shaped stimulation curve, with a clear suboptimal and supraoptimal stimulation range.

9. This test is now known as EXiLE test, for Ig*E* cross-linking (=*X*)-*i*nduced *L*uciferase *E*xpression [5].

10. In our lab, we have tested different types of multiwell plates. Clear plates are not recommended for final scans due to lower sensitivity than black or white plates. However, if there is no option but to use clear plates, light detection from below (bottom scans) will give higher sensitivity than top scans. Black plates give greatest sensitivity for fluorescence assays, and white plates give greatest sensitivity for luminescence assays. For opaque plates, for obvious reasons, light detection (and fluorescence excitation) must be from above. We found that opaque-walled, clear-bottomed plates do not greatly increase sensitivity. However, different plate readers may give different results. If you have the resources, it may be worthwhile to repeat these tests for the plate readers in your own lab.

11. If cells are sensitized in black/white plates, then there is no need to transfer cell lysates from clear to opaque plates; the entire experiment can be carried out in a single plate. However, we find it essential to examine the cells after an overnight incubation to check for cell death or contamination. A clear-bottomed plate is required for light microscopes.

12. Bubbles can be created by incorrect pipetting technique or sample evaporation, and may interfere with plate readings. Large bubbles can be removed by stabbing with a dry pipette tip (a wet pipette tip cannot burst bubbles). If there are many small bubbles throughout the plate, most can be removed by briefly centrifuging the plate.

Acknowledgements

This work was supported by the COST Action BM1007 Mast Cells and Basophils—Targets for Innovative Therapies.

References

1. Ricci G, Capelli M, Miniero R et al (2003) A comparison of different allergometric tests, skin prick test, Pharmacia UniCAPR and ADVIA CentaurR, for diagnosis of allergic diseases in children. Allergy 58:38–45
2. Sastre J (2010) Molecular diagnosis in allergy. Clin Exp Allergy 40:1442–1460
3. Taudou G, Varin-Blank N, Jouin H et al (1993) Expression of the alpha chain of human Fc epsilon RI in transfected rat basophilic leukemia cells: functional activation after sensitization with human mite-specific IgE. Int Arch Allergy Immunol 100:344–350
4. Miller L, Blank U, Metzger H, Kinet JP (1989) Expression of high-affinity binding of human immunoglobulin E by transfected cells. Science 244:334–337
5. Nakamura R, Uchida Y, Higuchi M et al (2010) A convenient and sensitive allergy test: IgE crosslinking-induced luciferase expression in cultured mast cells. Allergy 65:1266–1273
6. Wang X, Cato P, Lin H-C et al (2013) Optimisation and use of humanised RBL NF-AT-GFP and NF-AT-DsRed reporter cell lines suitable for high-throughput scale detection of allergic sensitisation in array format and identification of the ECM-integrin interaction as critical factor. Mol Biotechnol. doi:10.1007/s12033-013-9689-x
7. Lin J, Renault N, Haas H et al (2007) A novel tool for the detection of allergic sensitization combining protein microarrays with human basophils. Clin Exp Allergy 37:1854–1862

Chapter 14

Gene Silencing Approaches in Mast Cells and Primary Human Basophils

Vadim V. Sumbayev and Bernhard F. Gibbs

Abstract

The ability to silence gene expression is an invaluable tool for elucidating the importance of intracellular signaling proteins which contribute to the effector functions of mast cells and basophils. However, primary mast cells and their terminally differentiated blood counterpart, namely basophils, pose a difficult challenge for gene silencing approaches given not only their state of maturation and difficulty to transfect, but also because their functions are readily altered by cell-handling conditions. Here, we describe a method using lipofection which has been successfully employed to silence gene expression using siRNA in human LAD2 mast cells as well as primary human basophils.

Key words Transfection, siRNA, Lipofection, Electroporation, Nanofection

1 Introduction

Gene silencing is an epigenetic process which allows regulation of gene expression. The term "gene silencing" normally means "turning the gene off" without genetic modification. In other words, the gene which is expressed under normal circumstances is switched off by the cellular machinery. Gene silencing occurs when it is impossible to translate mRNA and can be performed on a transcriptional or a posttranscriptional level [1].

Transcriptional gene silencing is normally achieved by histone modifications. This involves creating an environment of heterochromatin around the target gene making it inaccessible for transcription factors or other components of the transcriptional machinery [1]. However, in most cases, gene silencing is performed at the posttranscriptional level. This is achieved by destruction or blocking of the mRNA transcribed from a target gene that normally encodes a specific target protein. The blocking of the target mRNA normally occurs through the activity of silencers which interact with repressor regions. However, a more reliable effect could be obtained upon destruction of the target mRNA [1].

Bernhard F. Gibbs and Franco H. Falcone (eds.), *Basophils and Mast Cells: Methods and Protocols*, Methods in Molecular Biology, vol. 1192, DOI 10.1007/978-1-4939-1173-8_14, © Springer Science+Business Media New York 2014

This is normally performed using RNA interference (RNAi), which is also known as posttranscriptional gene silencing (PTGS). During RNAi, specific RNA molecules inhibit the expression of the target gene, typically by inducing destruction of specific mRNA molecules [2].

This could be achieved by two ways:

1. Transfection of the cells with small interfering RNA (siRNA): Small interfering or silencing RNAs form a class of small double-stranded RNA molecules (max 20–25 base pairs in length) [2–4].

2. Use of small hairpin RNA or short hairpin RNA (shRNA) which makes a tight hairpin turn that can be used to silence target gene expression. shRNA is transfected into the cells in the form of plasmid DNA where it then undergoes transcription into shRNA [5].

In both cases, gene expression is ultimately silenced using siRNA. In the first case, the siRNA duplex is directly transfected into the cells; in the second, shRNA is produced on the matrix of transfected DNA and then processed by the intracellular machinery [2–5]. We will therefore consider the mechanisms of shRNA processing/action, since this will address both types of posttranscriptional mRNA destruction.

Plasmid DNA acts as a matrix for shRNA production. Generated shRNA is processed by the Dicer enzyme, an endoribonuclease of the RNase III family that cleaves double-stranded RNA (dsRNA) into short double-stranded RNA fragments of about 20–25 base pair length (duplexes), with a two-base overhang on the 3′ terminus. One of these duplexes is the siRNA of interest. This siRNA binds target mRNA and induces its degradation which is achieved by activation of the RNA-induced silencing complex (RISC) of endonucleases called "argonaute proteins," cleaving the target mRNA strand complementary to their bound siRNA. As the RNA fragments produced by Dicer are double stranded, each of them could, in theory, become converted into functional siRNA. However, only one of the two siRNA strands (guide strand) binds the argonaute protein and directs gene silencing [1, 2, 5]. These processes are summarized in Fig. 1.

Intracellular signaling networks occurring in human mast cells and basophils are poorly understood. In order to study the biological/biochemical activity of any signaling component it is necessary to specifically switch it off and monitor the affected processes. This would then allow conclusions to be made on the contribution of the signaling protein of interest to specific intracellular biochemical cascades or cycles as well as changes in overall cell function, such as mediator production and release. Such studies could be performed by gene silencing since pharmacological inhibitors of various signaling proteins often do not display absolute specificity. Additionally,

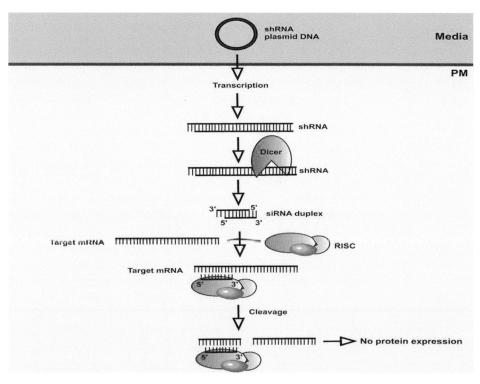

Fig. 1 Mechanism of siRNA activation and biochemical action. *Media* cell culture medium, *PM* plasma membrane

we face the problem that both mast cells and basophils are hematopoietic cells of myeloid lineage. These cells (myeloid hematopoietic cells) are notoriously difficult to transfect [6, 7] because of the following reasons:

1. They are highly differentiated and therefore these cells are not geared towards overexpressing plasmids.

2. They can often engulf and destroy foreign biologically active substances, including plasmids.

3. Their membrane is much less permeable compared to other cells and have substantially more proteins integrated into it, which hinders the ready uptake and diffusion of transfection material.

Currently, there are several methods of transfection which have been employed for human mast cells/basophils and other myeloid cells.

The first is *electroporation*. In this case, an electric current is used to deliver genetic material. The membrane becomes relatively conductive, thus allowing current to pass through the cell when the electric fields are intensified above a certain threshold. This leads to the transient formation of pores by electrical breakdown. Only the nucleic acid bound to plasma membrane is transferred into the cell. Another possible mechanism is that the electric pulse affects membrane stability where the appearance of unstable lipid bilayers results in the formation of vesicles containing nucleic acid which are then endocytosed. The potential problem with this technique is that biological responses of mast cells and basophils are regulated through plasma membrane-associated receptors. Electroporation could therefore affect the membrane potential by negatively influencing the ability of the inflammatory/immune receptors to recognize their ligands, which are vital in order to subsequently study their normal function [6, 7].

Another possible approach is a *lipofection* (a contraction of "liposome transfection"). This is a technique which allows delivery of nucleic acid into a cell by the use of liposomes. Liposomes are lipid-derived vesicles that can easily interact with the cell membrane since both binding partners are made of a phospholipid bilayer. Lipofection generally assumes the use of positively charged (cationic) lipid to form an aggregate (complex) with negatively charged (anionic) genetic material. A net positive charge of this aggregate increases the effectiveness of transfection through the negatively charged phospholipid bilayer of the plasma membrane. The main advantages of lipofection are the relatively high transfection efficiencies, the possibility of transfection of all types of nucleic acids into a wide range of cell types, and the relatively low toxicity of the transfection reagents [3, 4, 8].

Currently, a new approach is under development which uses nanomaterials/nanoparticles for the delivery of genetic materials. This approach, known as "nanofection," can result in very high transfection efficiencies but in terms of its application to mast cells or basophils it could be less effective since, upon endocytosis, nanomaterials often affect cytoskeleton elements. Upon degranulation, mast cells and basophils undergo major cytoskeleton alterations and this type of transfection could therefore affect the ability of mast cells/basophils to respond to stimuli normally and give rise to observations that are unrelated to specific silencing of a target gene [3, 9].

Given the above, lipofection is therefore currently deemed the best transfection approach which one could use to silence genes in human mast cells and basophils.

There are several commercial transfection reagents which could be used in this case: DOTAP, lipofectamine, Fugene 6, etc. These reagents allow for relatively high transfection efficiencies (up to 40 %) to be obtained whilst avoiding major cell damage or toxic effects on the target cells.

In our lab, we have successfully used DOTAP transfection reagent to deliver siRNA into LAD2 mast cells [4], primary human basophils [3], the monocyte cell line THP-1 [10], and the monocyte macrophage 6-cell line (MM6) as well as human myeloid leukaemia cells [11]. We will now present a protocol which describes the procedure for primary human basophils and LAD2 mast cells. The

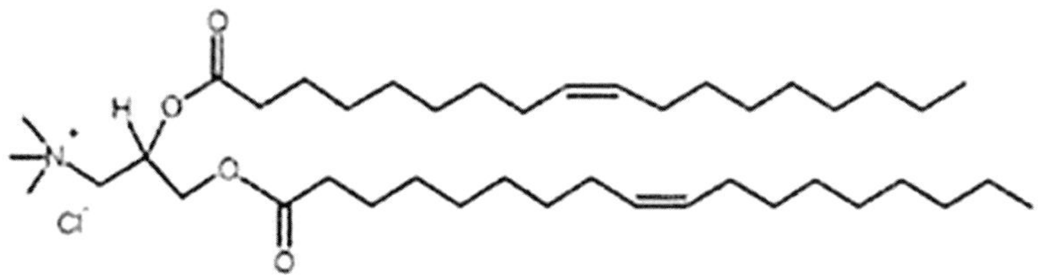

Fig. 2 Chemical structure of DOTAP chloride

method is based on the ability of DOTAP chloride (N-[1-(2,3-dioleoyloxy)propyl]-N,N,N-trimethylammonium chloride; *see* Fig. 2), a cationic liposome-forming compound, to interact with nucleic acid-forming aggregates which are endocytosed by target cells followed by a release of the genetic material inside the cell.

2 Materials

2.1 Cells

1. LAD2 human mast cells (*see* **Note 1** and Chapter 8): These cells are available from Prof. Dean Metcalfe and Dr. Arnold Kirshenbaum (NAID, NIH, USA). Cells should be cultured in the Stem-Pro-34 serum-free medium with supplements containing 2 mM L-glutamine, penicillin (100 U/mL), streptomycin (100 μg/mL), and recombinant human stem cell factor (SCF) (100 ng/mL) [12].

2. Primary human basophils (purified and handled as described in Chapter 2 of this book; *see* **Note 2**).

2.2 Reagents

1. DOTAP chloride reagent (can be purchased from various commercial sources).

2. HEPES (4-(2-hydroxyethyl)-1-piperazineethanesulfonic acid): Prepare HEPES-buffered saline: 20 mM HEPES, 150 mM NaCl, pH 7.4.

3. Nucleic acid, for example siRNA.

4. Ultrapure water suitable for molecular biology work.

3 Methods

3.1 Transfection Procedure

Using the above reagents, two solutions (solution A and solution B) are prepared (*see* **Note 3**).

1. *Solution A*: Dissolve 5 μg of siRNA (or DNA) in 50 μL of HBS (*see* **Note 4**).

2. *Solution B*: Gently mix 30 μL of the DOTAP reagent with 70 μL of the HBS.

3. Gently mix solutions A and B (avoid vortexing or centrifugation) and leave for 30 min at 15 ± 10 °C. This is your working reagent (WR).

4. Add 150 µL of the WR to 5 mL of the culture medium containing your cells and mix gently, for example by a careful swirling of the Petri dish (*see* **Note 5**).

5. Leave for 2–6 h for primary human basophils or overnight (~16 h for LAD2 mast cells or other types of myeloid cell lines).

6. Upon completion of the transfection change the culture medium. Your cells are then ready for experimentation (*see* **Note 6**).

3.2 Analysis of Gene Silencing

Gene silencing should always be confirmed using two approaches:

1. Measurement of the mRNA of the target gene (protein) using the method which is the most established in your laboratory. This could be reverse-transcription PCR or quantitative real-time PCR.

2. Detection of the actual amounts of your target protein. This should normally be done by Western blot analysis. However, if you are trying to silence the expression of plasma membrane-associated proteins (for example Toll-like receptors or IgE receptors), then flow cytometry could also be an excellent approach to test protein levels (*see* **Note 7**).

4   Notes

1. LAD2 mast cells are currently the best human mast cell line for studying IgE-dependent as well as IgE-independent mast cell responses (*see* Chapter 8). However, we have in the past noticed variations in responses (e.g., changes in the percentage of histamine release to anti-IgE stimulation after sensitization as well as very high spontaneous degranulation) while maintaining LAD2 cultures. It is advised that pilot experiments are first conducted to assess for acceptable functional responses before performing gene silencing studies.

2. It is essential to isolate and purify basophils in the shortest possible time in order to obtain viable cells after transfection. The current gene silencing methods, including the one described, can mainly be used in basophils for studying intracellular signaling processes and effects on de novo mediator generation. However, degranulation processes (e.g., histamine release), in our hands, appear to be more affected by the transfection reagent than we have seen with LAD2 mast cells.

3. Use sterile tubes to make both solutions.

4. It is recommended to optimize experimentally the amount of siRNA (or DNA) supplied, bearing in mind that DOTAP is normally nontoxic at concentrations below 150 µg/mL.

5. DOTAP allows for equal transfection quality in culture medium both in the presence or the absence of serum. Therefore, for transfection it is recommended to use the medium which you normally use to culture your cells [3, 4, 11].

6. It is essential to perform cell viability check in parallel to the main experiment or upon completion of the treatment. In this regard, an MTS (3-(4,5-dimethylthiazol-2-yl)-5-(3-carboxymethoxyphenyl)-2-(4-sulfophenyl)-2H-tetrazolium) test would be optimal. Additionally, ensure that you use a random or a mutated (scrambled—same overall nucleotide composition, but different sequence) siRNA control to certify that the effect you observe is specific and is a result of gene silencing. In addition, it is recommended to add a control for DOTAP reagent, thus making sure that it does not affect the pathways you study.

7. Gene silencing affects mRNA but it does not destroy the protein molecules which were already expressed. Therefore, the decrease in the constitutive levels of the silenced protein will depend not only on the mRNA levels but also on the stability of the actual protein in the cells.

References

1. Norata GD, Tibolla G, Catapano AL (2013) Gene silencing approaches for the management of dyslipidaemia. Trends Pharmacol Sci 34:198–205

2. Macrae I, Zhou K, Li F, Repic A, Brooks A, Cande W, Adams P, Doudna J (2006) Structural basis for double-stranded RNA processing by dicer. Science 311:195–198

3. Sumbayev VV, Nicholas SA, Streatfield CL, Gibbs BF (2009) Involvement of hypoxia-Inducible Factor-1 in IgE-mediated primary human basophil responses. Eur J Immunol 39:3511–3519

4. Sumbayev VV, Yasinska IM, Oniku AE, Streatfield CL, Gibbs BF (2012) Involvement of hypoxia-inducible factor-1 in the inflammatory responses of human LAD2 mast cells and basophils. PLoS One 7:e34259

5. Wang Z, Rao DD, Senzer N, Nemunaitis J (2011) RNA interference and cancer therapy. Pharm Res 28:2983–2995

6. Imai E, Isaka Y (2002) Gene electrotransfer: potential for gene therapy of renal diseases. Kidney Int 61:S37–S41

7. Vilarino N, MacGlashan D Jr (2005) Transient transfection of human peripheral blood basophils. J Immunol Methods 296:11–18

8. Burke B (2003) Macrophages as novel cellular vehicles for gene therapy. Expert Opin Biol Ther 3:919–924

9. Sumbayev VV, Yasinska IM, Gibbs BF (2013) Biomedical applications of gold nanoparticles. In: Said A, Tang CH, Oprisan S (eds) Recent advances in circuits, communications and signal processing, WSEAS Press, Athens, pp 342–348

10. Nicholas SA, Sumbayev VV (2009) The involvement of hypoxia-inducible factor 1 alpha in Toll-like receptor 7/8-mediated inflammatory response. Cell Res 19:973–983

11. Shatrov VA, Sumbayev VV, Zhou J, Bruene B (2003) Oxidized low density lipoprotein triggers HIF-1alpha protein via redox-dependent mechanism. Blood 101:4847–4849

12. Kirshenbaum AS, Akin C, Wu Y, Rottem M, Goff JP et al (2003) Characterization of novel stem cell factor responsive human mast cell lines LAD 1 and 2 established from a patient with mast cell sarcoma/leukemia; activation following aggregation of FcepsilonRI or FcgammaRI. Leuk Res 27:677–682

Chapter 15

Basophil Stimulation and Signaling Pathways

Edward F. Knol and Bernhard F. Gibbs

Abstract

Despite growing use of flow cytometry to analyze the functional characteristics of primary basophils the intracellular signaling cascades that control their ability to elaborate various inflammatory mediators and cytokines remain comparatively obscure. Additionally, some studies require the analysis of pro-allergic and inflammatory mediators, such as histamine, LTC_4, and various basophil-derived cytokines (e.g., IL-4 and IL-13). Elucidation of intracellular signaling proteins by Western blotting, cytosolic free calcium concentration by spectrofluorophotometry, and detection of mediator releases, as well as analysis of gene expressions by RT-PCR, generally require relatively large numbers of purified basophils. In selected assays, flow cytometry can enable the analysis of relatively low cell numbers and purity for the expression of intracellular signaling proteins or measurement of cytosolic free calcium concentrations by basophil-specific gating strategies. Unfortunately, many aspects of signal transduction relevant to human basophils cannot be readily extrapolated from the use of basophil or mast cell lines. This chapter therefore focuses on how to employ primary human basophils for studying mediator releases and signaling characteristics.

Key words Basophils, Signaling, IgE receptors, Western blotting, Flow cytometry, Inhibitors

1 Introduction

Human basophilic granulocytes are inflammatory cells that appear to be involved in the pathogenesis of a variety of allergic diseases (reviewed in [1]). Upon activation by various stimuli they release several biologically active mediators, such as histamine and leukotriene C_4, as well as cytokines such as IL-4 (*see* Chapter 10). Due to the limited availability of human basophils of high purity, precise knowledge of the signal transduction pathways leading to release reactions is still sparse. Activation of basophils through FcεRI signaling is mostly studied via anti-IgE or allergen-induced activation. Other receptor-mediated stimuli for human basophils include the bacterial peptide formyl-methionyl-leucyl-phenylalanine (fMLP) and the complement fragment C5a. Calcium ionophores A23187 or ionomycin as well as phorbol-myristate acetate (PMA) activate

Edward F. Knol and Bernhard F. Gibbs have contributed equally to this Chapter.

Bernhard F. Gibbs and Franco H. Falcone (eds.), *Basophils and Mast Cells: Methods and Protocols*, Methods in Molecular Biology, vol. 1192, DOI 10.1007/978-1-4939-1173-8_15, © Springer Science+Business Media New York 2014

basophils independent of cell membrane receptors. Priming of baso-phils can be achieved by interleukin-3 or platelet-activating factor which markedly potentiate mediator release caused by various stimuli.

It is clear that the receptor-mediated stimulation of basophils results in a strong donor-dependent activation determined, for instance, by histamine release. For FcεRI-induced degranulation the strength of activation of Syk has been hypothesized to be causal [2]. For many other stimuli this is not clear yet and we need better insights into basophil signal transduction cascades that control degranulation or the release of cytokines and other mediators.

2   Materials

2.1   Chemicals and Kits

1. Recombinant human IL-3: Prepare aliquots of a stock solution containing 10 μg/mL of IL-3 in Ca^{2+}-free HEPES-buffered Tyrode's solution to avoid repeated freeze-thaw cycles. Use at 0.1–1 ng/mL final concentration as a priming factor to enhance IgE-dependent basophil stimulation.

2. Anti-human IgE: Polyclonal IgG antibodies are most often employed. These need to be titrated in a pilot experiment to determine optimum basophil mediator release and concen-trated aliquots prepared accordingly and frozen at –20 °C for subsequent experiments. Note that some basophil mediators, e.g., IL-4, are released at five- to tenfold lower concentrations than those required for histamine release or CD63 expression. It is therefore advisable to use concentrations of anti-IgE (or other IgE-dependent stimuli) that are slightly suboptimal with respect to histamine release or CD63 expressions.

3. IgE-independent stimuli: 1 mM stock solutions in DMSO to avoid freeze-thaw issues (which are particularly of concern regarding cal-cium ionophores) and perform pilot basophil stimulation experi-ments to determine optimum (or suboptimum) basophil stimulation. For A23187 this is usually between 1 and 10 μM (note that there is a sharp bell-shaped response for this stimulus): for fMLP 100–1,000 nM, for C5a 1–10 nM, and for PMA 10–100 ng/mL. For C5a and IL-3, use either buffer or 0.9 % NaCl supple-mented with 1 mg/mL BSA to prepare stock solutions.

4. ELISA kits for histamine, LTC_4, and pro-allergic cytokines (e.g., IL-4): Note that for detection of cytokine release the most sensitive ELISA kits are usually required (i.e., mini-mum detection at ca. 1–3 pg/mL). Histamine releases also are mostly determined spectrofluorometrically based on the method described by Shore et al. [3].

5. Laemmli-lysis buffer for SDS-PAGE/Western blotting: Prepare lysis buffer consisting of 50 mM Tris–HCl pH 7.5, 5 mM EDTA, 10 mM EGTA, 5 mM DTT, 1 % Nonidet P-40,

1 mM PMSF, 100 μg/mL aprotonin, 20 μg/mL leupeptin, and 10 mM benzamidine and then mix with equal volumes of 2× concentrated Laemmli sample buffer (obtained from commercial sources). Freeze aliquots at –20 °C. Ensure complete dissolution of contents prior to use.

6. SDS-PAGE reagents: Tris base pH 8.8, Tris–HCl pH 6.8, 30 % acrylamide-Bis solution, glycerol, glycine, SDS, TEMED, APS. Blotting and transfer buffers.

7. Western blotting reagents: Tris-buffered saline and Tween-20 (TBST) solution (containing 20 mM Tris–HCl, pH 7.5, 137 mM NaCl, 0.1 % Tween 20), skimmed milk powder, antibodies to signaling proteins, secondary antibodies (e.g., labeled with either HRP or dyes if using LiCor imaging systems).

8. Calcium indicators: The free Ca^{2+} indicators indo-1 and fura-2 are acetoxy-methyl ester labelled. Basophils are incubated with approximately 1 μM in a Ca^{2+}-containing buffer. Within basophils the acetoxy-methyl ester, which can diffuse freely through the membrane, is cleaved by cytosolic esterases, resulting in a charged, cell-impermeable compound form of indo-1 and fura-2.

2.2 Buffers for Cell Culture and Stains

1. N-2-hydroxyethylpiperazine-N-2-ethanesulfonic acid (HEPES)-buffered Tyrode's solution (pH 7.4): NaCl 137.0 mM (8.0 g/L), glucose 5.6 mM (1.0 g/L), KCL 2.7 mM (201 mg/L), $CaCl_2 \cdot 2H_2O$ 1.0 mM (147 mg/L), $MgCl_2 \cdot 6H_2O$ 1.0 mM (203 mg/L), HEPES 10.0 mM (2.9 g/L), $NaH_2PO_4 \cdot 2H_2O$ 0.4 mM (62.5 mg/L). The pH is adjusted to 7.4 with NaOH (1 M). This buffer will keep for 1 week at 4 °C and may be used for brief periods (<1 h) of basophil stimulation.

2. HEPES-buffered Tyrode's solution (pH 7.4) without $MgCl_2$ and $CaCl_2$ (Ca^{2+}-free buffer): Used for washing basophils before experimentation and for terminating reactions at the end of incubation periods (though this is not usually done following long-term incubation periods, especially where ELISAs for LTC_4 and cytokine releases are required and dilution of samples must be avoided).

3. RPMI 1640 with L-glutamine, 1 % penicillin-streptomycin, and 1 mg/mL BSA: Used for experiments requiring long incubation periods (>1 h).

4. Alcian blue staining of basophils (adapted from [4]): Dissolve cetylpyridinium chloride (76 mg), lanthanum chloride (700 mg), NaCl (900 mg), Tween 20 (21 μL), and alcian blue (143 mg) in 100 mL distilled H_2O and stir for at least 2 h at room temperature. Filter using a 1 μm filter or, alternatively, centrifuge at $1,000 \times g$ for 15 min and carefully collect the supernatant. The solution is stable for at least 1 year at 4 °C.

To 10 μL of cell suspension add 65 μL of NaCl solution (1 mg/mL containing 0.1 % EDTA) followed by 65 μL of alcian blue solution (described above). Finally, add 5 μL of 1 M HCl, gently resuspend, and determine the total number and purity of basophils using a hemocytometer.

2.3 Basophils

1. Enrichment and purification of primary human basophils are described in detail in Chapter 2.

2. Ensure sufficient basophil purity and number using alcian blue stain and a hemocytometer (*see* Chapter 2, Subheading 2.2, **item 4**), or flow cytometer with basophil-discriminating antibodies (*see* Chapter 7). For determining mediator release, at least 100,000 basophils/vial are usually necessary. For RT-PCR and Western blotting, use at least 200,000–300,000 basophils/vial.

2.4 Equipment and Other Materials

1. Water purification system.

2. Microscope and hemocytometer.

3. CO_2 incubator or water bath set to 37 °C.

4. Centrifuges ($400–1,000 \times g$).

5. Heating block for 1.5 mL tubes.

6. ELISA plate reader.

7. LiCor Odyssey or comparable imaging system or darkroom for ECL detection using photographic film.

8. Flow cytometer.

9. Spectrofluorophotometer.

10. 50 and 10 mL test tubes (polypropylene) and 1.5 mL Eppendorf tubes.

11. Pipette tips.

3 Methods

The following methods describe the basic procedure for analyzing basophil responses as well as variations depending on whether the release of various mediator types is being assessed or signal transduction studies conducted. It is vital that cell handling and preparation of purified basophils are kept as short as possible.

3.1 Basophil Stimulation Assay: General Procedure

1. Wash basophils and resuspend in either Tyrode's buffer (short incubations) or RPMI 1640 medium (long incubations to determine cytokine release), at room temperature, and aliquot (400 μL) into test tubes at a density of ca. 50,000–150,000 basophils/mL. Include tubes for positive control (e.g., anti-IgE and/or IgE-independent stimulus) and negative control (buffer with cells alone).

2. Place all tubes in a water bath or culture cabinets set at 37 °C.

3. Add 50 μL of prewarmed buffer, priming factors (e.g., IL-3), or signal transduction inhibitors to the tubes and preincubate for 15 min. Avoid cooling.

4. Stimulate all tubes except negative control with 50 μL anti-IgE (or IgE-independent stimulus) for the required times (the total volume for each vial should now be 500 μL).

3.2 Histamine Release Analysis

1. Prepare and treat basophils as described above (Subheading 3.1; *see* **Note 1**) and stimulate for 30 min (unless release kinetics are being addressed, *see* **Note 2**).

2. Quench reactions by adding 1 mL of ice-cold Ca^{2+}-free HEPES-buffered Tyrode's solution into each tube and centrifuge immediately ($850 \times g$, 2 min, 4 °C).

3. Decant supernatants into fresh tubes and add 1.45 mL Ca^{2+}-free HEPES-buffered Tyrode's solution to the pellet tubes. For automated histamine analysis deplete proteins, including enzymes, in the supernatant by adding 2 % w/v perchloric acid. Lyse the pellet tubes by adding 50 μL perchloric acid (70 %) for automated analysis of histamine release according to the method described by Shore et al. [3]. Alternatively, freeze-thaw cell pellet samples (without perchloric acid) three times.

4. Briefly vortex pellet tubes and centrifuge ($850 \times g$, 10 min, 4 °C) to remove debris.

5. The tubes can be stored at −20 °C until ready for assay.

6. Assay for histamine (either using commercial kits or fluorometric analysis).

7. Histamine release is calculated as a percentage of the total content (present in the cell pellet and corresponding supernatant). Results are typically expressed as either relative percent releases (the % release into the supernatant for each condition/vial) or corrected percent release (the net % release after subtracting spontaneous releases obtained from the negative controls). Spontaneous release should be below 10 %, preferably below 5 %, to check for any nonspecific activation (e.g., caused by cell-handling issues).

3.3 Eicosanoid and Cytokine Release Analysis

1. Experimental conditions are the same as described in Subheading 3.1 except for the variable incubation periods and termination of reactions.

2. Unless the basophil density is very high (e.g., 200,000 basophils in 500 μL total reaction volume), it is not recommended to stop reactions using ice-cold Ca^{2+}-free HEPES-buffered Tyrode's solution since the mediators of interest may be diluted too much to detect. Instead, briefly place all tubes in ice water and then centrifuge ($850 \times g$, 2 min, 4 °C).

3. Decant supernatants into fresh vials and freeze immediately (−20 °C or lower) until ready for assay.

4. Eicosanoid (e.g., LTC$_4$) release is usually complete after 30-min stimulation and is measured only in the supernatants.

5. Optimum cytokine production from basophils varies from 4 h, for the detection of IL-4 release, to over 16 h for IL-13 releases. At the end of each stimulation period harvest the supernatants as described above and freeze immediately for storage prior to assaying cytokine content (*see* **Note 3**).

3.4 Measurement of Cytosolic Free Calcium Concentrations by Spectrofluorophotometer or Flow Cytometer

1. Prepare and treat basophils as described above (Subheadings 2.1, **item 8**, and 3.1).

2. For the spectrofluorophotometer and indo-1-loaded basophils excitation and emission wavelengths should be taken at 340 nm and 390 nm, respectively.

3. Before each measurement the cells are diluted in medium with 1 mM CaCl$_2$ to a density of approximately 1×10^6 cells/mL.

4. Calibration of the signal is obtained by permeabilization of the cells with 5 μM digitonin to obtain maximum fluorescence and then quenching with 0.5 mM MnCl$_2$ to obtain minimal fluorescence (*see* Fig. 1).

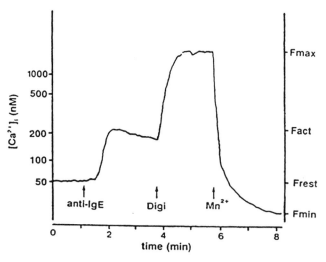

Fig. 1 Increase in [Ca^{2+}]$_i$ in a purified basophil suspension after anti-IgE stimulation. Basophils were loaded with indo-1 and fluorescence measurements were performed using a spectrofluorophotometer, as described in Subheading 3.4. In this recording the calibration of indo-1 fluorescence as a function of [Ca^{2+}]$_i$ was also carried out. All trapped indo-1 was saturated by permeabilization of the cells with 5 μm digitonin (Digi), resulting in a maximal fluorescence (F_{max}). Subsequently, the indo-1 signal was quenched by addition of 0.5 mM MnCl$_2$ (Mn^{2+}) resulting in minimal fluorescence (F_{min}). Fluorescence of the unstimulated population is marked as F_{rest} and the anti-IgE-stimulated population as F_{act} [5]

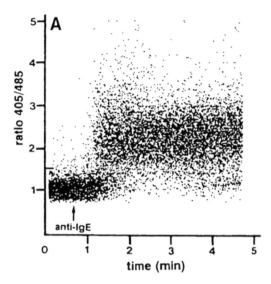

Fig. 2 Increase in [Ca^{2+}]$_i$ determined by flow cytometer in a purified basophil suspension after anti-IgE stimulation. Basophils were loaded with indo-1 and fluorescence measurements were performed in a flow cytometer, as described in Subheading 3.4. In contrast to the data shown in Fig. 1, the [Ca^{2+}]$_i$ in individual basophils is depicted [6]

5. Cytoplasmic free calcium concentration is calculated by the equation $[Ca^{2+}] = Kd \times ((F - F_{min})/(F_{max} - F))$, using 250 nM as the Kd for the Ca^{2+}/indo-1 complex.

6. For flow cytometry it is not possible to determine the precise $[Ca^{2+}]$ using the calibration strategy described above; only the relative ratio of $[Ca^{2+}]$ can be obtained (*see* Fig. 2).

7. Flow cytometry emission and excitation wavelengths are determined somewhat by the filters available, but should be within the range described above.

8. For flow cytometry, a sampling chamber with low magnetic stirring and heating at 37 °C is required.

9. Addition of EGTA (1.5 mM) or buffering Ca^{2+} concentrations in incubation buffers to about 100 nM selectively will prevent Ca^{2+} influx and will only show Ca^{2+} increase due to release from intracellular stores (*see* Fig. 3).

3.5 Determination of Activation Pathways by Flow Cytometry

1. Prepare and treat basophils as described above (Subheading 3.1). Depending on the system unprocessed blood, peripheral blood mononuclear cell preparation, or purified (partly or fully) basophils can be activated (*see* **Note 4**).

2. Stop reactions by adding ice-cold buffer with EDTA.

3. Antibodies to characterize basophils, such as CD123$^+$/CD203C$^+$/HLA-DR$^-$, or CCR3 are added together with CD63 (in order to estimate activated basophils) for about 30 min at 4 °C.

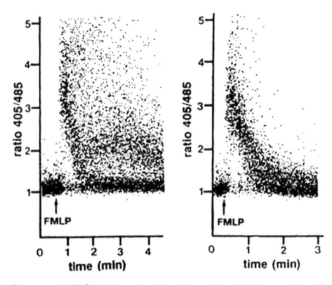

Fig. 3 Changes in $[Ca^{2+}]_i$ determined by flow cytometer in a purified basophil suspension following the addition of fMLP. Experiments were performed as described above. In the *right* panel, cells were stimulated without Ca^{2+}, but with 1.5 mM EGTA to deplete extracellular Ca^{2+}. The *right* panel depicts the increase in $[Ca^{2+}]_i$ from intracellular stores only [5]

4. If unprocessed blood was used, residual erythrocytes should be lysed.

5. To stain for intracellular proteins cells should be fixed and permeabilized by resuspending them in 300 μL of 0.3 % saponin and 3.7 % formaldehyde in PBS for 30 min at 4 °C.

6. Staining of phosphorylated (activation) proteins, such as phospho-p38 mitogen-activated protein kinase (p38 MAPK), is performed on the permeabilized cells at relatively early time points (e.g., 1, 3, 5, 10 min) following stimulation (*see* **Note 5**).

7. Control cells that are stored in ice-cold buffer are used to determine baseline phosphorylation.

8. Flow cytometric analysis should be performed on either labeled basophils or purified basophils.

3.6 Signal Transduction Experiments and Preparation of Samples for SDS-PAGE and Western Blotting

1. Prepare and treat basophils as described above (Subheading 3.1) and stimulate for the required times (*see* **Note 6**).

2. Stop cell incubations either by briefly placing tubes on ice water (if concentrated supernatants are required for mediator release assays) or by adding 1 mL of ice-cold Ca^{2+}-free HEPES-buffered Tyrode's solution.

3. Centrifuge immediately (850–1,000 × *g*; 2 min).

4. Remove supernatants and lyse cell pellets on ice by vigorous mixing in 15–30 μL of Laemmli-lysis buffer (*see* **Note** 7).

5. Immediately heat all tubes to over 95 °C for 3 min and either store at –70 °C for later analysis or proceed to SDS-PAGE.

6. Separate proteins by SDS-PAGE and transfer to nitrocellulose membranes. Include a molecular weight (MW) marker, e.g., pre-stained MW rainbow markers for each SDS-PAGE run.

7. Block membranes for 2 h in 5 % skimmed milk in TBST buffer.

8. Briefly wash twice with TBST and incubate membranes overnight at 4 °C with specific antibodies to either phosphorylated, total signaling proteins or beta-actin on a swirling platform.

9. Wash membranes 4–5 times in TBST for a total of 15 min.

10. Incubate with secondary antibodies (e.g., anti-mouse or anti-rabbit Ig horse radish peroxidase or LiCor-labeled antibodies for Odyssey imaging) for 1 h at room temperature.

11. Remove unbound secondary antibodies by washing membranes 4–5 times in TBST for a total of 15 min.

12. Visualize proteins either by chemiluminescence according to the manufacturer's instructions (e.g., ECL plus) or using a LiCor imaging system.

13. After detection, if additional signaling proteins require analysis, strip membranes for 15–25 min using commercial stripping reagents, wash in TBST (4×5 min), re-block, wash briefly and then re probe depending on the manufacturer's instructions.

4   Notes

1. If histamine release is being determined alone, i.e., without Western blotting or cytokine/LTC$_4$ releases, basophil preparations of lower purity may be used, especially for pilot experiments to gauge the optimum concentrations of stimuli required for subsequent experiments. In this case, even Ficoll-density enrichment may suffice for determining basophil histamine releases since, other than platelets in some donors, most of the blood histamine content is basophil derived.

2. Optimum kinetics for IgE-dependent histamine releases is usually around 30-min stimulation. However, this may vary if highly suboptimal or supraoptimal stimulus concentrations are used. IgE-independent stimuli, such as fMLP, display faster release kinetics. This is not usually a problem if a 30-min incubation period is employed (e.g., when fMLP or A23187 is being used as a positive control compared to anti-IgE or allergens) since the released histamine will not usually be broken down under the conditions described in this chapter.

When basophils are stimulated with PMA at least 60-min stimulation is required for maximal histamine release.

3. Optimum cytokine production from basophils varies from 4 h, for the detection of IL-4 release, to over 16 h for IL-13 release. However, since some preformed cytokines may be released very rapidly (within the first 30 min) it is recommended to initially use several stimulation periods, e.g., 30 min, 4 h, 8 h, 16 h, and more in order to gauge the kinetics of both preformed and de novo-generated cytokines as well as for assessing gene expressions by RT-PCR.

4. Analysis of basophil activation by flow cytometry enables to use basophil preparation of low purity, or even whole blood. In this case selective basophil markers (CD203c+, CD123+/ HLA-DR-, CCR3+/low side scatter) should be used.

5. Many signaling proteins are optimally phosphorylated within the first 15 min after basophil stimulation (e.g., Syk, p38 MAPK, ERK1 and 2). It is strongly advised to determine the optimal activity of the signal of interest by performing a kinetics experiment using basophils stimulated, for example, for 1, 5, 15, and 30 min. Other signaling proteins, e.g., HIF-1α, are maximally expressed at far greater periods (hours). Note that the concentrations of the stimulus and the degree of priming substantially affect signal transduction kinetics.

6. IgE-independent stimuli can be differentiated in receptor-dependent (e.g., fMLP, C5a) and receptor-independent (e.g., A23187) stimuli. The bacterial peptide fMLP serves as important positive control for basophil degranulation (especially in determining the so-called non-responders to IgE-dependent triggers; if the IgE-independent controls fail to elicit a response this may indicate cell-handling issues). C5a can be an alternative for fMLP for degranulation, but requires preceding stimulation with IL-3 for release of LTC$_4$. Calcium ionophores (e.g., A23187) or activators of protein kinase C (PKC), such as PMA, can be informative if receptor-mediated stimuli have no effect to check for the status of basophil function.

7. Care must be taken to immediately disrupt cell pellets with Laemmli-lysis buffer. On some occasions cell pellets are not clearly visible but cells are deposited on the sides of 1.5 mL tubes on fixed-angle rotors. Ensure, therefore, that Laemmli-lysis buffer comes into contact with this material. If pellet debris does not immediately disrupt (i.e., becomes turbid and difficult to resuspend) proceed to the next step of heating the vials and vortex after 30 s of the heating/boiling step. If protein concentrations need to be determined prior to SDS-PAGE and Western blotting disrupt the cells in lysis buffer alone on ice for 30 min before assessing protein concentrations

(Bradford Assay). The remaining lysed cells are then treated with Laemmli for SDS-PAGE and Western blotting. These procedures can also be carried out at a later date by freezing the lysed cells at −80 °C.

Acknowledgements

This work was supported by the COST Action BM1007 Mast Cells and Basophils—Targets for Innovative Therapies.

References

1. Falcone FH, Knol EF, Gibbs BF (2011) The role of basophils in the pathogenesis of allergic disease. Clin Exp Allergy 41:939–947
2. Miura K, Lavens-Phillips S, MacGlashan DW (2001) Piceatannol is an effective inhibitor of IgE-mediated secretion from human basophils but is neither selective for this receptor nor acts on Syk kinase at concentrations where mediator release inhibition occurs. Clin Exp Allergy 31:1732–1739
3. Shore PA, Burkhalter A, Cohn VH (1959) The detection of histamine, a new approach. J Pharmacol Exp Ther 127:182–186
4. Gilbert HS, Ornstein L (1975) Basophil counting with a new staining method using alcian blue. Blood 46:279–286
5. Knol EF (1991) Cellular mechanisms in the activation of human basophilic granulocytes. Chapter 5: Characterization of the role of Ca^{2+} in the degranulation of human basophilic granulocytes. Academic Thesis, University of Amsterdam
6. Knol EF, Mul FPJ, Kuijpers TW, Verhoeven AJ, Roos D (1992) Intracellular events in anti-IgE non-releasing human basophils. J Allergy Clin Immunol 90:92–103

Chapter 16

Identification and Immunophenotypic Characterization of Normal and Pathological Mast Cells

José Mário Morgado, Laura Sánchez-Muñoz, Cristina Teodósio, and Luís Escribano

Abstract

Mast cells (MCs) are secretory cells that are central players in human allergic disease and immune responses. With the exception of a few pathological situations, MCs are usually present at relatively low frequencies in most tissues. Since their first description, MCs in tissues were identified mostly using their morphological characteristics and their typical coloration when stained with aniline dyes. However, increasing availability of highly specific antibodies now permits the use of fluorescence-based flow cytometry as the method of choice for the quantification, characterization, and purification of cells in suspension. This technique allows for a rapid analysis of thousands of events and for the identification of cells present at frequencies as low as one event in 10^6 unwanted cells. This method also permits for simultaneous characterization of multiple antigens at a single-cell level, which is ideal in order to study rare populations of cells like MCs. Here we describe the basis of flow cytometry-based immunophenotyping applied to the study of MC. The protocol focuses on the study of human MCs present in body fluids (mainly bone marrow) but can easily be adapted to study MCs from other tissues and species.

Key words Mast cell, Mastocytosis, Flow cytometry, Immunophenotype

1 Introduction

Mast cells (MCs) are unique secretory cells which have gained notoriety over the years for their role as central players in human allergic disease and immune responses mediated by high-affinity IgE receptor (FcεRI) [1, 2]. Nowadays, MCs are known to participate in various cell-mediated reactions and in tissue repair processes after injury [reviewed in ref. 3]. MCs develop from CD34+ progenitors in the bone marrow (BM) [4, 5] but, unlike other leukocytes, they migrate through the bloodstream as precursors and are recruited to peripheral tissues where they begin their final maturation under the influence of cytokines and growth factors in the local microenvironment [6, 7].

Bernhard F. Gibbs and Franco H. Falcone (eds.), *Basophils and Mast Cells: Methods and Protocols*, Methods in Molecular Biology, vol. 1192, DOI 10.1007/978-1-4939-1173-8_16, © Springer Science+Business Media New York 2014

Before the onset of immunophenotyping techniques, the distinction between different cell types was dependent on morphological or functional differences between them. Since then, quantitative evaluation of MCs has been attempted in several tissues and pathological conditions using different techniques. The rise of antibodies highly specific for many different proteins potentiated the use of fluorescence-based flow cytometry; this technique became the method of choice for the quantification, characterization, and purification of cells in suspension, allowing the rapid analysis of thousands of cells [8–11]. Moreover, the use of a double-step acquisition procedure, in which an appropriate live-gate acquisition is performed, has largely contributed to the detection and study of small populations of cells present in single-cell suspension samples. This method allows identification of cells even when their frequency is as low as that of one event in up to a total of 10^6 unwanted cells [12].

In 1987 it was reported that a mouse monoclonal antibody (mAb) (YB5.B8) reacted with MCs without distinguishing mucosal from connective tissue MCs and did not bind to basophils [13]. This antibody was later demonstrated to be specific for the c-kit proto-oncogene product (KIT or CD117) [14] which was expressed not only by MCs but also on hematopoietic precursors in the bone marrow (BM; [15]).

In 1996, Orfao et al. demonstrated that BMMCs may be clearly identified by flow cytometry on the basis of their light scatter properties and strong CD117 expression [16]. In addition, these cells were shown to be negative for CD34, CD38, and BB4 antigens and displayed a high reactivity for anti-IgE and anti-CD33 (Siglec-3) mAbs. This technical advance was revealed to be of major value in the study of MC-related disorders like mastocytosis and other clonal mast cell diseases. Applying the same technical principles, Escribano et al. reported that BMMCs from patients with systemic mastocytosis (SM) display unique aberrant immunophenotypic characteristics, as compared to normal MCs [17]. Among other features, pathological MCs show aberrant expression of CD25 and CD2 together with abnormally high levels of CD11c and CD35 complement receptors, the CD59 complement regulatory molecule, the CD63 lysosomal membrane antigen, and the CD69 early-activation antigen [18–20]. More recently, three clearly different maturation-associated immunophenotypic profiles were found for BMMCs in SM [21] and related to both genetic markers of the disease and its clinical behavior.

Even though in situations like MC hyperplasia or SM a great number of MCs may be observed in tissues like BM or skin [22], under normal circumstances and in most SM cases, the number of MCs present in different tissues are, with few exceptions, considerably low [23]. For that reason, it is mandatory to analyze a high number of cells ($1–2 \times 10^6$ cells) in order to obtain information from sufficient MCs to correctly interpret their phenotypic characteristics.

Although flow cytometry is highly indicated for the study of cells and other particles in suspension, like those from peripheral blood (PB) and BM, when appropriate methods are employed to create cell suspensions from solid tissues these may also be efficiently studied using this technique. The protocols described in this chapter allow for the identification and enumeration of MCs using multiparametric flow cytometry on the basis of technical approaches used for the identification of cells present at low frequencies. This approach can be applied to virtually any cell suspension prepared from a wide range of human specimens, including BM, PB, organic fluids (e.g., ascitic fluid), and solid tissues, among others. In addition, the protocols described here allow for the study of surface membrane antigens and intracellular molecules, and are therefore particularly useful to study the typical MC granule contents stored within these cells. These protocols are mainly directed to study human MCs but the same principles may be easily applied to study other sources of MCs like animal model tissues or cell cultures.

2   Materials

1. 14–8 G biopsy needle for BM aspiration.
2. Vacutainer® tubes containing either tripotassium EDTA or heparin.
3. 25 G needle and syringe.
4. 50 mL conical bottom centrifuge tubes.
5. Phosphate-buffered saline (PBS, 1×): 137 mM NaCl, 2.7 mM KCl, 10 mM Na_2HPO_4, 1.8 mM KH_2PO_4, pH 7.4.
6. Hematological cell analyzer and/or other cell-counting system.
7. Cytospin centrifuge (optional).
8. Microscopy crystals and cover slips.
9. Toluidine blue 1 % (w/v) in methanol, pH 2.0–2.5.
10. Bright-field light microscope.
11. 12×75 mm polystyrene tubes.
12. Monoclonal antibodies directly conjugated with fluorochromes suitable to be detected by your flow cytometer (*see* **Note 1**) (Tables 1 and 2).
13. Red cell lysing solution [e.g., Facs Lysing solution 1× (Becton Dickinson): stock commercial 10× solution diluted 1/10 (v/v) in distilled water (dH_2O)] (*see* **Note 2**).

Table 1
Four color combinations recommended for immunophenotypic analysis of mast cells in the diagnosis of systemic mastocytosis

Tube #	FITC	PE	PerCP-Cy5.5	APC
Screening tubes[a]				
1	Control	Control	CD45	CD117
2	CD2	CD25	CD45	CD117
3	FcɛRI[b]	CD30	CD45	CD117
Further mast cell characterization[c]				
4	CD35	CD69	CD45	CD117
5	CD63	CD32	CD45	CD117
6	HLA-DR	CD123	CD45	CD117
7	cy Control	cy Control	CD45	CD117
8	cy Total tryptase (B12)[d]	CD34	CD45	CD117
9	cy CPA	CD203c	CD45	CD117

Control: Unstained negative control; CPA: carboxypeptidase A3; Cytoplasmic markers are preceded by "cy"; otherwise we refer to membrane markers
FITC Fluorescein isothiocyanate, *PE* Phycoerythrin, *PerCP* Peridinin chlorophyll protein complex, *Cy* Cyanin, *APC* Allophycocyanin
[a]Usually these combinations are enough to characterize the mast cell phenotype in the process of systemic mastocytosis diagnosis
[b]Indirectly observed by anti-IgE staining
[c]These combinations are merely suggestive and may be adapted according to the objective of the study
[d]This particular clone is not available commercially

14. PBS (1×) containing 0.5 % (w/v) of paraformaldehyde (optional).

15. Flow cytometer with at least four fluorescence detectors and appropriate filter sets.

16. Software for analysis of flow cytometry data.

17. Cell fixation and permeabilization reagents to assess the cytoplasmic expression of proteins [e.g., Fix&Perm (An der Grub, Bio Research GmbH, Vienna, Austria)] (*see* **Note 3**).

3   Methods

3.1   Cell Suspension Preparation

3.1.1   Specific Procedures for Bone Marrow Samples

1. Collect a minimum of 1.5–2 mL of BM aspirate using tubes containing EDTA or heparin as anticoagulant.

2. Prepare smears according to conventional methods taking special attention to prepare the smears with BM particles.

Table 2
Eight color combinations recommended for immunophenotypic analysis of mast cells in the diagnosis of systemic mastocytosis

Tube #	Pacific blue	Pacific orange	FITC	PE	PerCP-Cy5.5	PE-Cy7	APC	APC-H7
Screening tubes[a]								
1	Control	CD45	Control	Control	CD34	CD117	Control	Control
2	CD2	CD45	CD35	CD25	CD34	CD117	CD203c	CD69
3	HLA-DR	CD45	FcεRI[b]	CD30	CD34	CD117	CD123	CD38
Further mast cell characterization[c]								
3	HLA-DR	CD45	CD35	CD59	CD34	CD117	CD123	CD25[d]
4	HLA-DR	CD45	CD63	CD32	CD34	CD117	CD123	CD25[d]
5	HLA-DR	CD45	cy Control	cy Control	CD34	CD117	cy Control	CD25[d]
6	HLA-DR	CD45	cy Total tryptase (B12)[e]	cy Chymase	CD34	CD117	cy CPA	CD25[d]

Control: Unstained negative control; CPA: carboxypeptidase A3; cytoplasmic markers are preceded by "cy"; otherwise we refer to membrane markers

FITC Fluorescein isothiocyanate, *PE* Phycoerythrin, *PerCP* Peridinin chlorophyll protein complex, *Cy* Cyanin, *APC* Allophycocyanin, *H7* Analogue to Cy7

[a]Usually these combinations are enough to characterize the mast cell phenotype in the process of systemic mastocytosis diagnosis

[b]Indirectly observed by anti-IgE staining

[c]These combinations are merely suggestive and may be adapted according to the objective of the study

[d]To be included when a double population (CD25+ and CD25–) is observed in screening tubes

[e]This particular clone is not available commercially

3. Immerse air-dried preparations in 0.5 % toluidine blue solution during 4 min and then wash in water.

4. Mount with a cover slip and observe under the microscope to get an overall impression on whether MC numbers are low, normal, or high (Fig. 1) (*see* **Note 4**).

5. Pass the BM aspirate two or three times through a 25 G gauge needle in order to disaggregate the particles.

6. Quantify the amount of cells in the sample using a conventional hematological analyzer or other methods (e.g., Neubauer counting chamber).

3.1.2 Specific Procedures for High Diluted Samples (Organic Fluids)

1. Divide the sample into 40–45 mL aliquots (in 50 mL conical bottom tubes) and centrifuge for 10 min at $540 \times g$ at RT.

2. Discard the supernatant and resuspend the pellet in 1 mL of $1\times$ PBS.

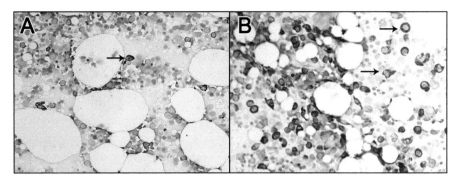

Fig. 1 Toluidine blue staining of two different BM smears. MCs may be identified based on their characteristic reddish violet color (*arrows*). The visual evaluation of a BM smear using this stain is of great help to determine the amount of sample to be stained for immunophenotyping by flow cytometry

3. Transfer all the samples to a single 50 mL conical bottom centrifuge tube.

4. Quantify the amount of cells in the sample using a conventional hematologic analyzer or other methods (e.g., Neubauer counting chamber).

3.1.3 Other Samples

As a general rule, any tissue susceptible of being turned into a cell suspension may be analyzed by flow cytometry. The process is relatively straightforward for some tissues which are, by definition, cell suspensions, like PB and BM blood. In the case of PB the number of MCs is usually very low and it is advisable to stain triplicates of each tube.

For solid tissues mechanical and/or enzymatic disaggregation must be employed in a process that may vary depending on the nature of the tissue.

3.2 Antigen Staining

Flow cytometry allows the detection of membrane-bound antigens and/or cytoplasmic contents of cells. After a cell suspension is obtained, the samples may be studied following the same general procedure regardless the origin of the sample. However, depending on the antigens to be assessed some variations of the protocol must be applied (i.e., membrane vs. cytoplasmic antigens) as detailed below.

If only membrane antigens are to be studied continue with the protocol in Subheading 3.2.1. If cytoplasmic antigens are meant to be studied proceed with the protocol in Subheading 3.2.2.

3.2.1 Staining Procedure for Surface Antigens Only

1. Label 12×75 mm polystyrene tubes according to the panel to be employed (Tables 1 and 2).

2. Pipette the volume of sample containing approximately 2.5×10^6 cells into each tube.

3. Add the appropriate volume of antibodies directed against cell surface markers to the tubes containing sample aliquots.

4. Incubate for 15 min at room temperature (RT) protected from light.

5. Add 2 mL of 1× red cell lysing solution and mix well by vigorous vortexing.

6. Incubate for 10 min at RT protected from light (*see* **Note 5**).

7. Centrifuge for 5 min at 540×g and discard the supernatant using a Pasteur pipette or vacuum system without disturbing the cell pellet, leaving approximately 50 µL residual volume in each tube.

8. Add 2 mL of 1× PBS to the cell pellet and mix well.

9. Centrifuge for 5 min at 540×g and discard the supernatant using a Pasteur pipette or a vacuum system without disturbing the cell pellet, leaving approximately 50 µL residual volume in each tube.

10. Resuspend the cell pellet in 300 µL of 1× PBS.

11. Acquire the cells after staining or store at 4 °C (in the dark) for a maximum of 3 h until measurement in the flow cytometer.

3.2.2 Combined Staining Protocol for Intracellular and Surface Membrane Antigens

1. Label 12×75 mm polystyrene tubes according to the panel to be employed (Tables 1 and 2).

2. Pipette the volume of sample containing approximately 2.5×10^6 cells into each tube.

3. Add the appropriate volume of antibodies directed against cell surface markers to the tubes containing sample aliquots.

4. Incubate for 15 min at RT protected from light.

5. Add 2 mL of 1× PBS to the cell pellet to rinse the unbound antibody and mix well.

6. Centrifuge for 5 min at 540×g and discard the supernatant using a Pasteur pipette or a vacuum system without disturbing the cell pellet, leaving approximately 50 µL residual volume in each tube.

7. Resuspend the cell pellet by mixing gently.

8. Add 100 µL of reagent A (fixation medium; Fix&Perm).

9. Incubate for 15 min at RT protected from light.

10. Add 2 mL of 1× PBS to the cell pellet and mix well.

11. Centrifuge for 5 min at 540×g and discard the supernatant using a Pasteur pipette or a vacuum system without disturbing the cell pellet, leaving approximately 50 µL residual volume in each tube.

12. Resuspend the cell pellet (*see* **Note 6**).

13. Add 100 µL of reagent B (permeabilizing solution; Fix&Perm) and mix well.

14. Add the appropriate volume of the antibodies directed against intracellular antigens and mix well.

15. Incubate for 15 min at RT protected from light.

16. Add 2 mL of 1× PBS to the cell pellet and mix well.

17. Centrifuge for 5 min at $540 \times g$ and discard the supernatant using a Pasteur pipette or a vacuum system without disturbing the cell pellet, leaving approximately 50 µL residual volume in each tube.

18. Resuspend the cell pellet in 500 µL of 1× PBS.

19. Acquire the cells after staining or store at 4 °C for a maximum of 3 h until measurement in the flow cytometer.

3.3 Instrument Setup and Data Acquisition

The sample acquisition should be performed using a two-step procedure. A first file is created with the information on enough total cells to have a general representation of the sample (i.e., 1×10^5 cells). For reference, we will name these files as "Step 1 files." Then, a second file is created and only the information is stored on those events falling inside a live gate drawn to include CD117$^+$ events. This will allow the analysis of a higher amount of cells while saving disc space and make the manipulation of the files easier. For reference we will name these files as "Step 2 files."

1. Run the quality control and compensation setup according to specific instructions from the manufacturer of the cytometer. Make sure that forward scatter (FSC) width (FSC-W), height (FSC-H), and area (FSC-A) parameters are enabled (*see* **Note 7**).

2. Create bivariate dot plots as represented in Fig. 2:

    (a) FSC versus SSC.

    (b) CD117 versus SSC.

    (c) CD117 versus CD45.

3. In the dot plot "CD117 versus SSC" display all events and draw a gate (R1) to include all CD117$^+$ events (*see* Fig. 2b).

4. In the dot plot "CD117 versus CD45" display R1 events and draw a gate (R2) to include all CD117^{high} events (*see* Fig. 2c).

5. For each tube create a "Step 1 file" by acquiring and storing the information on a total of at least 1×10^5 events.

6. Be sure that CD117^{high} cells (gate R2) can be clearly discriminated from CD117^{dim+} cells.

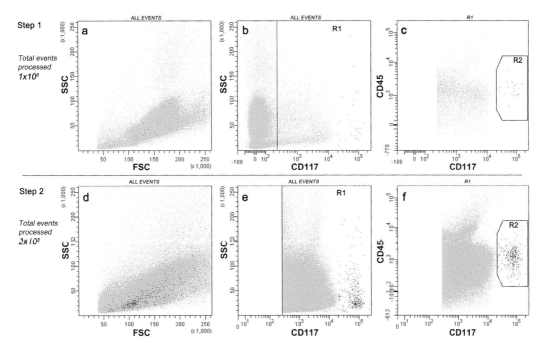

Fig. 2 Two-step acquisition procedure in a BM sample to study MCs. In Step 1 the information on all the events processed is stored to have general information on the sample studied. In Step 2 only the information on CD117+ events is stored; however it is important to register the number of total events processed in order to calculate the percentage of MCs in the sample

7. For each tube create a "Step 2 file" by acquiring and storing the information on the events falling inside the gate R1. Be sure to have a minimum of 100 CD117^{high} events (R2) for each tube.

8. Register the number of total processed events during the acquisition of "Step 2 files" for future calculation (usually this value is not saved by the acquisition software).

3.4 Data Analysis

Data analysis can be performed with any software capable of analyzing FCS 2.0 or FCS 3.0 files. In the examples shown, the Infinicyt software program (Cytognos) was used.

3.4.1 Mast Cell Identification and Enumeration

1. Create the following bivariate dot plots (Fig. 3):

   (a) FSC-A versus SSC-A.

   (b) FSC-A versus FSC-W.

   (c) CD117 versus SSC.

   (d) CD45 versus CD117.

   (e) If other "identification markers" are included create CD117 versus "identification marker" dot plots to improve MC identification.

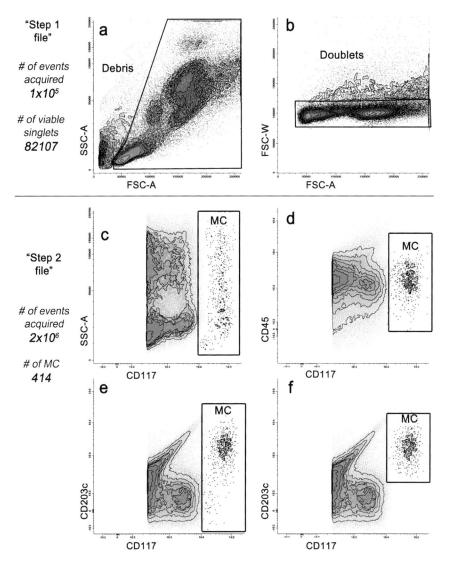

Fig. 3 Analysis procedure to identify MCs. In "Step 1 files" the number of viable singlets (events remaining after discarding doublets and debris) and the number of total events processed must be registered (Panels **a** and **b**). In "Step 2 files" the number of events fulfilling the phenotype of MCs and the number of total events processed must be registered. The use of extra identification markers may help to correctly identify MCs (Panels **c–f**)

2. Analyze "Step 1 files":

   (a) Exclude cell debris (*see* Fig. 3a) and doublets (*see* Fig. 3b and **Note 8**).

   (b) Register the number of events that remain after excluding debris and doublets for each file (viable singlets).

3. Analyze "Step 2 files":

   (a) Select and register the number of events fulfilling the phenotype of MC based on the identification markers used excluding cell debris and doublets (*see* **Note 9**).

4. Recall the following values registered during the process of acquisition and analysis of data from each tube:

    (a) Number of total events processed in "Step 1 files."

    (b) Number of viable singlets (events in "Step 1 files" after removing debris and doublets).

    (c) Number of total events processed in "Step 2 files."

    (d) Number of events fulfilling the phenotype of MC in "Step 2 files."

5. Calculate the percentage of MC (*see* **Note 10**):

    (a) Apply the following formula using the values obtained from each tube:

$$\%MC = \frac{D}{C \times \left(\dfrac{B}{A}\right)} \times 100$$

    (b) Calculate the mean value among the different tubes.

3.4.2 Mast Cell Phenotype Assessment

1. For each tube analyzed register the information of fluorescence intensity for MCs in each channel including the fluorescence intensity values from the control tube to control the autofluorescence of MCs (*see* **Note 11**).

2. One may use the raw fluorescence intensity values to compare different samples or correct the values of each marker with the autofluorescence in the corresponding channel (*see* **Note 12**).

3. Positivity must be established taking the autofluorescence in each channel (control tube) as a negative reference (Fig. 4).

4. Record the phenotypic profile of MCs identified on the samples studied.

3.5 Expected Results

MCs display distinct immunophenotypes depending on their stage of maturation, tissue environment, and activation status [24]. For this reason, and for the correct interpretation of the distinct profiles detected in MC-related disorders, it is essential to know the normal immunophenotypic profile of MCs in each situation. Since the BM is the most common source of MCs to study by flow cytometry, mainly for diagnostic purposes, we present here the most common immunophenotypic features of MC in this tissue under normal and pathological situations (Table 3).

3.5.1 Mast Cell-Committed Precursors

MCs mature from hematopoietic precursors which, based on in vitro experiments, were shown to be CD34+, c-kit+, CD14−, CD17− [25, 26], FcεRI− [27], CD38 often positive, HLA-DR often negative [28], and CD13+ [29]. Recent ex vivo studies, using BM from both healthy controls and patients with myelodysplastic syndrome (MDS), suggest that MC-committed precursors may be

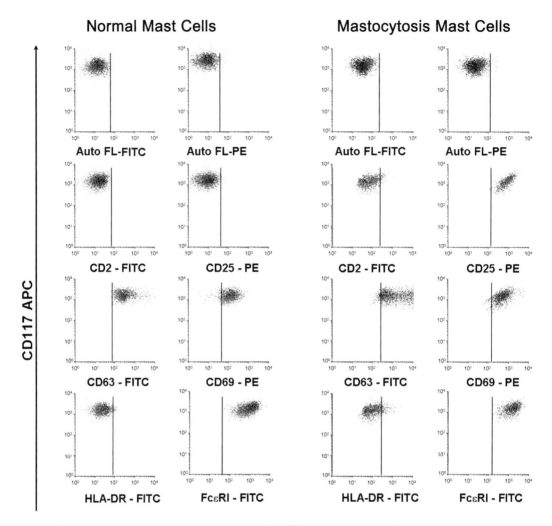

Fig. 4 MC phenotype assessment in two representative BM samples obtained from a nonmastocytosis case and from one patient with mastocytosis. The use of a "control" tube allows for the correction of autofluorescence of MCs which is variable among samples and is detected in the different channels. The autofluorescence levels in the corresponding channel must be used to determine the positivity and the relative intensity of expression for each antigen studied

identified within the BM CD34+ HPC compartment as being CD117hi/HLA-DR−/int [30]. Nevertheless, these precursors are extremely infrequent in normal BM [0 ± 0.005 % (range 0–0.02 %)] [30] and, consequently, our knowledge on the normal pattern of MC maturation is mainly based on in vitro-differentiated MCs [31–34]. More recently, it has been reported that both immature MC-committed progenitors and mature MCs express CD117, CD58, CD63, CD147, CD151, CD203c, and CD172a independently of the growth factors used, but that the expression of IL-3Rα (CD123) and of the granulocyte-macrophage colony-stimulating factor receptor (GM-CSFR) is restricted to early MC

Table 3

Qualitative and semiquantitative patterns of expression of individual markers on normal, reactive, and systemic mastocytosis bone marrow mast cells. Adapted from [17–21, 36, 41, 49, 50, 52–54, 70]

Functional group	Antigen	CD	Normal BM	Reactive BM	Overall SM	ISM	WDSM	ASM/MCL
Cytokine receptor	IL-2Rα	CD25	–	–	–/+ (93 %)	+ (100 %)	–/+dim (27 %)	+ (100 %)
	IL-3Rα	CD123	–	NR	–/+ (72 %)	–/– (84 %)	–	–/++ (80 %)
	c-Kit	CD117	+++ (100 %)	+++ (100 %)	++/+++ (100 %)	++/+++ (100 %)	+++ (100 %)	++ (100 %)
Adhesion-related molecules	LFA-2	CD2	–	–	–/+ (72 %)	–/– (82 %)	–/+dim (9 %)	–/+ (18 %)
	Integrin alpha-L	CD11a	–/+ (20 %)	NR	–	NR	NR	NR
	Integrin alpha-M	CD11b	–/+ (50 %)	–/+ (50 %)	–/+ (50 %)	NR	NR	NR
	Integrin alpha-X	CD11c	–/+ (71 %)	NR	+/++ (100 %)	NR	NR	NR
	Integrin beta-2	CD18	+ (65 %)	NR	–/+ (44 %)	NR	NR	NR
	Siglec-2	CD22	–/+ (60 %)	–/+ (50 %)	–/+ (96 %)	–/+ (95 %)	+/++ (100 %)	+/+ (100 %)
	Integrin beta-1	CD29	++ (100 %)	++ (100 %)	+ (100 %)	NR	NR	NR
	Siglec-3	CD33	++/+++ (100 %)	++/+++ (100 %)	+++ (100 %)	NR	NR	NR
	HPCA-1	CD34	–	–	–	–	–	–
	Pgp-1	CD44	++ (100 %)	++ (100 %)	++ (100 %)	NR	NR	NR
	Integrin alpha-4	CD49d	+/++ (100 %)	NR	–/+ (80 %)	NR	NR	NR
	Integrin alpha-5	CD49e	+ (100 %)	NR	–/+ (30 %)	NR	NR	NR
	Integrin alpha-V	CD51	+ (100 %)	+	–/+ (45 %)	NR	NR	NR
	ICAM-1	CD54	–/+ (75 %)	NR	++ (100 %)	NR	NR	NR
Complement-related molecules	CR1	CD35	–	+	+ (100 %)	NR	NR	NR
	Complement decay-accelerating factor	CD55	+ (100 %)	+ (100 %)	+/++ (100 %)	NR	NR	NR
	Membrane attack complex inhibition factor	CD59	+ (100 %)	+ (100 %)	+/++ (100 %)	++ (100 %)	+ (100 %)	++ (100 %)
	C5aR	CD88	–/+ (18 %)	NR	–/+ (54 %)	NR	NR	NR

(continued)

Table 3
(continued)

Functional group	Antigen	CD	Normal BM	Reactive BM	Overall SM	ISM	WDSM	ASM/MCL
Immunoglobulin receptors	FcεRI	NA	++/+++ (100 %)	++/+++ (100 %)	++/+++ (100 %)	+/+++ (100 %)	+++ (100 %)	+/++ (100 %)
	FcγRIIIB	CD16	-/+ (13 %)	-/+ (13 %)	-/+ (69 %)	-/+ (75 %)	-/+ (22 %)	-/+ (18 %)
	FcγRII	CD32	+ (100 %)	+ (100 %)	+/+++ (100 %)	++ (100 %)	+ (100 %)	++ (100 %)
	FcγRI	CD64	-/+ (4 %)	-/+ (4 %)	-/+ (84 %)	-/+ (87 %)	-/+ (40 %)	-/+ (18 %)
MHC-related molecules	HLA-I	NA	++ (100 %)	++ (100 %)	+/+++ (100 %)	++/+++ (100 %)	++	+/+++ (100 %)
	HLA-DR	NA	-/+ (25 %)	-/+ (25 %)	-/+ (85 %)	-/+ (90 %)	-/+dim (50 %)	-/+ (82 %)
Tetraspanins	CD9 antigen	CD9	+++ (100 %)	+++ (100 %)	++/+++ (100 %)	NR	NR	NR
	LAMP3	CD63	++ (100 %)	++/+++[a] (100 %)	++/+++ (100 %)	++/+++ (100 %)	++ (100 %)	++/+++ (100 %)
Mast cell proteases	Tryptase	NA	++ (100 %)	++ (100 %)	+/+++ (100 %)	+/++ (100 %)	+++ (100 %)	+ (100 %)
	Carboxypeptidase A	NA	++ (100 %)	++ (100 %)	+/+++ (100 %)	+/++ (100 %)	+++ (100 %)	+ (100 %)
Activation markers	Early activation antigen CD69	CD69	+ (100 %)	+ (100 %)	+/++ (100 %)	++ (100 %)	+ (100 %)	+/++ (100 %)
	E-NPP 3	CD203c	+ (100 %)	NR	+/++ (100 %)	++ (100 %)	+ (100 %)	+/++ (100 %)
Other	LCA	CD45	+ (100 %)	+ (100 %)	+/++ (100 %)	++ (100 %)	+ (100 %)	+ (100 %)
	Transferrin receptor protein 1	CD71	+ (100 %)	NR	-/+ (38 %)	NR	NR	NR
	Bcl-2	NA	-/+ (94 %)	-/+ (94 %)	-/+ (87 %)	-/++ (81 %)	+/++ (100 %)	+/++ (100 %)

NA not applies, *NR* not reported, *ISMs* indolent systemic mastocytosis, *WDSM* well-differentiated systemic mastocytosis, *ASM* aggressive systemic mastocytosis, *MCL* mast cell leukemia

Symbols: −/+: expressed in a subset of patients (percentage of positive cases); −: absent expression; +: moderate positive expression; ++: positive expression; +++: strong positive expression. Mixed symbols indicate variable reactivity, either among cases or among cells from the same individual. Values within parentheses represent the percentage of positive cases

[a]Expression of CD63 is increased in BM mast cells from myelodysplastic syndromes

precursors [32]. There is a general consensus in the literature indicating that proteins typically associated with MCs, like the FcεRI, MC proteases (chymase and tryptase), or histamine, are only expressed in late stages of the maturation process and are absent in CD34+ MC precursors [5, 27, 33, 35]. The exception seems to be tryptase which, based on unpublished observations of our group from ex vivo studies, may be dimly expressed in a small proportion of CD34+ MC-committed precursors.

3.5.2 Mature Resting BMMC Phenotype Under Normal and Reactive Conditions

Normal MCs display high light scatter and autofluorescence and express a broad set of proteins, including myeloid-related antigens (e.g., CD33), proteins related with the initiation of the MC inflammatory response (e.g., FcεRI) [16, 36], or MC proteases (e.g., cytoplasmic carboxypeptidase and cytoplasmic total tryptase), displaying relatively high amounts of cytoplasmic immature tryptase [21]. Other proteins are described in the majority of normal/reactive MCs, like bcl2 (94 %) or cytoplasmic mature tryptase [21], while others are only detected in a restricted number of them, like the IgG Fc receptors CD16 or CD64 [16, 17, 36, 37]. Furthermore, normal/reactive BMMCs constantly lack the expression of several proteins, some of them relevant from an SM diagnosis point of view, like CD2 or CD25 [16, 17, 36].

3.5.3 Activated Immunophenotype of Normal MCs

MCs undergo the final stages of their differentiation/maturation after the migration of their precursors into those vascularized tissues or serosal cavities in which they ultimately reside [38]. Mature tissue MCs are heterogeneous, and specific subpopulations with varied mediator profiles and different functional properties are observed in the different tissues [39] where they have an important role in the recognition of pathogens or other signs of infection [40]. A variety of stimuli can activate MCs to release a diverse array of biologically active products (reviewed in [38]) and MC activation by IgE-dependent stimuli or other triggers is associated with significant changes in antigen expression. These antigens include β2 integrins, cytokine receptors, complement receptors, and members of the tetraspan antigen family [41], like the lysosomal glycoprotein CD63 which is constitutively expressed on MCs, and upregulated by IgE receptor cross-linking [41, 42]. Likewise, both the ectonucleotide pyrophosphatase/phosphodiesterase 3 (CD203c) and the CD69 activation-linked cell surface antigen are upregulated upon IgE activation [26, 41, 43, 44]. Other antigens, like MHC class II, are not expressed on resting MCs, but their expression on MCs isolated from pathogen-infected tissues and/or stimulated by tumor necrosis factor (TNF), INFγ, or bacterial lipopolysaccharide (LPS) reflects a role for MCs in adaptive immune responses since they may contribute in the presentation of antigens to T-cells [45–47].

Although MCs express multiple direct receptors for pathogens and their products, the indirect activation of MCs during infection allows them to respond to a wider range of organisms [39]. As previously referred, MCs constitutively express the high-affinity IgE receptor (FcεRI) and the IgG receptor (FcγRII, CD32). Nevertheless, expression for both FcγRI (CD64) and FcγRIII (CD16) is only induced after exposure to INFγ [48]. This Fc-receptor-mediated activation generally leads to production of lipid mediators, the generation of various cytokines and chemokines and degranulation, as well as a decrease in cytoplasmic contents of MC proteases such as tryptase [39].

3.5.4 MC Immunophenotype in Systemic Mastocytosis

Early studies on the immunophenotypic features of SM BM MC reported several aberrant phenotypes that allowed for a clear discrimination from normal and reactive MC [17, 49–55] (Table 3). These studies reported the aberrant expression for CD2 and CD25 as a hallmark for SM, since these proteins were absent in normal/reactive BMMCs but expressed in the great majority of SM patients [17, 50, 51]. From these two markers, CD25 has been described to be the most sensitive, specific, and less variable, since positivity for CD2 has been described to vary depending on the fluorochrome used in the study [56].

Apart from the aberrant expression of CD2 and CD25, SM BM MC displays abnormally high expression of CD33 [52, 53] and of the CD2 ligand—CD58– [54]. Increased expression for activation markers such as CD69 [20] or CD63 [19], and complement-associated molecules, like CD11c, CD35 [19], CD59, or CD88, are also found in SM BM MC. In contrast, expression of CD117 [54], the CD71 transferrin receptor, and CD29 integrin is abnormally downregulated in these patients [17] (Table 3).

Despite the fact that SM is a group of heterogeneous diseases regarding both clinical behavior and prognosis [57–64], the immunophenotypic profiles of the distinct subtypes of SM have only recently been studied individually [21]. Three different patterns were identified, which correlated with prognostic and molecular subtypes of SM and reflected the maturation status of the cells [21].

The most frequently detected immunophenotypic profile, an activated phenotype, is associated to the majority of ISM patients with (s+) or without (s–) skin lesions [59], usually associated with a good prognosis [61]. BMMCs from these patients showed a mature profile (CD34-, CD117hi, FcεRI^{hi}) associated with the typical CD2$^+$/CD25$^+$ aberrant SM phenotype [21]. Furthermore, an activated phenotype with increased expression of CD63, CD69, and CD203c proteins, associated with expression of both CD64 and the MHC class II molecules –HLA-DR and HLA-DQ–, was detected in these patients. Such aberrant overexpression of some proteins could be related, at least in part, to the constitutive activation induced by the D816V KIT mutation, which virtually all these

SM patients carry [21, 65] (Fig. 2). Interestingly, BMMC burden in ISM patients can be extremely low [0.07 % (range: 0.04–1.4 %) on ISM– and 0.06 (range: 0.00001–1.7 %) on ISM+ cases]. The coexistence of both normal and pathological MCs in the same patient is relatively frequent in these disease categories (33 % of ISM– patients without skin lesions and 18 % of ISM+ patients). Furthermore, aberrant MCs can be as few as 20 % of the total BMMCs (personal observation), which raises the need of studying a large amount of cells so as to have enough sensitivity in order to avoid false-negative results.

A small group of patients, provisionally classified as well-differentiated SM (WDSM), do not have BMMC with the typical aberrant $CD2^+/CD25^+$ phenotype [21, 57, 58]. Most of these patients do not carry the D816V KIT mutation [65] and their BMMCs display a mature ($CD34$–, $CD117^{hi}$, $Fc\epsilon RI^{hi}$) resting immunophenotype presenting only few immunophenotypic changes such as overexpression of bcl2, carboxypeptidase, or total tryptase [21]. The lack of an aberrant phenotype, as clear as the CD25 expression, on these patients, and the fact that their phenotype resembles that found in normal BMMC, leads to a lower sensitivity in the detection of WDSM cases by flow cytometry [21]. However, we recently found that the BMMCs of these patients aberrantly express CD30, a receptor belonging to the TNF family, and present a typical $CD30^+/CD25^-$ phenotype; in contrast, ISM cases may present a $CD25^+/CD30^-$ or a $CD25^+/CD30^+$ phenotype, this being later found in virtually all the aggressive forms of SM (results accepted for publication).

In contrast to the other groups of patients, poor-prognosis SM patients typically show a $CD2^-/CD25^+$ phenotype, which has been associated with a decreased expression of antigens acquired during MC maturation/differentiation, like CD117, FcεRI, or HLA-I; increased positivity for antigens present in early stages of MC differentiation, like CD123, HLA-DR, or HLA-DQ; and low levels of cytoplasmic tryptase and carboxypeptidase in association with low light scatter features [21]. This immunophenotypic profile reflects a more immature phenotype [21, 27, 30, 32, 37], which could be explained on the basis of the degree of clonal hematopoiesis, opposing to ISM patients, who usually carry the D816V KIT mutation restricted to MC compartment. These patients typically display a multilineage involvement [21, 65].

4   Notes

1. The combinations of antibodies to be used depend on the objective of the study and the equipment available. Despite this, some basic principles must be followed to identify and study MCs like the selection of identification markers and

selection of sensitive fluorochromes. Tables 1 and 2 show basic combinations recommended for immunophenotypic analysis of MC in systemic mastocytosis studies and may serve as a basis for the establishment of other panels according to the goal of each investigator. Four-color (Table 1) and eight-color (Table 2) versions are shown.

2. Other red cell lysing solutions may be used if validated to study MC.

3. The fixation solution is usually formalin based while the permeabilization solution is saponin based (commercial formulations unrevealed). The protocol indicated here assumes the usage of a commercial kit for fixation and permeabilization such a as Fix&Perm (An der Grub, Bio Research GmbH, Vienna, Austria) or similar. However, other commercial or homemade formulations may be employed after validation to study MCs.

4. Perform BM aspiration in posterior iliac spine, using an 11 to 8 G biopsy needle in order to obtain enough BM particles. Since MCs are attached to the stroma and stromal cells, BM aspiration should be performed firmly and quickly. The harvest of higher volumes of sample in a single aspirate will not increase the number of MCs collected.

5. The red blood cells present in samples anticoagulated with heparin are more difficult to lyse. For this reason, the time of incubation may be adjusted according to the anticoagulant used: usually 10 min for samples containing EDTA and 15 min for those with heparin.

6. In this step the clot formed may be difficult to dissolve. Complete disaggregation is critical for correct permeabilization of cell membranes and particular attention must be paid to avoid false-negative results for cytoplasmic antigens.

7. The light that reaches each photomultiplier tube generates an electronic pulse and up to three different measures of that pulse may be available: pulse width (W), pulse maximum intensity (height; H), and pulse area (A). The width of the pulse depends on the "time" that a particle takes to pass in front of the laser beam while the amount of fluorescence is given by the maximum intensity (H) and reflects on the pulse area; these latter two measures should be proportional (if not consider revising the calibration of the equipment) and both can be used to quantify the fluorescence in each channel; usually pulse height is used in analogue equipment and pulse area is used in digital cytometers.

8. "Doublet discrimination" is a process whereby the area of the fluorescence light pulse is plotted against the width. Doublets will have greater pulse width than a single cell, as they take longer to pass through the laser beam, and therefore can be

excluded from the analysis. The area of the fluorescence light pulse may also be plotted against the pulse height in order to exclude doublets.

9. MCs strongly express CD117, CD203c, and FcɛRI. Nevertheless, none of these antigens is a specific marker for MCs; for instance, CD117 is also detected on a major fraction of hematopoietic precursor cells (HPC), CD56⁺bright NK cells, and neoplastic cells from patients diagnosed with gammopathies, acute leukemia, and myelodysplastic syndromes, among other hematologic malignancies, and in cells derived from other non-hematopoietic tissues (reviewed in [66]); CD203c and FcɛRI are also expressed on basophils [67–69]. The use of a CD117^{high}/CD45^{low} combination can accurately identify BMMC [21, 56] but further refinement may be done. The strong reactivity for CD117 in the absence of expression for CD38 and CD34 allows discriminating between MC and CD34 HPC and CD117⁺ plasma cells, while the expression of Fcɛ-RI and CD33 together with a strong expression for CD117 allows discriminating between MC and basophils [16].

10. MCs are present at low frequencies in most tissues. In both normal and SM BM samples, MCs usually represent less than 0.2 % of nucleated cells [16, 17, 36]. Interestingly, despite the fact that in systemic MC disorders, like SM, these values are significantly increased, low and overlapping frequencies are still found on these patients, compared to normal BM [0.21 % ± 0.27 % (range: 0.001 %–1.7 %) vs. 0.02 % ± 0.02 % (range: 0.001 %–0.09 %), respectively] [16, 37]. Furthermore, it is also known that increased BMMCs can also be detected in reactive BM (0.087 ± 0.12 % [range: 0.0021–0.54 %]) [37] or in patients with other hematological disorders like Waldenström macroglobulinemia (0.095 ± 0.11 % [range: 0.01–0.47 %]) or myelodysplastic syndromes (0.099 ± 0.12 % [range: 0.002–0.47 %]) [37].

11. This is particularly important when studying MC since they present high autofluorescence and it may significantly vary between samples. Usually one measure of central tendency (i.e., mean, median, geometric mean) and a measure of dispersion (i.e., standard deviation, interquartile range, coefficient of variation) should be recorded.

12. The fluorescence intensity is reported in arbitrary units and most of the fluorochrome-conjugated antibodies available do not have a stoichiometric amount of fluorochrome. Thus, the fluorescence intensity is directly proportional to the amount of protein but in order to make comparisons one must use the same reagents and the same procedures. Despite this, stoichiometric conjugates of fluorochrome antibodies are available which allow the quantification of the number of molecules identified using fluorescence standards.

References

1. Ishizuka T, Okajima F, Ishiwara M et al (2001) Sensitized mast cells migrate toward the antigen: a response regulated by p38 mitogen-activated protein kinase and Rho-associated coiled-coil-forming protein kinase. J Immunol 167:2298–2304

2. Kitaura J, Kinoshita T, Matsumoto M et al (2005) IgE- and IgE + Ag-mediated mast cell migration in an autocrine/paracrine fashion. Blood 105:3222–3229

3. Moon TC, St Laurent CD, Morris KE et al (2010) Advances in mast cell biology: new understanding of heterogeneity and function. Mucosal Immunol 3:111–128

4. Kitamura Y, Ito A (2005) Mast cell-committed progenitors. Proc Natl Acad Sci U S A 102: 11129–11130

5. Shimizu Y, Sakai K, Miura T et al (2002) Characterization of "adult-type" mast cells derived from human bone marrow CD34(+) cells cultured in the presence of stem cell factor and interleukin-6. Interleukin-4 is not required for constitutive expression of CD54, Fc epsilon RI alpha and chymase, and CD13 expression is reduced during differentiation. Clin Exp Allergy 32:872–880

6. Austen KF, Boyce JA (2001) Mast cell lineage development and phenotypic regulation. Leuk Res 25:511–518

7. Jamur MC, Oliver C (2011) Origin, maturation and recruitment of mast cell precursors. Front Biosci (Schol Ed) 3:1390–1406

8. Gross HJ, Verwer B, Houck D, Recktenwald D (1993) Detection of rare cells at a frequency of one per million by flow cytometry. Cytometry 14:519–526

9. Gross HJ, Verwer B, Houck D et al (1995) Model study detecting breast cancer cells in peripheral blood mononuclear cells at frequencies as low as 10(-7). Proc Natl Acad Sci U S A 92:537–541

10. Leary JF (1994) Strategies for rare cell detection and isolation. Methods Cell Biol 42(Pt B):331–358

11. Leary JF, Schmidt DF, Gram JG et al (1994) High-speed flow cytometric analysis and sorting of human fetal cells from maternal blood for molecular characterization. Ann N Y Acad Sci 731:138–141

12. Sánchez ML, Almeida J, Vidriales B et al (2002) Incidence of phenotypic aberrations in a series of 467 patients with B chronic lymphoproliferative disorders: basis for the design of specific four-color stainings to be used for minimal residual disease investigation. Leukemia 16:1460–1469

13. Mayrhofer G, Gadd SJ, Spargo LD, Ashman LK (1987) Specificity of a mouse monoclonal antibody raised against acute myeloid leukaemia cells for mast cells in human mucosal and connective tissues. Immunol Cell Biol 65: 241–250

14. Lerner NB, Nocka KH, Cole SR et al (1991) Monoclonal antibody YB5.B8 identifies the human c-kit protein product. Blood 77: 1876–1883

15. Ashman LK, Cambareri AC, To LB et al (1991) Expression of the YB5.B8 antigen (c-kit proto-oncogene product) in normal human bone marrow. Blood 78:30–37

16. Orfao A, Escribano L, Villarrubia J et al (1996) Flow cytometric analysis of mast cells from normal and pathological human bone marrow samples: identification and enumeration. Am J Pathol 149:1493–1499

17. Escribano L, Orfao A, Díaz-Agustin B et al (1998) Indolent systemic mast cell disease in adults: immunophenotypic characterization of bone marrow mast cells and its diagnostic implications. Blood 91:2731–2736

18. Núñez-López R, Escribano L, Schernthaner G-H et al (2003) Overexpression of complement receptors and related antigens on the surface of bone marrow mast cells in patients with systemic mastocytosis. Br J Haematol 120: 257–265

19. Escribano L, Orfao A, Díaz-Agustín B et al (1998) Human bone marrow mast cells from indolent systemic mast cell disease constitutively express increased amounts of the CD63 protein on their surface. Cytometry 34: 223–228

20. Díaz-Agustín B, Escribano L, Bravo P et al (1999) The CD69 early activation molecule is overexpressed in human bone marrow mast cells from adults with indolent systemic mast cell disease. Br J Haematol 106:400–405

21. Teodosio C, García-Montero AC, Jara-Acevedo M et al (2010) Mast cells from different molecular and prognostic subtypes of systemic mastocytosis display distinct immunophenotypes. J Allergy Clin Immunol 125:719–726

22. Alvarez-Twose I, Matito A, Sanchez-Munoz L et al (2012) Contribution of highly sensitive diagnostic methods to the diagnosis of systemic mastocytosis in the absence of skin lesions. Allergy 67:1190–1191

23. Sánchez-Muñoz L, Morgado JMT, Alvarez-Twose I et al (2013) Flow cytometry criteria for systemic mastocytosis: bone marrow mast cell counts do not always count. Am J Clin Pathol 139:404–406

24. Schernthaner GH, Jordan JH, Ghannadan M et al (2001) Expression, epitope analysis, and functional role of the LFA-2 antigen detectable on neoplastic mast cells. Blood 98:3784–3792

25. Agis H, Willheim M, Sperr WR et al (1993) Monocytes do not make mast cells when cultured in the presence of SCF. Characterization of the circulating mast cell progenitor as a c-kit+, CD34+, Ly-, CD14-, CD17-, colony-forming cell. J Immunol 151:4221–4227

26. Agis H, Füreder W, Bankl HC et al (1996) Comparative immunophenotypic analysis of human mast cells, blood basophils and monocytes. Immunology 87:535–543

27. Rottem M, Okada T, Goff JP, Metcalfe DD (1994) Mast cells cultured from the peripheral blood of normal donors and patients with mastocytosis originate from a CD34+/Fc epsilon RI- cell population. Blood 84:2489–2496

28. Kempuraj D, Saito H, Kaneko A et al (1999) Characterization of mast cell-committed progenitors present in human umbilical cord blood. Blood 93:3338–3346

29. Kirshenbaum AS, Goff JP, Semere T et al (1999) Demonstration that human mast cells arise from a progenitor cell population that is CD34(+), c-kit(+), and expresses aminopeptidase N (CD13). Blood 94:2333–2342

30. Matarraz S, López A, Barrena S et al (2008) The immunophenotype of different immature, myeloid and B-cell lineage-committed CD34+ hematopoietic cells allows discrimination between normal/reactive and myelodysplastic syndrome precursors. Leukemia 22:1175–1183

31. Dahl C, Hoffmann HJ, Saito H, Schiøtz PO (2004) Human mast cells express receptors for IL-3, IL-5 and GM-CSF; a partial map of receptors on human mast cells cultured in vitro. Allergy 59:1087–1096

32. Schernthaner G-H, Hauswirth AW, Baghestanian M et al (2005) Detection of differentiation- and activation-linked cell surface antigens on cultured mast cell progenitors. Allergy 60:1248–1255

33. Tedla N, Lee C-W, Borges L et al (2008) Differential expression of leukocyte immunoglobulin-like receptors on cord-blood-derived human mast cell progenitors and mature mast cells. J Leukoc Biol 83:334–343

34. Yokoi H, Myers A, Matsumoto K et al (2006) Alteration and acquisition of Siglecs during in vitro maturation of CD34+ progenitors into human mast cells. Allergy 61:769–776

35. Shimizu Y, Suga T, Maeno T et al (2004) Detection of tryptase-, chymase + cells in human CD34 bone marrow progenitors. Clin Exp Allergy 34:1719–1724

36. Escribano L, Orfao A, Villarrubia J et al (1998) Immunophenotypic characterization of human bone marrow mast cells. A flow cytometric study of normal and pathological bone marrow samples. Anal Cell Pathol 16:151–159

37. Escribano L, Garcia-Montero AC, Núñez R, Orfao A (2006) Flow cytometric analysis of normal and neoplastic mast cells: role in diagnosis and follow-up of mast cell disease. Immunol Allergy Clin North Am 26:535–547

38. Galli SJ, Nakae S, Tsai M (2005) Mast cells in the development of adaptive immune responses. Nat Immunol 6:135–142

39. Marshall JS (2004) Mast-cell responses to pathogens. Nat Rev Immunol 4:787–799

40. Abraham SN, St John AL (2010) Mast cell-orchestrated immunity to pathogens. Nat Rev Immunol 10:440–452

41. Valent P, Schernthaner GH, Sperr WR et al (2001) Variable expression of activation-linked surface antigens on human mast cells in health and disease. Immunol Rev 179:74–81

42. Furuno T, Teshima R, Kitani S et al (1996) Surface expression of CD63 antigen (AD1 antigen) in P815 mastocytoma cells by transfected IgE receptors. Biochem Biophys Res Commun 219:740–744

43. Bühring HJ, Simmons PJ, Pudney M et al (1999) The monoclonal antibody 97A6 defines a novel surface antigen expressed on human basophils and their multipotent and unipotent progenitors. Blood 94:2343–2356

44. Ghannadan M, Baghestanian M, Wimazal F et al (1998) Phenotypic characterization of human skin mast cells by combined staining with toluidine blue and CD antibodies. J Invest Dermatol 111:689–695

45. Frandji P, Oskéritzian C, Cacaraci F et al (1993) Antigen-dependent stimulation by bone marrow-derived mast cells of MHC class II-restricted T cell hybridoma. J Immunol 151:6318–6328

46. Henz BM, Maurer M, Lippert U et al (2001) Mast cells as initiators of immunity and host defense. Exp Dermatol 10:1–10

47. Wong GH, Clark-Lewis I, McKimm-Breschkin JL, Schrader JW (1982) Interferon-gamma-like molecule induces Ia antigens on cultured mast cell progenitors. Proc Natl Acad Sci U S A 79:6989–6993

48. Woolhiser MR, Okayama Y, Gilfillan AM, Metcalfe DD (2001) IgG-dependent activation of human mast cells following up-regulation of FcgammaRI by IFN-gamma. Eur J Immunol 31:3298–3307

49. Bodni RA, Sapia S, Galeano A, Kaminsky A (2003) Indolent systemic mast cell disease:

immunophenotypic characterization of bone marrow mast cells by flow cytometry. J Eur Acad Dermatol Venereol 17:160–166

50. Escribano L, Orfao A, Villarrubia J et al (1995) Expression of lymphoid-associated antigens in mast cells: report of a case of systemic mast cell disease. Br J Haematol 91:941–943

51. Escribano L, Orfao A, Villarrubia J et al (1997) Sequential immunophenotypic analysis of mast cells in a case of systemic mast cell disease evolving to a mast cell leukemia. Cytometry 30: 98–102

52. Escribano L, Díaz-Agustín B, Bravo P et al (1999) Immunophenotype of bone marrow mast cells in indolent systemic mast cell disease in adults. Leuk Lymphoma 35:227–235

53. Escribano L, Díaz-Agustín B, Bellas C et al (2001) Utility of flow cytometric analysis of mast cells in the diagnosis and classification of adult mastocytosis. Leuk Res 25:563–570

54. Escribano L, Díaz-Agustín B, Núñez R et al (2002) Abnormal expression of CD antigens in mastocytosis. Int Arch Allergy Immunol 127: 127–132

55. Pardanani A, Kim Linger T, Reeder T et al (2004) Bone marrow mast cell immunophenotyping in adults with mast cell disease: a prospective study of 33 patients. Leuk Res 28:777–783

56. Escribano L, Diaz-Agustin B, López A et al (2004) Immunophenotypic analysis of mast cells in mastocytosis: when and how to do it. Proposals of the Spanish Network on Mastocytosis (REMA). Cytometry B Clin Cytom 58:1–8

57. Akin C, Escribano L, Nuñez R et al (2004) Well-differentiated systemic mastocytosis: a new disease variant with mature mast cell phenotype and lack of codon 816 c-Kit mutations. J Allergy Clin Immunol 113:S327

58. Akin C, Fumo G, Yavuz AS et al (2004) A novel form of mastocytosis associated with a transmembrane c-kit mutation and response to imatinib. Blood 103:3222–3225

59. Alvarez-Twose I, González de Olano D, Sánchez-Muñoz L et al (2010) Clinical, biological, and molecular characteristics of clonal mast cell disorders presenting with systemic mast cell activation symptoms. J Allergy Clin Immunol 125:1269–1278

60. Bonadonna P, Perbellini O, Passalacqua G et al (2009) Clonal mast cell disorders in patients with systemic reactions to Hymenoptera stings and increased serum tryptase levels. J Allergy Clin Immunol 123:680–686

61. Escribano L, Alvarez-Twose I, Sánchez-Muñoz L et al (2009) Prognosis in adult indolent systemic mastocytosis: a long-term study of the Spanish Network on Mastocytosis in a series of 145 patients. J Allergy Clin Immunol 124: 514–521

62. Lim K-H, Tefferi A, Lasho TL et al (2009) Systemic mastocytosis in 342 consecutive adults: survival studies and prognostic factors. Blood 113:5727–5736

63. Valent P, Horny HP, Escribano L et al (2001) Diagnostic criteria and classification of mastocytosis: a consensus proposal. Leuk Res 25: 603–625

64. Valent P, Akin C, Escribano L et al (2007) Standards and standardization in mastocytosis: consensus statements on diagnostics, treatment recommendations and response criteria. Eur J Clin Invest 37:435–453

65. Garcia-Montero AC, Jara-Acevedo M, Teodosio C et al (2006) KIT mutation in mast cells and other bone marrow hematopoietic cell lineages in systemic mast cell disorders: a prospective study of the Spanish Network on Mastocytosis (REMA) in a series of 113 patients. Blood 108:2366–2372

66. Escribano L, Ocqueteau M, Almeida J et al (1998) Expression of the c-kit (CD117) molecule in normal and malignant hematopoiesis. Leuk Lymphoma 30:459–466

67. Gane P, Pecquet C, Crespeau H et al (1995) Flow cytometric monitoring of allergen induced basophil activation. Cytometry 19: 361–365

68. Valent P, Majdic O, Maurer D et al (1990) Further characterization of surface membrane structures expressed on human basophils and mast cells. Int Arch Allergy Appl Immunol 91:198–203

69. Valent P, Bettelheim P (1992) Cell surface structures on human basophils and mast cells: biochemical and functional characterization. Adv Immunol 52:333–423

70. Valent P, Cerny-Reiterer S, Herrmann H et al (2010) Phenotypic heterogeneity, novel diagnostic markers, and target expression profiles in normal and neoplastic human mast cells. Best Pract Res Clin Haematol 23:369–378

Part IV

Whole Organism: Disease and Knockout Models

Chapter 17

Identification of Murine Basophils by Flow Cytometry and Histology

Christian Schwartz and David Voehringer

Abstract

Here we describe how murine basophils can be detected in vivo by flow cytometry and immunofluorescence staining. Basophils constitute a homogeneous population of CD4⁻CD19⁻CD49b⁺IgE⁺ cells in flow cytometric analysis. When IgE levels are low one can also use anti-FcεRI or anti-CD200R3 antibodies instead of anti-IgE. For immunofluorescence staining we use an anti-Mcpt8 antibody since Mcpt8 is a specific marker for murine basophils. We describe how to prepare the tissue to cut cryo-sections and how to perform the staining using a tyramide-based amplification kit.

Key words Basophils, Mcpt8, Flow cytometry, Immunofluorescence staining, Tyramide amplification

1 Introduction

Basophils are the rarest of granulocytes, comprising only 0.5 % of blood leukocytes. Basophils were first identified 130 years ago by Paul Ehrlich using basic anilin dyes to stain the contents of their cytoplasmic granules [1]. In mice, basophils were not detected until 1981 [2]. Due to their rarity and the lack of appropriate staining techniques, murine basophils were thought to be a redundant cell type. Only 22 years later, new techniques allowed the detection of basophils in mice and led to a renaissance of basophil research [3–6]. Instead of hematologic stainings and electron microscopy, detection of basophils by fluorochrome-labeled antibodies directed to surface antigens came to the fore. Over the past years, new flow cytometric and immunofluorescence stainings of basophils in mice have been developed. In this chapter, we outline the routine identification of murine basophils using both methods.

Flow cytometric analysis and fluorescence microscopy, both using fluorochrome-conjugated antibodies against cell surface antigens, are two of the most commonly used techniques of today's immunologist and allow the researcher to detect small cell populations. Flow cytometry is primarily used to quickly analyze

Bernhard F. Gibbs and Franco H. Falcone (eds.), *Basophils and Mast Cells: Methods and Protocols*, Methods in Molecular Biology, vol. 1192, DOI 10.1007/978-1-4939-1173-8_17, © Springer Science+Business Media New York 2014

vast numbers of cells, distinguish different cell populations, and characterize a specific cell type. While flow cytometry analyzes the composition of different organs, immunofluorescence is often used to determine the localization of a distinct cell type within tissues.

In contrast to mice, four monoclonal antibodies directed against human basophils are available for flow cytometry and immunohistochemistry [7–13]. Unfortunately, they cannot be used for the detection of murine basophils. Furthermore, CD63 and CD203c, activation markers for human basophils, have not been described for mouse basophils (reviewed in [14, 15]). Therefore combinations of other markers are needed to reliably identify basophils in mice.

Among other surface markers, murine basophils express the Fc receptor for immunoglobulin (Ig)E, IL-3Rα, CD49b, CD90.2, CD200R3, and CD244 [16]. Although they are not exclusively expressed on basophils, a combination of the integrin CD49b and Fc receptor-bound IgE is routinely used to detect basophils [17–20]. In the first part of Subheading 3, we want to explain the routine staining procedure for the flow cytometric detection of murine splenic basophils using this combination of anti-CD49b and anti-IgE antibodies. Since basophils do not express markers specific for other major cell populations, like CD4 and CD19, we use these markers to gate out T and B cells and thereby get a more distinct CD4$^-$CD19$^-$CD49b$^+$IgE$^+$ basophil population.

In the second part of Subheading 3, we want to describe the immunofluorescence staining of murine basophils with an antibody directed against the basophil-specific mast cell protease 8. Despite its name, this protease is exclusively expressed in mouse basophils and has been used for the generation of basophil-deficient and -reporter mice [16, 18, 21–24]. Here, we describe how to prepare the tissue for cryo-sections and how we perform the staining using a tyramide-based amplification kit. The cryo-sections are stained with the anti-Mcpt8-antibody, followed by a peroxidase-conjugated secondary antibody. The peroxidase activity catalyzes covalent deposition of fluorophores in the immediate environment of the enzyme, thereby amplifying weak signals and thereby allowing the detection of murine basophils.

2   Materials

2.1 Flow Cytometry Components

1. FACS buffer: 2 L Dulbecco's PBS (phosphate-buffered saline; 9.55 g/L), 50 mL FCS (fetal calf serum), 0.2 g NaNO$_3$. Prepare 2 L and store at 4 °C (*see* **Note 1**).

2. ACK (ammonium-chloride-potassium) lysing buffer: 1 L H$_2$O, 8.29 g NH$_4$Cl, 1 g KHCO$_3$, 0.037 g EDTA. Store at 4 °C.

3. Consumables: Plastic petri dish (9 cm), plastic syringe (5 mL), cell strainer or nylon mesh (70 μm), FACS tubes (5 mL), conical tubes (15 mL).

4. Counting chamber, Trypan Blue.

5. Antibodies: Anti-CD16/32: clone 2.4G2 (BioXCell), Alexa647-conjugated anti-CD49b: clone HMα2 (Biolegend), PE-conjugated anti-IgE: clone 23G3 (eBioscience), PerCP/Cy5.5-conjugated anti-CD4: clone RM4-5 (eBioscience), PerCP/Cy5.5-conjugated anti-CD19: clone ebio1D3 (eBioscience).

6. DAPI (4′,6-diamidino-2-phenylindole).

2.2 Histology Components

Components for tissue and slide preparation:

1. 4 % PFA (paraformaldehyde): Dissolve 4 g paraformaldehyde (Roth) at 65 °C in 50 mL ddH$_2$O and 1 mL 1 M NaOH. Add 10 mL 10× PBS (95.5 g/L). Cool to room temperature. Adjust pH 7.4 with 1 M HCl. Add H$_2$O to 100 mL. Filter through 0.45 μm filter. Store at –20 °C.

2. Tissue freezing medium.

3. Disposable Vinyl Specimen Molds (15 × 15 × 5 mm) (Sakura Finetek).

4. Slides: SuperFrost Plus Gold (Thermo Scientific).

5. Cover slides.

6. Liquid barrier marker or Pap pen.

7. Fluoromount-G (Southern Biotech).

Components for staining procedure:

8. Tyramide Signal Amplification Cyanine 3 Tyramide Reagent Pack (Perkin Elmer).

9. Blocking buffer: 0.1 M Tris–Cl, pH 7.5, 0.15 mL NaCl, 0.5 % Blocking Reagent (Perkin Elmer included in Reagent Pack). Dissolve at 60 °C. Aliquot at 3 mL and store at –20 °C. Do not freeze after thawing.

10. PBS, pH 7.4.

11. H$_2$O$_2$.

12. Humid chamber.

13. Slide staining rack.

14. Antibodies: Anti-CD16/32: clone 2.4G2 (BioXCell), rat serum (Sigma), mouse serum (Sigma), anti-Mcpt8: clone TUG8 (BioLegend), Horseradish-peroxidase-conjugated goat-anti-rat-IgG (Jackson ImmunoResearch).

15. DAPI.

3   Methods

3.1   Flow Cytometry

Always work on ice unless stated otherwise.

1. Prepare a single-cell suspension from a freshly isolated spleen in 10 mL FACS buffer. Use the plunger of a 5 mL syringe to grind the organ through a 70 µm cell strainer into a petri dish. Collect the cell suspension in a 15 mL Falcon tube.

2. Pellet the cells by centrifugation for 5 min at $400 \times g$ at 4 °C. Discard the supernatant and loosen the pellet.

3. Add 1 mL ACK buffer to lyse the erythrocytes for 2 min at room temperature. Add 9 mL FACS buffer to stop the reaction and centrifuge ($400 \times g$, 5 min, and 4 °C). Resuspend the pellet in FACS buffer.

4. Count the cells using a counting chamber by mixing 20 µL of the cell suspension with 180 µL trypan blue.

5. Adjust cells to 3×10^7 cells/mL.

6. Transfer 100 µL (3×10^6 cells) into a separate 5 mL FACS tube (*see* **Notes 2** and **3**).

7. Add 2 µg anti-CD16/32 antibody to the cells for 5 min at room temperature to block unspecific Fc receptor-binding sites.

8. Prepare antibody master mix in FACS buffer (4 °C) and keep on ice in the dark.

   (a) For every sample use 100 µL FACS buffer.

   (b) Add anti-CD4-PerCP/Cy5.5 (1:800 or 0.25 µg/mL), anti-CD19-PerCP/Cy5.5 (1:400 or 0.5 µg/mL), anti-CD49b-Alexa647 (1:200 or 2.5 µg/mL), and anti-IgE-PE (1:200 or 0.5 µg/mL) (*see* **Notes 4** and **5**).

   (c) Vortex.

   (d) Add 100 µL to each sample.

9. Incubate for 20 min on ice in the dark.

10. Fill FACS tube with FACS buffer and centrifuge ($400 \times g$, 5 min, 4 °C). Discard the supernatant and loosen the pellet (*see* **Note 6**).

11. Just before analysis on the flow cytometer, add 0.5 µg DAPI to the sample to discriminate live and dead cells (*see* **Note 7**).

12. At the cytometer gate for all leukocytes, exclude doublets, and gate on DAPI negative, non-T-non-B cells (CD4⁻CD19⁻). The basophils constitute the CD49b⁺IgE⁺ population (*see* **Notes 8** and **9**) (*see* Fig. 1).

3.2   Histology

1. Put freshly isolated organ (e.g., spleen) directly into 4 % PFA and incubate for 2 h at 4 °C (*see* **Note 10**).

2. Transfer fixed tissue in 50 mL PBS and incubate overnight at 4 °C.

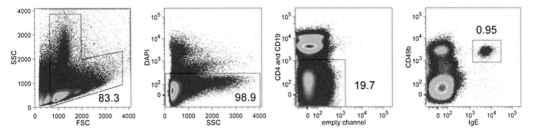

Fig. 1 Flow cytometric staining of basophils. From *left* to *right*: Cells gated on leukocytes (FSC/SSC), DAPI-negative, non-B-non-T cells (CD4⁻CD19⁻), CD49b⁺IgE⁺ basophils. Cells were measured on a FACS Canto II instrument (BD Biosciences, CA) and analyzed with FlowJo software (Treestar, OR)

3. Embed tissue in cryomolds in tissue freezing medium, slowly freeze in liquid nitrogen, and store at −80 °C (*see* **Note 11**).

4. Cut sections at 6 μm, circle with liquid barrier marker, and let dry slides for at least 3 h or overnight at room temperature.

5. Wash slides 2 × 5 min in PBS using a slide staining rack (*see* **Note 12**).

6. Incubate in 1 % H_2O_2 in PBS for 1 h at room temperature. Carefully flick off gas bubbles from sections.

7. Wash slides 2 × 5 min in PBS (*see* **Note 13**).

8. Add 100 μL blocking buffer containing 1 % mouse serum onto each section and incubate for 30 min at room temperature (*see* **Note 14**).

9. Wash slides 2 × 5 min in PBS.

10. Add 100 μL of 1:100 diluted unlabeled anti-Mcpt8-antibody (0.5 μg) to each section. Incubate for 2 h at room temperature (*see* **Notes 15** and **16**).

11. Wash 2 × 5 min in PBS.

12. Add 100 μL of 1:500 diluted horseradish-peroxidase-conjugated goat-anti-rat antibody (0.16 μg) to each section. Incubate for 45 min at room temperature in the dark.

13. Wash 2 × 5 min in PBS.

14. Prepare 1:100 dilution of tyramide-Cy3 in amplification buffer (supplied in the kit). Add 100 μL to each section and incubate for 7 min at room temperature in the dark (*see* **Note 17**).

15. Wash 2 × 5 min in PBS.

16. Add 100 μL of DAPI (2 μg) to each section and incubate for 20 min in the dark (*see* **Notes 18** and **19**).

17. Wash 2 × 5 min in PBS.

18. Take slides and briefly put the edge of each slide onto a paper towel to remove PBS. Add one drop of fluoromount G onto each section and cover with cover slide (*see* **Note 20**).

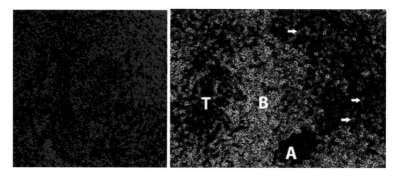

Fig. 2 Immunofluorescence staining of basophils (anti-Mcpt8, *red*) in spleens from C57BL/6 mice. *Left*: Nuclei were counterstained with DAPI (*blue*). *Right*: B cells were counterstained with anti-B220 (*green*). *White arrows* indicate basophils encircling the white pulp. *T* T cell zone, *B* B cell zone, *A* artery. Photomicrographs were taken on a Laser Scanning Microscope LSM 700 (Carl Zeiss, Jena, Germany) and analyzed with ZEN lite 2011 software (Carl Zeiss)

19. Store slides at 4 °C in the dark and let them dry for at least 3 h before analysis on a fluorescence microscope (*see* **Notes 21** and **22**). Representative pictures are shown in Fig. 2.

4 Notes

1. For the staining of blood basophils, heparin (2,000 U/L) should be added to the buffer until erythrocytes have been lysed.

2. Dependent on which organ is used for analysis, basophil numbers can be very low. Therefore, more cells should be used for the staining procedure.

3. When analyzing many samples, we find it useful to stain in a 96-well plate, reducing antibody cocktails to 50 μL/well, and an additional washing step with 200 μL FACS buffer after the antibody staining.

4. There are some situations when Fc receptor-bound IgE might not be detectable. This is dependent on the age of the mouse and the hygiene status of the animal facility, and some knock-out mouse strains are not able to produce IgE (Stat6-KO, IL-4/IL-13-KO) or the receptor (FcR-γ-chain-KO, FcεRI-KO). To stain basophils in these situations, other antibodies must be used. Suitable antibodies are listed in Table 1.

5. There are currently two clones for the anti-CD49b antibody available from commercial sources. In our hands the HMα2 clone gives a brighter CD49b⁺ population compared to the DX-5 clone.

Table 1
Other markers suitable for detection of basophils in flow cytometry

Surface marker	Expression on basophils	Also expressed on	Clone	Company
FceRIα	++	Mast cells, subset of DCs	MAR-1	BioLegend
CD49b	++	NK, NKT, subset of T cells	HMα2	BioLegend
CD200R3	++	Mast cells	Ba13	Biolegend
CD90.2 (depends on mouse strain)	+	T cells, NKT, thymocytes, stem cells	53-2.1	eBioscience
IgE	- to +++	B cells, mast cells	23G3	Southern Biotech
CD16/32	++	Macrophages, NK cells, B cells	2.4G2	eBioscience
CD244	++	NK cells, T cells, mast cells	2B4	eBioscience

6. Cells can be fixed for later analysis or intracellular staining in 4 % PFA for 30 min at 4 °C followed by two washing steps in PBS and the appropriate intracellular staining. For live/dead discrimination use fixable viability dyes.

7. We find that stained samples should be analyzed quickly, to reduce apoptosis of granulocytes.

8. During flow cytometric analysis, always acquire enough cells to gain a distinct basophil population. A good way to do so is to set the stopping gate to the basophil population and acquire at least 500 cells in this gate.

9. Basophils are somewhat autofluorescent; therefore when analyzing cell surface markers an isotype control is essential.

10. Be careful not to fix the tissue for too long.

11. The embedded tissue can also be frozen on dry ice.

12. To reduce background of some tissues, pretreat the slides with sodium citrate buffer (2.94 g trisodium citrate, 1 L distilled water, adjust pH to 6.0 with 1 M HCl, add 0.5 mL Tween-20; store at 4 °C). Heat the buffer to 95 °C and incubate the slides for 10 min. This also de-masks some antigens.

13. Never let the slides run dry. Work in a moist chamber. Always use blocking solution to dilute antibodies and DAPI. As a humid chamber we use a box with a lid, line it with wet paper towels, and put the slides on two plastic pipettes, so that they do not touch the wet paper towels.

14. When adding any solution to the sections, be careful not to wash away the section. Best pipette it next to the tissue and always use the same spot to add the solution.

15. Instead of staining at room temperature for 2 h, staining overnight at 4 °C is also applicable.

16. Instead of using the anti-Mcpt8 staining, basophils can be identified as c-kit⁻IgE⁺, c-kit⁻FcεRI⁺, or IL-4⁺c-kit⁻MBP⁻CD4⁻ cells in immunofluorescence microscopy.

17. Other companies also offer signal amplification kits (Vector, Invitrogen). In addition, there are also other conjugates for the tyramide available. When a biotin-conjugated antibody is involved it is mandatory to perform a block of endogenous biotin-binding sites. Therefore, we use the Streptavidin/Biotin Blocking Kit (Vector Laboratories). After the first block with serum, wash and add one drop of streptavidin-blocking solution to each section. Incubate for 15 min at room temperature. Rinse briefly in PBS. Add one drop of biotin-blocking solution onto each section and incubate for 15 min. Wash 2×5 min and continue with the appropriate antibody.

18. At this point a second staining can be integrated. Do not forget to block free antibody-binding sites.

19. If there is no violet laser installed in the fluorescence microscope, other viability dyes can be used. Propidium iodide gives a bright signal, but cannot be used together with Cy3-conjugated antibodies.

20. To apply one drop we normally cut off the tip of a blue 1,000 µL pipette tip.

21. Control the immunofluorescence staining by using an isotype control and a biological control. As biological control basophil-deficient mice (Mcpt8Cre, Mcpt8DTR) or basophil-depleted mice (MAR-1, Ba103) can be used.

22. Fluorescence fades over time, so timely analysis is recommended.

Acknowledgements

This work was supported in part by an ERC starting grant (PAS_241506) from the European Union.

References

1. Ehrlich P (1879) Beiträge zur Kenntnis der granulierten Bindegewebszellen und der eosinophilen Leukozyten. Arch Anat Physiol 3(166)

2. Urbina C, Ortiz C, Hurtado I (1981) A new look at basophils in mice. Int Arch Allergy Appl Immunol 66:158–160

3. Gessner A, Mohrs K, Mohrs M (2005) Mast cells, basophils, and eosinophils acquire constitutive IL-4 and IL-13 transcripts during lineage differentiation that are sufficient for rapid cytokine production. J Immunol 174:1063–1072

4. Min B et al (2004) Basophils produce IL-4 and accumulate in tissues after infection with a Th2-inducing parasite. J Exp Med 200:507–517

5. Mukai K et al (2005) Basophils play a critical role in the development of IgE-mediated

chronic allergic inflammation independently of T cells and mast cells. Immunity 23:191–202

6. Voehringer D, Shinkai K, Locksley RM (2004) Type 2 immunity reflects orchestrated recruitment of cells committed to IL-4 production. Immunity 20:267–277

7. Bodger MP et al (1987) A monoclonal antibody reacting with human basophils. Blood 69:1414–1418

8. Gane P et al (1993) Flow cytometric evaluation of human basophils. Cytometry 14:344–348

9. Han X et al (2008) Immunophenotypic study of basophils by multiparameter flow cytometry. Arch Pathol Lab Med 132:813–819

10. Irani AM et al (1998) Immunohistochemical detection of human basophils in late-phase skin reactions. J Allergy Clin Immunol 101:354–362

11. Kepley CL, Craig SS, Schwartz LB (1995) Identification and partial characterization of a unique marker for human basophils. J Immunol 154:6548–6555

12. McEuen AR et al (1999) Development and characterization of a monoclonal antibody specific for human basophils and the identification of a unique secretory product of basophil activation. Lab Invest 79:27–38

13. McEuen AR et al (2001) Mass, charge, and subcellular localization of a unique secretory product identified by the basophil-specific antibody BB1. J Allergy Clin Immunol 107:842–848

14. Buhring HJ, Streble A, Valent P (2004) The basophil-specific ectoenzyme E-NPP3 (CD203c) as a marker for cell activation and allergy diagnosis. Int Arch Allergy Immunol 133:317–329

15. Kleine-Tebbe J et al (2006) Diagnostic tests based on human basophils: potentials, pitfalls and perspectives. Int Arch Allergy Immunol 141:79–90

16. Ohnmacht C, Voehringer D (2009) Basophil effector function and homeostasis during helminth infection. Blood 113:2816–2825

17. Liu AY et al (2013) Mast cells recruited to mesenteric lymph nodes during helminth infection remain hypogranular and produce IL-4 and IL-6. J Immunol 190:1758–1766

18. Ohnmacht C et al (2010) Basophils orchestrate chronic allergic dermatitis and protective immunity against helminths. Immunity 33:364–374

19. Nabe T et al (2013) Roles of basophils and mast cells infiltrating the lung by multiple antigen challenges in asthmatic responses of mice. Br J Pharmacol 169:462–476

20. Torrero MN et al (2009) CD200R surface expression as a marker of murine basophil activation. Clin Exp Allergy 39:361–369

21. Lunderius C, Hellman L (2001) Characterization of the gene encoding mouse mast cell protease 8 (mMCP-8), and a comparative analysis of hematopoietic serine protease genes. Immunogenetics 53:225–322

22. Lutzelschwab C et al (1998) Characterization of mouse mast cell protease-8, the first member of a novel subfamily of mouse mast cell serine proteases, distinct from both the classical chymases and tryptases. Eur J Immunol 28:1022–1033

23. Wada T et al (2010) Selective ablation of basophils in mice reveals their nonredundant role in acquired immunity against ticks. J Clin Invest 120:2867–2875

24. Sullivan BM et al (2011) Genetic analysis of basophil function in vivo. Nat Immunol 12:527–535

Chapter 18

Mast Cell-Mediated Reactions In Vivo

Vladimir Andrey Giménez-Rivera, Martin Metz, and Frank Siebenhaar

Abstract

Mast cells are involved in many physiological reactions in which their functions can be very diverse. Models of allergic skin inflammation and systemic anaphylactic reactions in mice are validated methods in which the role of mast cells is well established. In this chapter, we therefore present protocols for passive cutaneous anaphylaxis and contact hypersensitivity, i.e., models which can be used to identify and characterize the role of mast cells as well as mast cell mediators and receptors in allergic IgE-dependent and -independent skin inflammation, and for passive systemic anaphylaxis, a model ideally suited to characterize the systemic effects of mast cell-derived mediators and mast cell receptors.

Key words Mast cells, Passive cutaneous anaphylaxis, Passive systemic anaphylaxis, Contact hypersensitivity

1 Introduction

Passive cutaneous anaphylaxis (PCA) and passive systemic anaphylaxis (PSA) in mice are classical models mimicking type I allergic responses. Here, mast cells are passively loaded with antigen-specific IgE and mice are then subsequently challenged with the respective allergen. This leads to the cross-linking of IgE, activation of FcεRI receptors, and degranulation of mast cells and release of various mediators [1]. In PCA, this reaction occurs locally at the site of IgE injection in the skin and will lead to measurable extravasation and increase in skin thickness. In contrast, PSA reflects a systemic anaphylaxis resulting in cardiovascular and respiratory symptoms and in a pronounced drop in body temperature. Both models are ideally suited to characterize mediators and receptors involved in allergic type I responses and to identify and characterize the effects of drugs aimed at affecting mast cell function [2–4].

It has to be noted, however, that other factors besides mast cells can potentially modulate some or all aspects of the observed reaction, for example basophils, complement factors, or strain and age of mice [5].

Bernhard F. Gibbs and Franco H. Falcone (eds.), *Basophils and Mast Cells: Methods and Protocols*, Methods in Molecular Biology, vol. 1192, DOI 10.1007/978-1-4939-1173-8_18, © Springer Science+Business Media New York 2014

Contact hypersensitivity (CHS) is a classical type IV allergic reaction with a delayed skin reaction elicited by a hapten [6, 7]. This model is used to understand the pathophysiology of allergic contact dermatitis in humans and to identify and characterize interaction between immune cells in the skin and lymph nodes. The key players in the sensitization and elicitation phases of type IV reactions are T cells and dendritic cells. Therefore, this model is well suited to dissect the role of mast cells in the modulation of adaptive immune responses.

2 Materials

2.1 PCA

1. Mice between 6 and 12 weeks old (*see* **Note 1**).
2. Monoclonal IgE anti-DNP (Sigma-Aldrich) (*see* **Notes 2** and **3**).
3. Dinitrophenyl-human serum albumin (DNP-HSA) (Sigma-Aldrich).
4. Evans blue.
5. Dimethylformamide.
6. Caliper (e.g., Mitutoyo Thickness Gage).
7. Micro-fine syringes for insulin 0.3 mL (e.g., Becton Dickinson).
8. 27G and 30G needles.
9. Micro-dissecting forceps (e.g., Braun, Harvard Apparatus) (2×).
10. Chirurgical scissors (e.g., Braun, Harvard Apparatus).
11. 96-Well flat-bottom plate for ELISA.

2.2 PSA

1. Mice between 6 and 12 weeks old (*see* **Note 1**).
2. Monoclonal IgE anti-DNP (Sigma-Aldrich) (*see* **Notes 2** and **3**).
3. Dinitrophenyl-human serum albumin (DNP-HSA) (Sigma-Aldrich).
4. Mouse restrainer (e.g., LABART).
5. Micro-fine syringes for insulin 0.3 mL (e.g., Becton Dickinson).
6. Needles: 27G and 30G.
7. Microprobe thermometer with a rectal probe for mice (e.g., Physitemp Instruments) (*see* **Note 4**).

2.3 CHS Materials

1. Mice between 6 and 12 weeks old (*see* **Note 1**).
2. Hapten and appropriate solvent and vehicle (Table 1).
3. Caliper (Mitutoyo Thickness Gage).
4. 1–10 μL pipette.
5. Hair shaver.

Table 1
Haptens in CHS

Abbreviation	Vehicle	Type of reaction	Sensitization area	Challenge area	Sensitization dose	Challenge dose
OXA	Acetone	Th1	Belly	Ear	1–6 % w/v	0.4–0.6 % w/v
DNFB	Acetone	Th1	Belly	Ear	0.3–0.5 % v/v	0.1–0.2 % v/v
TNCB	Acetone-olive oil [3:1]	Th1	Belly	Ear	30 mg/mL	3 mg/mL
FITC isomer I	Acetone-DBP [1:1]	Th2	Belly	Ear	2 % v/v	0.2 % v/v

Substance name
OXA: 4-Ethoxymethylene-2-phenyl-2-oxazolin-5-one (Oxazolone)[a]
DNFB: 1-Fluoro-2,4-dinitrobenzene
TNCB: 2-Chloro-1,3,5-trinitrobenzene
FITC isomer I: Fluorescein isothiocyanate isomer I
DBP: Dibutyl phthalate

[a]Storing at –20 °C increases the time of use

3   Methods

3.1   PCA

3.1.1   Day 0 (Passive Sensitization)

1. Prepare and pre-warm the IgE anti-DNP working solution before injection: 20 μL of IgE anti-DNP (5 μg/mL) per animal is required. IgE anti-DNP concentration is ideally kept as a stock solution, i.e., at 2 mg/mL. To get a working solution dilute the antibody 1:400 from the stock in saline (*see* **Note 3**).

2. Prepare antigen solution: 100 μL of Dinitrophenyl-human serum albumin (DNP-HSA) (4 mg/mL) per animal is required. The concentration of DNP-HSA stock solution recommended is 100 mg/mL. To get working solution dilute the stock in proportion 1:25 in saline or 1 % Evans blue if the interest is oedema quantification (*see* **Note 5**).

3. Perform an ear intradermal injection with a 30G needle of 20 μL of IgE anti-DNP or vehicle (saline alone) in the ear pinna of each animal (*see* **Notes 6** and **7** and **Fig. 1**).

3.1.2   Day 1 (Cutaneous Anaphylaxis Elicitation)

1. Measure the ear thickness baseline (*see* **Notes 7** and **8** and **Fig. 2**).

2. Perform a tail vein injection with a 27 g needle of 100 μL of DNP-HSA or saline. For simple ear swelling or histology, the DNP-HSA should be diluted in saline. For extravasation assessment the DNP-HSA should be diluted in Evans blue (*see* **Note 9**).

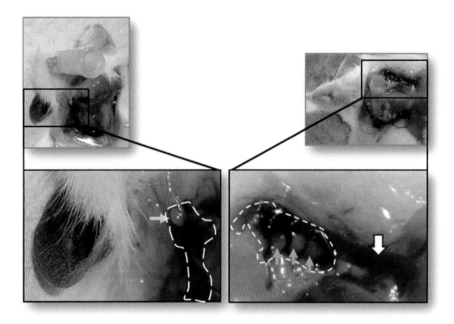

Fig. 1 Leakage of fluid injected in the ear pinnae. 50 μL of 10 % Evans blue injected i.d. in the ear pinnae (*red arrow*) generates reflux through extraperitoneal cavity (*dotted white line*) to the superficial cervical lymph nodes (*yellow/green arrows*). The dye was not delivered to the lymph nodes via blood flow; hence, neither the jugular vein (*white arrow*) nor the microvasculature is stained with the dye. That picture was taken immediately after injection

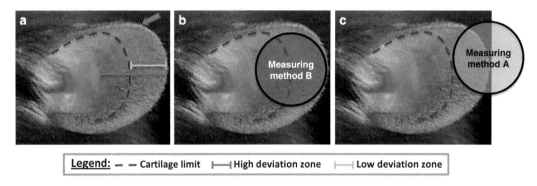

Fig. 2 Two different methods for ear swelling measurements. (**a**) Cartilage location in the mice ear, area of high and low deviation, and starting point to place the caliper spindle (*blue arrow*). (**b**) Including the cartilage (high deviation area) in the measured area may provoke high variability in the measurements (10–23 %). (**c**) Excluding the cartilage enhances the sensitivity and diminishes the variability (10–3 %)

3.1.3 Assessment of Ear Swelling

1. Repeat the ear thickness measurement as described for the baseline (*see* **Note** 7 and Fig. 2). The recommended time points are 30 min and 1, 2, 4, and 6 h after the challenge.

2. For analysis of ear swelling, ear thickness at baseline has to be subtracted from the ear thickness at each time point after elicitation (*see* **Note** 7).

3.1.4 Quantifying Evans Blue Dye Extravasation

This technique is used to assess the extent of extravasation which is mainly responsible for the swelling process.

1. Euthanize the animal at desired time point after elicitation (1–2 h).

2. Excise the ears from each animal.

3. Make a 6 μm punch biopsy.

4. Split the two halves.

5. Place each biopsy in a 2 mL vial filled with 0.5 mL of dimethylformamide (DMF).

6. Incubate for 3–5 h at 55 °C and shake at $52 \times g$.

7. Pass the whole-ear exudate through a 40 μm cell strainer.

8. Pipette 150 μL of each ear exudate on the NUNC 96-well flat-bottom plate.

9. Perform optical density measurement at 650 nm.

10. To perform the quantification of Evans blue, compare absolute values obtained within the different groups (*see* **Notes 10** and **11**).

3.2 PSA

3.2.1 Day 0 (Passive Sensitization)

1. Prepare monoclonal IgE anti-DNP working solution: 200 μL of IgE anti-DNP (200 μg/mL) per animal is required. The concentration of the IgE anti-DNP stock solution recommended is 2 mg/mL. To get working solution dilute the antibody 1:10 from the stock in 0.9 % NaCl. IgE anti-DNP could be obtained from hybridoma cells (*see* **Note 3**). The stock is normally stored at 2 mg/mL at –80 °C. Once diluted to working concentration it may be stored at 4 °C and used within 2 weeks or discarded.

2. Perform an intraperitoneal injection of 200 μL of IgE anti-DNP or vehicle (saline alone).

3.2.2 Day 1 (Systemic Anaphylaxis Elicitation)

1. Prepare antigen working solution: 100 μL of Dinitrophenyl-human serum albumin (DNP-HSA) (Sigma-Aldrich) (10 mg/mL) per animal is required. The concentration of DNP-HSA stock solution recommended is 100 mg/mL. To get the working solution dilute the stock in proportion 1:10 in saline (*see* **Note 5**).

2. Baseline: Measure and note the initial body temperature by immobilizing the animal and register the rectal temperature.

3. Warming the animal: Place the animal under a warming lamp for 5 min before the injection leading to the enhancement of the superficial blood flow. It may facilitate the injection.

4. Perform a tail vein injection with a 30G needle of 100 μL of DNP-HSA or saline.

3.2.3 Body Temperature Measurement

1. Measure rectal temperature at 10-min intervals for the first hour, and then at 90, 120, and 180 min following the challenge.

*3.2.4 Assessment
of Mast Cell Mediator
Release*

1. Sacrifice the mice after the first temperature measurement (10 min after induction of anaphylaxis).

2. Collect whole blood (for example by cardiac puncture) and peritoneal lavage fluid (PLF).

3. Leave blood sample for at least 1 h to clot.

4. Centrifuge the sample at $3,300 \times g$ for 20 min, and remove the serum from the clot by gently pipetting off into a clean tube.

5. To assess mast cell activation, measure mMCP-1 and/or histamine by ELISA in serum and/or PLF.

3.3 CHS (*See* Note 12)

*3.3.1 Day 5
(Sensitization)*

1. Hapten reconstitution: Perform accordingly to Table 1. For FITC, the hapten must be stored at 4 °C after reconstitution. The recommended stock concentration is 16 % w/v in acetone. Perform a dilution 1:4 in acetone thereafter; dilute 1:2 in DBP to obtain the sensitizing concentration. For TNCB, prepare 1 mL of vehicle mixture (proportion 1:3 olive oil/acetone). Weigh and reconstitute 30 mg of TNCB per 1 mL of vehicle to get the sensitizing dose. For DNFB and oxazolone, weigh 0.5 mg or 6 mg of hapten, respectively, per 1 mL of acetone to obtain the sensitizing dose (*see* Table 1 for additional concentrations, and **Notes 13–15** to increase the performance of the hapten application.

2. Shave the abdominal region of the mice (around 1.5 cm^2).

3. Apply twice 10 μL of sensitizing solution over the shaved area by pipetting and smearing with the pipette tip (*see* **Note 16**).

4. Wait for 10 s to let the solution dry on the skin. Keep the animal under sedation during that time.

3.3.2 Day 0 (Challenge)

1. Hapten reconstitution: Perform according to Table 1. For FITC, perform a dilution 1:40 in acetone. Thereafter, dilute 1:2 in DBP to obtain the challenging concentration. For TNCB, prepare 1 mL of vehicle mixture (proportion 1:3 olive oil/acetone), weigh, and reconstitute 3 mg of TNCB per 1 mL of vehicle to get the challenging dose. For DNFB and oxazolone, reconstitute 0.1 mg or 0.6 mg of hapten, respectively, per 1 mL of acetone to obtain the challenging dose (*see* Table 1 for additional concentrations). To increase the performance of the hapten application, *see* **Notes 13–15**.

2. Place the animal under isoflurane sedation.

3. Measure and record the baseline of ear thickness baseline (*see* **Note** 7 and Fig. 2).

4. Apply 10 μL of challenging solution on the inner side of the ear and 10 μL on the dorsal side of the ear (*see* **Notes 16** and **17**).

5. Let dry for a minimum of 10 s. Keep the animal under sedation.

6. Perform ear measurement as needed for 2–5 days. The recommended time points are every 24 h for 5 days (*see* **Note 18**).

4   Notes

1. The number of mast cells increases along the life-span of the mice and different strains of mice have different mast cell numbers. This may result in altered responses in older mice or mice of different strain backgrounds. Furthermore, female mice are to be preferred, as male mice might have injured/inflamed ears due to fighting.

2. IgE specific for alternative antigens, e.g., TNP, may also be used but need close adjustment in terms of concentration.

3. Sigma-Aldrich distributes both the IgE anti-DNP (IgE clone: SPE-7) and the hybridoma cells (IgE clone: SP2). It is important to titrate the optimal concentration every time the lot is renewed. The aliquots of IgE should be stored in high concentrations and in small volume aliquots. In our lab it is storage at 2 mg/mL in saline at –80 °C. Aliquots diluted to working concentration may be stored at 4 °C, used in the next 2 days, and discarded afterwards.

4. Alternatively, the use of subcutaneous transponder can be used to monitor the temperature over time (e.g., BMDSBio Medic Data Systems).

5. The stock solution should be stored at –20 °C (100 mg/mL) in DMEM-Pipes.

6. The site of injection should be approximately 2–4 mm under the distal end of the ear pinnae and we highly recommend a volume of 20 µL per ear (*see* Fig. 1).

7. An established method to perform ear injection or measurement is to maintain the animal under isoflurane sedation (21 % of O_2 and 2 % isoflurane) using an isoflurane exsiccator.

8. Recommended guidelines for ear swelling:

   (a) Subtract the baseline ear thickness with the ear thickness at each time point after the elicitation of the reaction. Animals may differ to some extent in the baseline ear thickness.

   (b) Measure always in the same place. Place the edge of the caliper-spindle in the beginning of the upper ear folded area (*see* blue arrow in Fig. 1). If there is appearance of necrosis or other relevant signs outside of the measured area, it should be documented but not measured instead of the originally selected area.

   (c) Methods of ear swelling: During the measurement process, the exclusion of the cartilage is preferred (*see* Fig. 2). Thus, excluding the cartilage by measuring the edges of the ear will reduce the variability within groups (Method A, Fig. 2.

9. The use of restrainers to perform intravenous tail injection is preferred over sedation with isoflurane since under sedation the blood pressure decreases and the tail vein diameter is reduced, making it more difficult to inject.

10. Collecting histological samples is an additional method to analyze mast cell morphology after the treatment (degranulation, localization, and numbers). We recommended semi-thin sections (1 μm) and staining with alkaline Giemsa.

11. Evans blue extravasation can be also applied to other skin areas, e.g., back skin, if PCA is elicited in those areas.

12. Reports of mast cell involvement in that model are controversial. That is mainly due to three reasons. (a) The contribution of mast cells in CHS may vary depending on the applied model. (b) Small variations in the protocol generate striking differences in the outcome (i.e., ear thickness). Such variations include type of hapten, dose, area of sensitization, and even measuring method and (c) the lot-dependent variation in the biological activity of the haptens. Table 1 summarizes the main experimental haptens used and other information.

13. Use always fresh reconstituted compounds. Haptens have a high tendency to be reduced. Use within 30 min after reconstitution.

14. Use tubes resistant to acetone degradation like polypropylene (PP) and high-density polyethylene (HDPE) tubes, for example 1 and 2 mL Eppendorf tubes. Other plastics like current FACS tubes are not suitable for use with organic solvents such as acetone.

15. Some haptens like FITC create insoluble precipitates after reconstitution in the vehicle; therefore it is necessary to filter the solution before application.

16. The grade of sensitization is depending on the contact area. A larger contact area may result in a higher rate of sensitization.

17. Place the animal in dorsal position. Pipette following the exterior edge of the ear and let the liquid drop down towards the head. Avoid ear movements of the animal by keeping the animal in deep sedation with isoflurane. Sudden movements may reduce the amount of total hapten per unit area.

18. The topical application of substances in animals can have a disadvantage in the cross-contamination by the cleaning behavior of the mice. Normally, for measurement of ear swelling, it does not represent a major problem as little of the substances will be transferred from one ear to the other ear. However, it may have an effect on the systemic immunologic response. Figure 3 shows the inflammatory signal using a reporter system 24 h after application of a hapten in the left ear. Mouth, forepaws, and even the right ear are indeed showing an inflammatory signal.

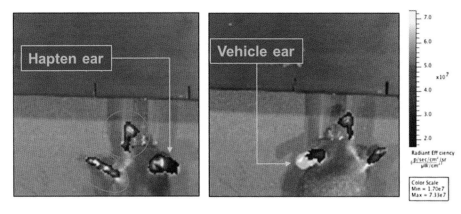

Fig. 3 Cross-contamination after hapten painting. The following day after hapten painting the mice show inflammatory signal in forepaws, mouth (*orange circles*), and contralateral ear

References

1. Verdier F, Chazal I, Descotes J (1994) Anaphylaxis models in the guinea-pig. Toxicology 93:55–61
2. Siebenhaar F, Magerl M, Peters EM, Hendrix S, Metz M, Maurer M (2008) Mast cell-driven skin inflammation is impaired in the absence of sensory nerves. J Allergy Clin Immunol 121:955–961
3. Mori T, Kabashima K, Fukamachi S, Kuroda E, Sakabe J, Kobayashi M, Nakajima S, Nakano K, Tanaka Y, Matsushita S, Nakamura M, Tokura Y (2013) D1-like dopamine receptors antagonist inhibits cutaneous immune reactions mediated by Th2 and mast cells. J Dermatol Sci 71:37–44
4. Han SY, Bae JY, Park SH, Kim YH, Park JH, Kang YH (2013) Resveratrol inhibits IgE-mediated basophilic mast cell degranulation and passive cutaneous anaphylaxis in mice. J Nutr 143:632–639
5. Miyajima H, Watanabe N, Ovary Z, Okumura K, Hirano T (2002) Rat monoclonal anti-murine IgE antibody removes IgE molecules already bound to mast cells or basophilic leukemia cells, resulting in the inhibition of systemic anaphylaxis and passive cutaneous anaphylaxis. Int Arch Allergy Immunol 128:24–32
6. Christensen AD, Haase C (2012) Immunological mechanisms of contact hypersensitivity in mice. APMIS 120:1–27
7. Popov A, Mirkov I, Kataranovski M (2012) Inflammatory and immune mechanisms in contact hypersensitivity (CHS) in rats. Immunol Res 52:127–132

INDEX

Bernhard F. Gibbs and Franco H. Falcone (eds.), *Basophils and Mast Cells: Methods and Protocols*, Methods in Molecular Biology,
vol. 1192, DOI 10.1007/978-1-4939-1173-8, © Springer Science+Business Media New York 2014